# DRUG RECEPTORS

BIOLOGICAL COUNCIL

The Coordinating Committee for Symposia
on Drug Action

# DRUG RECEPTORS

## *A Symposium*

*Edited by*

H. P. RANG

*Department of Physiology and Biochemistry*
*University of Southampton*



University Park Press
Baltimore · London · Tokyo

*First published 1973 by*

THE MACMILLAN PRESS LTD
*London and Basingstoke*
*Associated companies in New York, Melbourne,*
*Dublin, Johannesburg and Madras*

*Published in North America by*
UNIVERSITY PARK PRESS
*Chamber of Commerce Building*
*Baltimore, Maryland 21202*

**Library of Congress Cataloging in Publication Data**

Main entry under title:

A Symposium on drug receptors.

At head of title: Biological Council, The Coordinating Committee for Symposia on Drug Action.

"Report of a symposium held on 17 and 18 April 1972 in London at Middlesex Hospital Medical School; sponsored by British Pharmacological Society [and others]"

1. Drug Receptors—Congresses. I. Rang, Humphrey Peter, ed. II. Biological Council. Coordinating Committee for Symposia on Drug Action. III. British Pharmacological Society. IV. Title: Drug receptors.
RM301.S898 615'.7 73-8807

ISBN 0-8391-0713-7

Printed in Great Britain

Biological Council

Coordinating Committee for Symposia on Drug Action

*Report of a symposium held on 17 and 18 April 1972*
*in London*
*at The Middlesex Hospital Medical School*

Sponsored by
British Pharmacological Society
and
Biochemical Society
British Society for Immunology
Physiological Society
Royal Society of Medicine
Society for Drug Research
Society for Endocrinology
Society for Experimental Biology
Society of Chemical Industry (*Pesticides Group*)
Society of Chemical Industry (*Physicochemical and Biochemical Panel*)

*Organized by a symposium committee consisting of*

H. P. Rang (*Chairman and Hon. Secretary*)
Edith Bülbring
A. W. Cuthbert
L. T. Potter

# FOREWORD

The idea of a symposium on *Drug Receptors* was suggested to me in 1971 by the Biological Council's Coordinating Committee for Symposia on Drug Action. At that time the field had been rather static for several years but a few preliminary notes had just appeared which suggested that cholinergic receptors could be specifically labelled by means of radioactive snake toxins (cobra toxin and α-bungarotoxin in particular). Moreover, the electric organs of various fish, such as the eel (*Electrophorus*) and the ray (*Torpedo*) had been shown to provide a much richer source of cholinergic receptor material than was available hitherto. The unholy alliance of these two war-like creatures, the cobra and the electric eel (which Nature has mercifully contrived to keep apart) seemed certain to lead to rapid developments in the time intervening between the planning stage and the meeting itself in April 1972. We were not disappointed. In the final session Dr J.-P. Changeux withdrew with a flourish from his breast pocket a tiny glass tube with a distinct blue band across it—the receptor protein displayed before our very eyes!

Our aim in planning the programme was to try to bring together the various separate approaches that have been used to study drug receptors.

The symposium therefore includes work by pharmacologists on the classification of receptors by the use of antagonists, by electrophysiologists on the characterization of the ionic permeability changes caused by neuro-transmitters, and by biochemists on the labelling and isolation of receptor macromolecules. One of the most promising meeting-points is, in my opinion, the application to drug-receptor mechanisms of ideas that have been developed in relation to enzyme regulation. Ten years ago, in spite of the fact that the algebraic description of drug–receptor interactions was virtually identical to that of enzyme kinetics, the two problems seemed to be a long way apart, because enzyme molecules were thought of as rigid structures which acted on, but did not respond to, substrate molecules. Receptors, on the other hand, had to be flexible and responsive to the binding of small molecules. During the last few years, though, the two have converged to the point of collision, mainly because of the increasing emphasis in enzymology of the importance of flexibility in enzyme molecules, and of conformational changes brought about by the attachment of small molecules. This coming together of biochemistry and pharmacology, and the use of theories developed for allosteric enzyme regulation to explain certain kinds of drug action, is a recurring theme of the papers that were presented.

The symposium is entitled *Drug Receptors*, but the word 'drug' does not really convey the meaning properly. What we need is a word for any small molecule—whether it be a neurotransmitter, a hormone, an allosteric regulatory substance or a synthetic drug—which reacts with a specific site on a macromolecule and thereby modifies the macromolecule so as to alter its functional properties. Perhaps some spare-time lexicographer will present us with the *mot juste*, so that we can communicate more freely. Until then, 'drug' at least has the merit of being short.

This symposium was one of a highly successful series organized by the Biological Council. It attracted an audience of nearly six hundred, and I must here express my thanks, particularly to Miss G. M. Blunt for organizing this large and complicated meeting virtually single-handed, and also to the Wellcome Trust for their generosity in providing a grant which enabled us to invite speakers from many parts of the world.

H. P. RANG
Southampton
*November 1972*

# CONTENTS

# LIST OF PARTICIPANTS

E. A. Barnard, Department of Biochemical Pharmacology, State University of New York, Buffalo, N.Y. 14214, U.S.A.

J. W. Black, Research Institute, S.K.F. Ltd, Welwyn, Herts., England.

T. B. Bolton, Department of Pharmacology, University of Oxford, Oxford OX1 3QT, England.

E. Bülbring, Physiological Laboratory, University of Oxford, Oxford OX1 3PT, England.

A. S. V. Burgen, National Institute for Medical Research, Mill Hill, London NW7 1AA, England.

J.-P. Changeux, Unité de Neurobiologie Moléculaire, Département de Biologie Moléculaire, Institut Pasteur, Paris 15e, France.

D. Colquhoun, Department of Physiology and Biochemistry, University of Southampton, Southampton SO9 3TU, England.

E. De Robertis, Instituto de Anatomía General y Embriología, Facultad de Medicina, Universidad de Buenos Aires, Buenos Aires, Argentina.

C. M. S. Fewtrell, Department of Physiology and Biochemistry, University of Southampton, Southampton SO9 3TU, England.

H. M. Gerschenfeld, Laboratoire de Neurobiologie, Ecole Normale Supérieure, 46, rue d'Ulm, Paris 5e, France.

B. L. Ginsborg, Department of Pharmacology, University of Edinburgh, Edinburgh, Scotland.

D. H. Jenkinson, Department of Pharmacology, University College London, London WC1E 6BT, England.

A. Karlin, Department of Neurology, College of Physicians and Surgeons, Columbia University, New York, N.Y. 10032, U.S.A.

B. Katz, Department of Biophysics, University College London, London WC1E 6BT, England.

J. S. Kehoe, Laboratoire de Neurobiologie, Ecole Normale Supérieure, 46, rue d'Ulm, Paris 5e, France.

G. A. Kerkut, Department of Physiology and Biochemistry, University of Southampton, Southampton SO9 3TU, England.

L. G. Magazanik, Sechenov Institute of Evolutionary Physiology and Biochemistry, Academy of Sciences of the USSR, Leningrad, Soviet Union.

R. D. O'Brien, Section of Neurobiology and Behavior, Cornell University, Ithaca, N.Y. 14850, U.S.A.

T. R. Podleski, Section of Neurobiology and Behavior, Cornell University, Ithaca, N.Y. 14850, U.S.A.

L. T. Potter, Department of Biophysics, University College London, London WC1E 6BT, England.

H. P. Rang, Department of Physiology and Biochemistry, University of Southampton, Southampton SO9 3TU, England.

H. O. Schild, Department of Pharmacology, University College London, London WC1E 6BT, England.

S. J. Singer, Department of Biology, University of California at San Diego, La Jolla, California, U.S.A.

S. Thesleff, Institute of Pharmacology, University of Lund, Lund, Sweden.

# ACTION OF CATECHOLAMINES ON THE SMOOTH MUSCLE CELL MEMBRANE

EDITH BÜLBRING

*Physiological Laboratory, University of Oxford, Oxford OX1 3PT, England*

At a previous symposium on drug action, entitled *Adrenergic Mechanisms*, the dual action of adrenaline was one of the problems discussed. The observations then available led to the idea (Bülbring, 1960) that adrenaline had two actions, one a direct action on the cell membrane and another action affecting the membrane only indirectly, the primary action being metabolic. The direct action on the membrane ($\alpha$-action)—presumably an increase in permeability to one or several ions—would depolarize the membrane and make it more excitable. The metabolic action ($\beta$-action) on the other hand, would affect the functional state of the cell by making more metabolic energy available. It was assumed that this energy could be used, not only for the contractile mechanism, but also for metabolic processes which stabilize the cell membrane, making it less excitable.

The hypothesis implied that the response of every smooth muscle to adrenaline was the result of the two opposing actions and that the final response observed was determined by which of the two actions was dominant. The hypothesis did not provide an answer to the question why the $\alpha$- and $\beta$-actions, which in most smooth muscles were antagonistic, could in some tissues be synergistic. It did, however, offer a line of approach for the explanation of Dale's early work on the action of ergot. Dale had shown how the presence of a $\beta$-effect could be unmasked when the $\alpha$-effect had been blocked with ergotoxine (Dale, 1913). Dale had also described (Dale, 1906) the change of the response of the cat uterus to the adrenergic transmitter during pregnancy, a change brought about not by adrenergic blocking agents but under the influence of hormones.

In nonpregnant uterus the $\beta$-action is dominant and hence hypogastric nerve stimulation causes relaxation. In early pregnancy the $\alpha$-action is dominant and hence hypogastric nerve stimulation causes uterine contraction.

Since the nature of the adrenergic transmitter does not undergo any change (Vogt, 1965) it is clear that the properties of the smooth muscle cells must change. In order to investigate these changes the electrophysiological approach was necessary.

It is not surprising that progress has been slow and that our understanding of the mode of action of adrenaline is still far from complete since, for a start, the electrical properties of each tissue on which adrenaline acts have to be established. Perhaps, the first step towards understanding the behaviour of smooth muscle has been the definition of the factors which determine smooth muscle tone, namely, the demonstration of a close correlation between the membrane potential, the rate of spontaneous spike discharge and the development of mechanical tension (Bülbring, 1955). If there is no tone, adrenaline cannot relax it but can only cause contraction. If a moderate background of activity exists, adrenaline can either reduce this and relax the muscle or it can cause further contraction.

The majority of visceral smooth muscles exhibit some spontaneous activity which is periodically interrupted by silent periods of varying duration. The membrane potential is set just above or just below the firing level. As a result, the slightest change in membrane potential may either accelerate or stop spontaneous spike activity. Nevertheless, observations on the effect of catecholamines on the membrane potential are by themselves insufficient to throw much light on the actual mechanism of the drug action. However, in recent years (see Bülbring, Brading, Jones & Tomita, 1970) a thorough investigation of the electrical properties of the smooth muscle cell membrane has been carried out, and important information is now available on the fine structure of different smooth muscles, the spread of current throughout the tissue, and the ion distribution and ion movement across the cell membrane. We are beginning to understand the ionic basis for the resting potential and the action potential, as well as various other mechanisms responsible for the presence or absence of spontaneous activity. It is possible to identify the ionic nature of the changes in membrane conductance underlying the changes in membrane potential which may be produced by catecholamines.

From these studies a picture has emerged which, at first sight, appears to provide a relatively simple explanation not only for the α- and β-action, but also for the fact that the α-action by itself can cause depolarization or hyperpolarization of the cell membrane thus being either excitatory or inhibitory, depending on the type of tissue.

The 'type of tissue' can be defined, not only by the organ of which it is a part, but by the state of the smooth muscle cell in that tissue, namely, whether it has a high or a low membrane potential, whether it is in a state of rest or activity, and what is the relative contribution of the different ions to its membrane conductance. In fact, it is probably the state of the smooth muscle cell itself which determines the character of the final response to the catecholamines.

The membrane potential of smooth muscles is determined mainly by the ratio $[K]_i/[K]_o$ (Holman, 1958). The great variation of membrane potential in different muscles appears to be largely due to the great variation in potassium permeability. For example, the taenia coli of the guinea-pig has a low membrane potential, associated with a relatively low potassium permeability. Besides, chloride contributes significantly to the total membrane conductance (Kuriyama, 1963; Ohashi, 1970). The membrane potential is unstable, close to the firing threshold, and the taenia is perhaps the most spontaneously active visceral smooth muscle.

The response of most intestinal smooth muscle to any catecholamines, including the adrenergic transmitter, noradrenaline, is the sum of the $\alpha$- and $\beta$-effects, each of which can be revealed in the presence of the appropriate blocking agent. In these muscles (and the taenia is a perfect example) the $\alpha$- and $\beta$-actions of catecholamines are synergistic. Both produce relaxation and block spontaneous spike discharge. However, this is achieved by two entirely different mechanisms (Bülbring & Tomita, 1968).

The block produced by the $\alpha$-action is the result of the membrane hyperpolarization (Fig. 1a) which is caused by an increase in potassium conductance (Bülbring & Tomita, 1969a). The actual spike mechanism is not affected. In fact, a larger and faster action potential can be evoked if, during the phase of hyperpolarization, a sufficiently strong stimulus is applied.

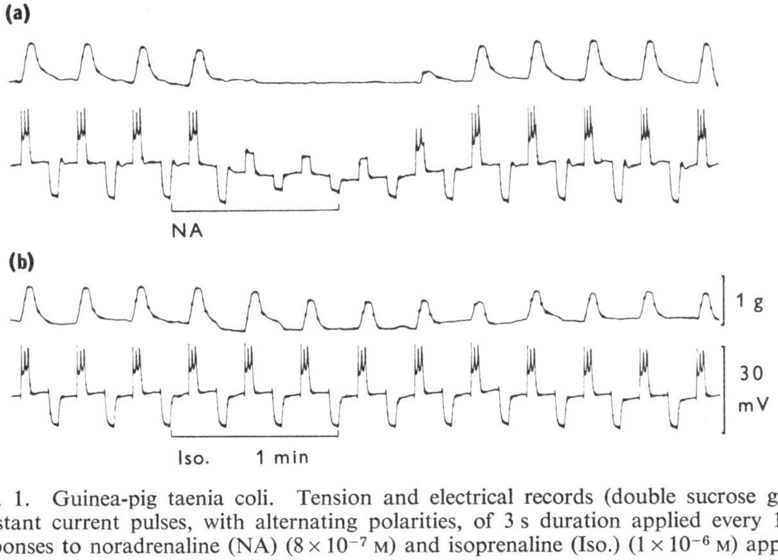


FIG. 1. Guinea-pig taenia coli. Tension and electrical records (double sucrose gap). Constant current pulses, with alternating polarities, of 3 s duration applied every 10 s. Responses to noradrenaline (NA) ($8 \times 10^{-7}$ M) and isoprenaline (Iso.) ($1 \times 10^{-6}$ M) applied for 1 min, as indicated by horizontal bar. (a), Noradrenaline hyperpolarizes the membrane and increases its conductance (as shown by the decrease in the amplitude of the voltage deflections produced by constant current pulses). Depolarizing current no longer generates action potentials, and consequently produces no mechanical response. (b), Isoprenaline diminishes the mechanical response without affecting the electrical properties of the membrane.

The block produced by the $\beta$-action is due to the suppression of the slow depolarization, or pacemaker potential, which generates the spontaneous spike (Bülbring & Tomita, 1969b). The $\beta$-action on membrane activity affects only the spontaneous spike generation. There is no change in membrane potential or membrane resistance, and no increase in stimulus intensity is necessary to evoke a spike. However, the tension response to the spike is diminished (Fig. 1b). This interference with excitation–contraction coupling seems to be the same in all smooth muscles. It will not be further discussed here, since this paper is mainly concerned with the action of catecholamines on the cell membrane.

While the $\beta$-effect seems to be uniform in all smooth muscles, the $\alpha$-effect, that is, the change in membrane conductance, is different in different tissues.

Dale's observations (Dale, 1906) of the changing uterine response to sympathetic nerve stimulation during pregnancy have already been mentioned. What then happens to the state of the smooth muscle cells in the pregnant uterus? The most striking change is a rise of the membrane potential to a level about 20 mV higher than that in nonpregnant uterus (Casteels & Kuriyama, 1965; Bülbring, Casteels & Kuriyama, 1968). This change is brought about by an increase in the membrane permeability to potassium. Naturally, this is associated with a change in the pattern of spontaneous activity, from almost continuous activity in the nonpregnant uterus to near inactivity during pregnancy, varying with the animal species.

In addition to the increased potassium permeability of the membrane, two further changes take place during pregnancy which are important for the response to catecholamines (Bülbring, Casteels & Kuriyama, 1968). One is a change in sensitivity to alterations in the external calcium concentration to which I shall refer later. The other is a change in the chloride distribution, which is particularly great in the cat uterus on which Dale made his early observations. The intracellular chloride content in the cat uterus in early pregnancy is nearly twice that in nonpregnant uterus and hence the chloride equilibrium potential shifts from $-25$ mV in the virgin cat to $-11$ mV in the pregnant cat. In all smooth muscles so far investigated chloride appears to be actively transported into the cell (Casteels, 1965), so that the chloride equilibrium potential is less negative than the membrane potential. Any increase in chloride conductance will thus cause depolarization and, consequently, excitation. This effect is enhanced as a result of the increase in the intracellular chloride concentration in the pregnant cat uterus. Other animal species do not show the same change in chloride distribution as the cat, or only to a lesser extent.

We have so far only investigated the membrane conductance changes caused by catecholamines in guinea-pig uterus (Bülbring & Szurszewski, 1971) using immature animals injected with oestrogen and progesterone. The $\alpha$-effect consists of depolarization, acceleration of spontaneous spike discharge and increased membrane conductance. Superficially this effect resembles that of acetylcholine. However, latency and duration are longer and the ions involved in the conductance change are different (Fig. 2).

The depolarization produced by acetylcholine is due to increased sodium conductance, while the depolarization by noradrenaline is mainly due to an increase in chloride conductance. If chloride is replaced by an impermeant anion the depolarization may be transiently increased but is then rapidly abolished and may be reversed to hyperpolarization. The contribution of

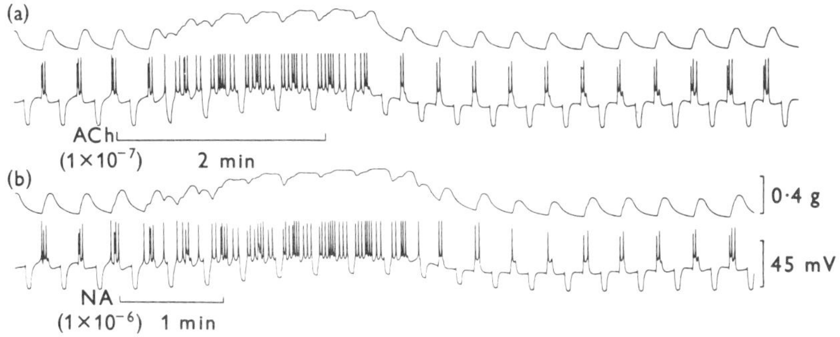


FIG. 2. Guinea-pig uterus, oestrogen+progesterone dominated. (a), Effects of acetylcholine (ACh) applied for 2 min and (b), of noradrenaline (NA) applied for 1 min. Note longer latency and longer duration of the response to noradrenaline than of that to acetylcholine which was applied for a longer period, as indicated by horizontal bars (Szurszewski, 1971).

potassium ions to the increase in membrane conductance can also be revealed by the reversal of the depolarization to hyperpolarization after reducing the external potassium concentration (Fig. 3). Moreover, it has been shown that adrenaline increases $^{42}$K-efflux in these tissues (Brading, unpublished observations). The depolarization may still be observed in sodium-free solution in which sodium is substituted with Tris, but the repetitive spike discharge, which is generated by the depolarization, depends on the presence of sodium. If both sodium and chloride are absent, the depolarization and excitation are both abolished. Sodium is thus clearly involved in the α-effect on the uterus, though the increase in chloride conductance seems to be the primary cause for the depolarization.

In the vas deferens chloride conductance is also increased by catecholamines, but the dominant ion involved in the conductance change is sodium (Magaribuchi, Ito & Kuriyama, 1971). In sodium-free solution the effect of noradrenaline on the vas deferens is abolished. This is particularly interesting since this tissue is in physiological conditions activated by the release of noradrenaline from sympathetic nerves and the excitatory junction potential is sodium dependent (though the spike depends on calcium influx).

Some more data concerning the ionic basis of the increase in membrane conductance caused by catecholamines is summarized in Table 1.

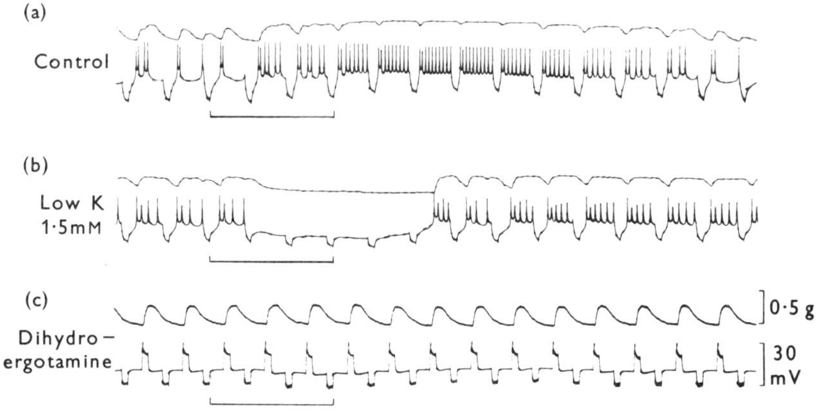


FIG. 3. Guinea-pig uterus, oestrogen + progesterone dominated. Propranolol ($2 \times 10^{-6}$ M) present throughout. Effect of adrenaline (Adr.) ($1 \times 10^{-6}$ M) (a), applied for 1 min (bar) in the presence of 5·9 mM potassium (Control); (b), in the presence of 1·5 mM potassium; (c), after addition of dihydroergotamine ($2 \times 10^{-6}$ M). Note that, in low external potassium, adrenaline causes hyperpolarization (as in taenia, see Fig. 1) which is abolished by an α-blocking agent.

TABLE 1. *Ions contributing to the increase in membrane conductance by catecholamines (α-action)*

| Tissue | $K^+$ | $Cl^-$ | $Na^+$ | Author |
|---|---|---|---|---|
| Guinea-pig taenia coli | ++ | | | Shuba & Klevets, 1967 |
| | ++ | + | 0 | Bülbring & Tomita, 1968, 1969 |
| Guinea-pig uterus (oestrogen + progesterone-dominated) | (+) | ++ | + | Bülbring & Szurszewski, 1971 |
| Guinea-pig vas deferens | (+) | + | ++ | Magaribuchi, Ito & Kuriyama, 1971 |
| Rat portal vein | (+) | ++ | 0 | Wahlström, 1972 |
| Rabbit common carotid artery | | + | + | Mekata & Niu, 1972 |

In the guinea-pig taenia potassium is the dominant ion contributing to the total change in membrane conductance caused by catecholamines; in the uterus it is chloride, and in the vas deferens, sodium. In the portal vein the main evidence has been obtained by measuring ion fluxes (Wahlström, 1972). It was found that, as in other tissues, there is some increase in potassium efflux. However, the increase is no greater than 10–20%, and is not proportional to the concentration of noradrenaline. In contrast, the chloride efflux may be doubled and this effect is proportional to the dose of noradrenaline. The chloride permeability may be increased 3·3 times. As in the taenia coli, sodium does not seem to contribute to the conductance change.

The observations shown in Table 1 present a complicated picture and there are too few observations to allow a general conclusion concerning the reason for the difference in ion species to which the membrane permeability is increased by catecholamines. One clue may be provided by the observation that, in gencral, catecholamines increase both potassium and chloride conductance. If the membrane potential of the tissue is low (as in the taenia) the increase of membrane conductance to potassium is dominant; if the membrane potential is high (as in the pregnant uterus) the increase in chloride conductance is dominant.

A possible explanation for the diversity may be found in the different calcium-binding capacity of the tissues. As mentioned earlier, a change occurs during the course of pregnancy in the sensitivity of the myometrium to reduction or increase of the external calcium concentration (Coutinho & Csapo, 1959; Bülbring, Casteels & Kuriyama, 1968). The nonpregnant uterus is rapidly depolarized by exposure to calcium-deficient solution. The pregnant uterus, however, is rather insensitive to the removal of calcium and excess calcium causes little or no hyperpolarization but often initiates activity.

Our knowledge of the processes which determine the membrane potential by controlling the ion permeability of the cell membrane, by influencing the movement of ions across, or their binding at the cell membrane, is still very limited. These processes include (a) various ion pumping mechanisms and (b) the many ways by which calcium is involved in the functions of the smooth muscle cell.

At the symposium on *Adrenergic Mechanisms* the evidence then available led to the conclusion that 'sympathomimetic effects are the result of two, often opposing actions, one on the cell membrane ($\alpha$) and the other on cell metabolism ($\beta$)'. Today I would like to extend this hypothesis by proposing that both actions may be metabolic, and that both may be intimately involved in the cellular distribution of calcium.

In order to evaluate the evidence supporting this idea we have to remember that calcium has at least two distinct functions at the smooth muscle cell membrane. As in many other tissues, calcium controls the membrane permeability to other ions. But, in contrast to other excitable tissues, where sodium carries the action current, the action potential of smooth muscle is produced by the entry of calcium ions. Though sodium seems to contribute to a varying extent to membrane activity, especially to the slow components, the spike itself appears to be a calcium spike in all visceral smooth muscles (Bülbring & Kuriyama, 1963; Kuriyama, Osa & Toida, 1966; Brading, Bülbring & Tomita, 1969b; Bülbring & Tomita, 1970a,b).

Though catecholamines do affect the slow generator potential they do not affect the actual spike mechanism. On the other hand, the activity of a host of enzymes is probably responsible for the distribution of calcium at the outer membrane as well as inside the cell. These enzyme systems which control the binding and the release of calcium may well be influenced by catecholamines.

The observations of the effects of changing the external calcium concentration on membrane resistance of taenia coli have been surprising (Bülbring & Tomita, 1969c). Excess calcium hyperpolarizes the membrane, but this is associated with a reduction of the electrotonic potential indicating an increase in potassium conductance. On the other hand, when the calcium concentration is reduced to one-fifth or even one-tenth of the normal concentration, the membrane is depolarized, as expected, but the electrotonic potential is increased, indicating a decrease in potassium conductance. Only when the external calcium is reduced further to zero does the membrane potential fall to a low value with a reduction of the electrotonic potential indicating an increase in sodium conductance (Bülbring & Tomita, 1970a,b). That this is so is shown by the observation that membrane potential and membrane resistance recover if, in calcium-free solution, sodium is also removed. A similar restoration can be achieved by an increase of the external magnesium concentration. Various divalent ions can substitute for calcium, either for the spike (barium, strontium) or for membrane stabilization (magnesium). It has been suggested that there may be two different calcium-binding sites at the cell membrane of the taenia coli at which calcium controls the permeability to other ions (Bülbring & Tomita, 1970a,b; Brading, Bülbring & Tomita, 1969a). For example, calcium bound at the outer layer of the cell membrane might control sodium permeability, while inside the cell membrane calcium might control potassium permeability.

In the taenia coli, or in the nonpregnant uterus, the calcium binding by the membrane is probably much weaker than in the pregnant uterus. This greater calcium binding during pregnancy may be one factor causing the low sodium and high potassium permeability of the membrane (Casteels, 1965). Moreover, the guinea-pig taenia is normally rather insensitive to tetraethylammonium (TEA). However, in the presence of excess calcium, TEA becomes effective. In contrast, the fundus of the guinea-pig stomach, whose membrane potential is much higher than that of the taenia, is completely quiescent and a spike can be evoked by electrical stimulation only in the presence of TEA (Osa & Kuriyama, 1970; Ito, Kuriyama & Sakamoto, 1970).

Finally, what is the supporting evidence for the involvement of calcium in the action of catecholamines? (1) Excess calcium mimics the $\alpha$-action on the membrane. In the taenia excess calcium causes hyperpolarization and inhibition of spontaneous activity (Fig. 4), and in the uterus depolarization and excitation (Fig. 5). Both appear to be due to the same changes in membrane conductance as those produced by the $\alpha$-action of catecholamines (Bülbring & Tomita, 1969c). (2) Excess calcium potentiates the $\alpha$-effect. Removal of calcium abolishes the $\alpha$-effect (Bülbring & Tomita, 1969c).

It is difficult to assess the $\alpha$-action of catecholamines in calcium-free

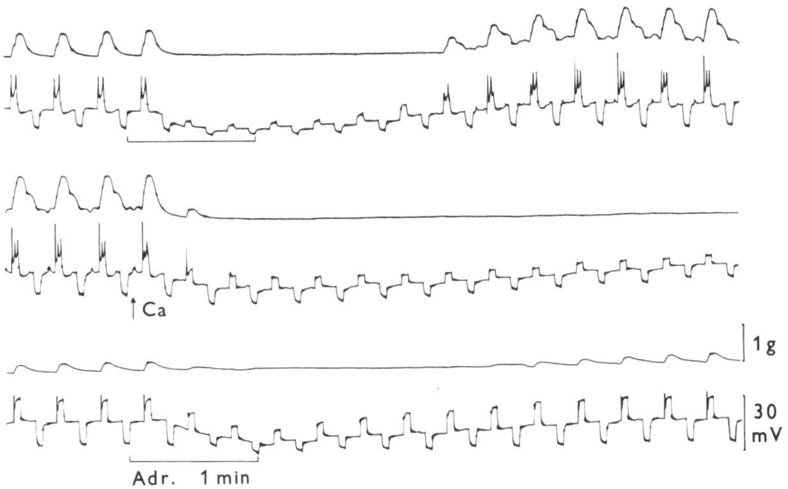


FIG. 4. Guinea-pig taenia coli. Effect of adrenaline (Adr.) ($2 \times 10^{-6}$ M), applied for 1 min (bar), before (top) and after (bottom) raising the external calcium concentration from 2·5 mM to 15 mM (at arrow). (In the bottom record the current intensity was increased to evoke a spike.)

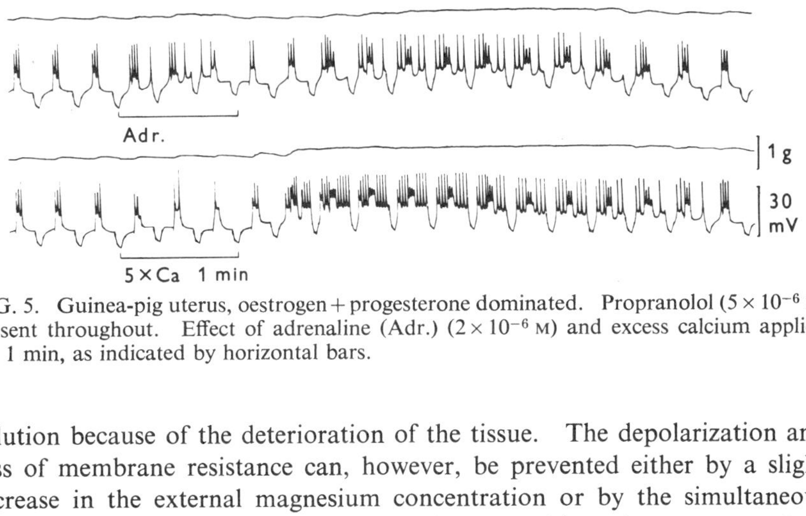


FIG. 5. Guinea-pig uterus, oestrogen + progesterone dominated. Propranolol ($5 \times 10^{-6}$ M) present throughout. Effect of adrenaline (Adr.) ($2 \times 10^{-6}$ M) and excess calcium applied for 1 min, as indicated by horizontal bars.

solution because of the deterioration of the tissue. The depolarization and loss of membrane resistance can, however, be prevented either by a slight increase in the external magnesium concentration or by the simultaneous removal of calcium and sodium as well. In neither circumstances does adrenaline produce any change in membrane conductance. But addition of calcium restores the α-action (Bülbring, 1970). No other divalent cation can substitute for calcium in supporting the effect of catecholamines on membrane conductance (Bülbring & Tomita, 1969c).

While excess calcium mimics the inhibitory and excitatory α-effects of catecholamines and potentiates both, it affects the β-action in the opposite direction. Excess calcium restores the tension response after it has been

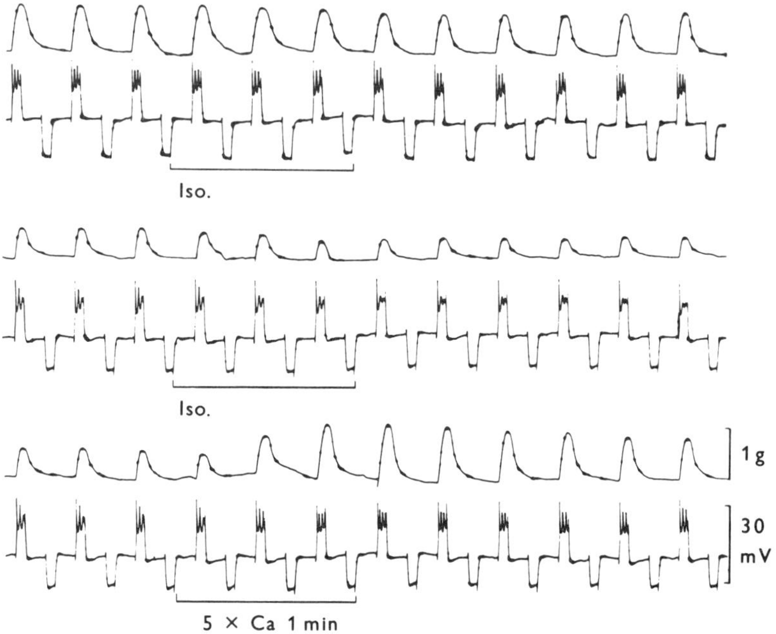


FIG. 6. Guinea-pig taenia coli. The effect of isoprenaline (Iso.) ($1 \times 10^{-6}$ M) applied for 1 min (bar) upper record: in the absence; middle record: in the presence of theophylline ($5 \times 10^{-4}$ M). Note that theophylline reduced the tension response and potentiated the effect of isoprenaline. Lower record: exposure to excess calcium for 1 min (bar) restored the tension response transiently to the original size.

depressed as a result of the β-action (Fig. 6). A similar antagonism can also be observed between isoprenaline and noradrenaline.

Robison, Butcher & Sutherland (1971) believe that 'the adrenergic β-receptor is probably an integral component of the adenyl cyclase system . . . and that β-adrenergic effects in general result from an increase in the intracellular level of cyclic AMP'. In all smooth muscles the β-effect appears to be a reduction of the tension development in response to membrane excitation. This interference with excitation–contraction coupling is thought to be the result of a reduction of the availability of calcium ions for the activation of the contractile protein, because the calcium is taken up into intracellular storage sites. The enzyme involved in this binding of calcium is believed to be activated by cyclic AMP.

On the other hand, Robison, Butcher & Sutherland (1971) point out that 'catecholamines also have the ability to reduce the level of cyclic AMP' and that 'the receptors for this type of effect . . . have the characteristics of adrenergic α-receptors'. They proposed a possible model of the situation of adrenergic receptors in the cell membrane as part of a regulatory subunit bonded to a catalytic subunit in such a way that the α-action decreases and the β-action increases the activity of adenyl cyclase. They emphasize, however, that an inhibitory effect on adenyl cyclase activity by a catecholamine in a broken cell preparation has never been observed. Moreover, observations that both types of receptors can mediate superficially similar effects (as in the taenia for example) are not compatible with this model.

We have seen that, indeed, the α- and β-effects on the taenia are only superficially similar, both causing relaxation, but that the two mechanisms are totally different.

Robison, Butcher & Sutherland (1971) have considered the possibility that the α-receptor may interact with a different enzyme system from that which is activated by β-receptors. 'If such an enzyme system were to compete for the same substrate pool utilized by adenyl cyclase, then it is easy to imagine how the stimulation of such a system could reduce the level of cyclic AMP without affecting the catalytic potential of adenyl cyclase.'

The same concept of competition has been put forward by Born (1971) to explain the inhibition of platelet aggregation by cyclic AMP. The aggregating effect of ADP depends on protein phosphorylation. Born assumes that cyclic AMP accelerates the phosphorylation of other proteins at the expense of the phosphoprotein involved in aggregation. ATP is necessary for the phosphorylations caused by both ADP and cyclic AMP. Their opposing effect could then be accounted for by assuming competition for a limited pool of ATP.

I believe that this concept would be compatible with the observations of α- and β-effects on smooth muscle whether they are synergistic or antagonistic.

It has been shown that the two essential requirements for the action of catecholamines are (1) metabolic energy supply (Bueding, Bülbring, Gercken, Hawkins & Kuriyama, 1967), and (2) calcium (Bülbring & Tomita, 1969c; Bülbring, 1970).

One can assume that the β-action (which is similar in all smooth muscles) involves the phosphorylation of a protein, a process which is activated by cyclic AMP and which leads to the accumulation of calcium at intracellular membrane structures. The main result is a reduction of the intracellular calcium ion concentration so that less calcium is available for the contractile mechanism.

Continuing the analogy with the observations on platelets (Born, 1971) it may be assumed that the α-action involves the phosphorylation of another protein which does not depend on cyclic AMP. This enzyme system would utilize ATP from the same pool as the adenyl cyclase system, but it would cause the release of calcium from storage sites. The responses to catecholamines obtained from different tissues would then depend, firstly, on the location, on the amount and on the availability of bound calcium and, secondly, on the ion species whose contribution to membrane conductance is controlled by bound calcium and is chiefly influenced by the release of calcium.

Romero & Whittam (1971) showed recently that an increase in the intracellular calcium concentration caused an increase in the potassium permeability of the red blood cell membrane. If the same mechanism also operates in the taenia, then the α-action of catecholamines, by releasing calcium from stores, could increase the intracellular calcium concentration and thus increase the potassium permeability. This increase in potassium permeability by catecholamines is their dominant effect on the taenia and produces hyperpolarization which stops spike discharge. Therefore, in contrast to most visceral muscles, the α-action on taenia and other intestinal muscles is inhibitory.

The hypothesis that catecholamines produce their action indirectly by influencing calcium binding and calcium release requires much more experimental evidence. Concerning the metabolic action of catecholamines, a recent paper by Panet & Selinger (1972) may be relevant. They describe the synthesis of ATP coupled to calcium release from sarcoplasmic reticulum. This may be part of the mechanism by which, in the taenia coli, adrenaline increases the tissue content of ATP and CP (Bueding, Bülbring, Gercken, Hawkins & Kuriyama, 1967). In addition, Bueding, Butcher, Hawkins, Timms & Sutherland (1966) described an increase in the level of cyclic AMP. The increases in ATP and in cyclic AMP were both extremely small. However, the very small changes might indicate yet another control mechanism which the body provides by circulating a hormone, adrenaline, which is capable of exerting simultaneously two competitive actions. The two demands on the common ATP pool may parallel the preponderance of either an α- or a β-response of the tissue which is determined by the metabolic state of the cells.

## REFERENCES


BORN, G. V. R. (1971). In: *Effects of Drugs on Cellular Control Mechanisms*, Biological Council Symposium, ed. Rabin, B. R. & Freedman, R. B., p. 237. London: Macmillan.

BRADING, A. F., BÜLBRING, E. & TOMITA, T. (1969a). *J. Physiol., Lond.*, **200**, 621.

BRADING, A. F., BÜLBRING, E. & TOMITA, T. (1969b). *J. Physiol., Lond.*, **200**, 637.

BUEDING, E., BÜLBRING, E., GERCKEN, G., HAWKINS, J. T. & KURIYAMA, H. (1967). *J. Physiol., Lond.*, **193**, 187.

BUEDING, E., BUTCHER, R. W., HAWKINS, J., TIMMS, A. R. & SUTHERLAND, E. W. (1966). *Biochim. biophys. Acta*, **115**, 173.

BÜLBRING, E. (1955). *J. Physiol., Lond.*, **128**, 200.

BÜLBRING, E. (1960). *Adrenergic Mechanisms.* Ciba Foundation Symposium, p. 275. London: Churchill.

BÜLBRING, E. (1970). *Rendic. R. Gastroenterol.*, **2**, 197.

BÜLBRING, E., BRADING, A. F., JONES, A W. & TOMITA, T. (1970). *Smooth Muscle.* London: Edward Arnold.

BÜLBRING, E., CASTEELS, R. & KURIYAMA, H. (1968). *Br. J. Pharmac. Chemother.*, **34**, 388.

BÜLBRING, E. & KURIYAMA, H. (1963). *J. Physiol., Lond.*, **166**, 29.

BÜLBRING, E. & SZURSZEWSKI, J. H. (1971). *J. Physiol., Lond.*, **217**, 39P.

BÜLBRING, E. & TOMITA, T. (1968). *J. Physiol., Lond.*, **194**, 74.

BÜLBRING, E. & TOMITA, T. (1969a). *Proc. R. Soc.*, B, **172**, 89.

BÜLBRING, E. & TOMITA, T. (1969b). *Proc. R. Soc.*, B, **172**, 103.

BÜLBRING, E. & TOMITA, T. (1969c). *Proc. R. Soc.*, B, **172**, 121.

BÜLBRING, E. & TOMITA, T. (1970a). *J. Physiol., Lond.*, **210**, 217.

BÜLBRING, E. & TOMITA, T. (1970b). In: A Symposium on *Calcium and Cellular Function* ed. Cuthbert, A. W., p. 249. London: Macmillan.
CASTEELS, R. (1965). *J. Physiol., Lond.*, **178**, 10.
CASTEELS, R. & KURIYAMA, H. (1965). *J. Physiol., Lond.*, **177**, 263.
COUTINHO, E. M. & CSAPO, A. (1959). *J. gen. Physiol.*, **43**, 13.
DALE, H. H. (1906). *J. Physiol., Lond.*, **34**, 163.
DALE, H. H. (1913). *J. Physiol., Lond.*, **46**, 291.
HOLMAN, M. E. (1958). *J. Physiol., Lond.*, **141**, 464.
ITO, Y., KURIYAMA, H. & SAKAMOTO, Y. (1970). *J. Physiol., Lond.*, **211**, 445.
KURIYAMA, H. (1963). *J. Physiol., Lond.*, **166**, 15.
KURIYAMA, H., OSA, T. & TOIDA, N. (1966). *Br. J. Pharmac. Chemother.*, **27**, 366.
MAGARIBUCHI, T., ITO, Y. & KURIYAMA, H. (1971). *Jap. J. Physiol.*, **21**, 691.
MEKATA, F. & NIU, H. (1972). *J. gen. Physiol.*, **59**, 92.
OHASHI, H. (1970). *J. Physiol., Lond.*, **210**, 405.
OSA, T. & KURIYAMA, H. (1970). *Jap. J. Physiol.*, **20**, 626.
PANET, R. & SELINGER, Z. (1972). *Biochim. biophys. Acta*, **255**, 34.
ROBISON, G. A., BUTCHER, R. W. & SUTHERLAND, E. W. (1971). *Cyclic AMP.* New York & London: Academic Press.
ROMERO, P. J. & WHITTAM, R. (1971). *J. Physiol., Lond.*, **214**, 481.
SHUBA, M. F. & KLEVETS, M. Y. (1967). *Sechenov. Physiol. J., USSR*, **13**, 1.
SZURSZEWSKI, J. H. (1971). B.Sc. Thesis, University of Oxford.
VOGT, M. (1965). *J. Physiol., Lond.*, **179**, 163.
WAHLSTRÖM, B. (1972). *J. Physiol., Lond.*, **226**, 63P.

# ACTIONS OF CATECHOLAMINES ON THE MEMBRANE PROPERTIES OF LIVER CELLS

D. G. HAYLETT AND D. H. JENKINSON

*Department of Pharmacology, University College London, London WC1E 6BT, England*

Most of our knowledge of the properties and mode of action of receptors has come from work with nerve and muscle rather than with non-excitable tissues such as the liver and the various salivary glands. This is not because of any lack of interest in these organs but reflects rather the difficulty of applying certain experimental procedures (for example, the measurement of changes in membrane conductance) to tissues which are structurally complex, and in which the cells are often interconnected to form a three-dimensional syncytium. Another complication is that the cells in such tissues are generally rather small, certainly compared with skeletal muscle fibres, or with many neurones.

The aim of the work to be described was to learn something more of the mode of action of the adrenergic receptors in the liver. In particular, we wished to test whether catecholamines alter the permeability of hepatic cells to inorganic ions, a point of interest in view of the growing evidence that changes in membrane permeability are concerned in the responses of several other tissues to adrenaline and noradrenaline. This has been studied in most detail in the longitudinal muscle of the intestine in which the permeability change has been shown to be mediated by α-receptors, and to involve potassium (Jenkinson & Morton, 1965, 1967a,b; Bülbring & Tomita, 1968, 1969a,b) and to a lesser extent chloride ions (Ohashi, 1971; see also Bogach & Klevets, 1967). Also, it has been known for some time that adrenaline, in addition to accelerating hepatic glycogenolysis, produces a transient increase in plasma potassium concentration in many species by causing the release of potassium from the liver (D'Silva, 1934, 1937), and it seemed possible that this could be a consequence of a change in the potassium permeability of the parenchymal cell membrane.

The choice of a suitable preparation with which to test this hypothesis was influenced by the need to be able to make substantial changes in the composition of the fluid bathing the cells. This suggested the use of either tissue slices or isolated cells. Although both approaches proved feasible, the experiments to be described were made with slices (for a preliminary account of results obtained with isolated cells under short-term tissue culture conditions, see Green, Dale & Haylett, 1972). The slices (thickness c. 300 μm) were prepared from the median lobe of the liver of guinea-pigs, and were first incubated for 3 h at 38° C in a bathing fluid of the following composition (mM): NaCl, 125; KCl, 6; $CaCl_2$, 1·0; $MgSO_4$, 1·2; $NaH_2PO_4$, 1·0; $NaHCO_3$, 15; Na pyruvate, 2 (pH 7·4 when equilibrated with 5% $CO_2$ in $O_2$). Further details are given in other publications (Haylett & Jenkinson, 1972a,b) where it is also shown that the slices could maintain a stable ionic composition for several hours after the initial incubation period.

It proved possible to follow the exchange of labelled potassium in the slices, and an experiment to determine the effect of noradrenaline on both

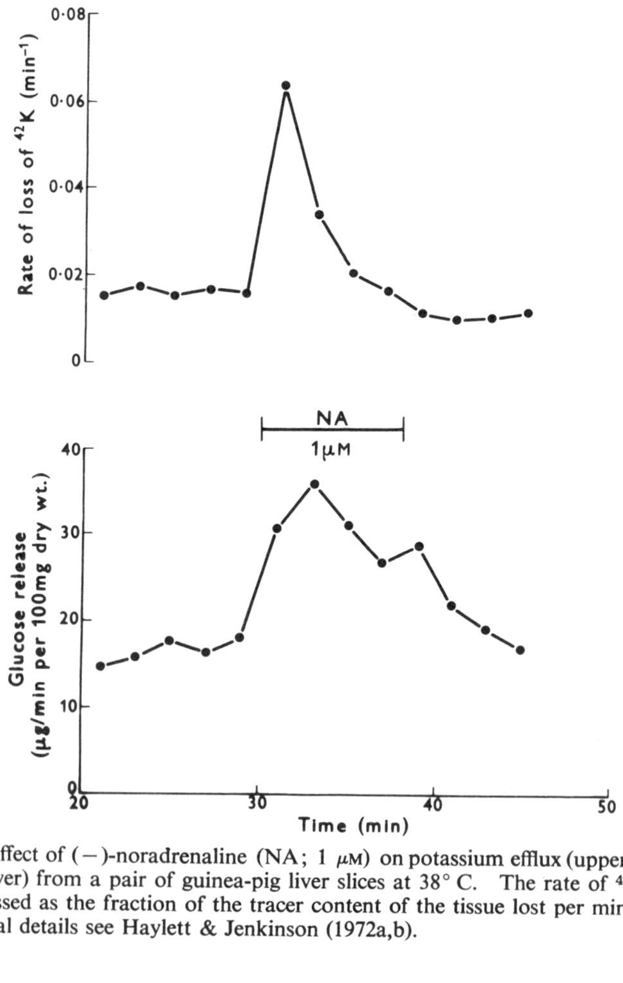


FIG. 1. Effect of (−)-noradrenaline (NA; 1 μM) on potassium efflux (upper) and glucose release (lower) from a pair of guinea-pig liver slices at 38° C. The rate of $^{42}K$ efflux has been expressed as the fraction of the tracer content of the tissue lost per min. For other experimental details see Haylett & Jenkinson (1972a,b).

potassium efflux and glucose release is illustrated in Fig. 1. The marked increase in the rate of loss of $^{42}K$ suggests that a change in membrane permeability may have occurred. If this effect were specific to potassium ions, or nearly so, the membrane potential of the cells would also be expected to increase, since analyses of the slices had suggested that the potassium equilibrium potential of the parenchymal cells is likely to have been at least −80 mV, that is, much greater than the resting potential which under the present experimental conditions lay between −30 and −40 mV (mean 36·2 ± 0·8 mV, S.E. of 30 observations). Hyperpolarization was indeed observed, as illustrated in Fig. 2 (see also later).

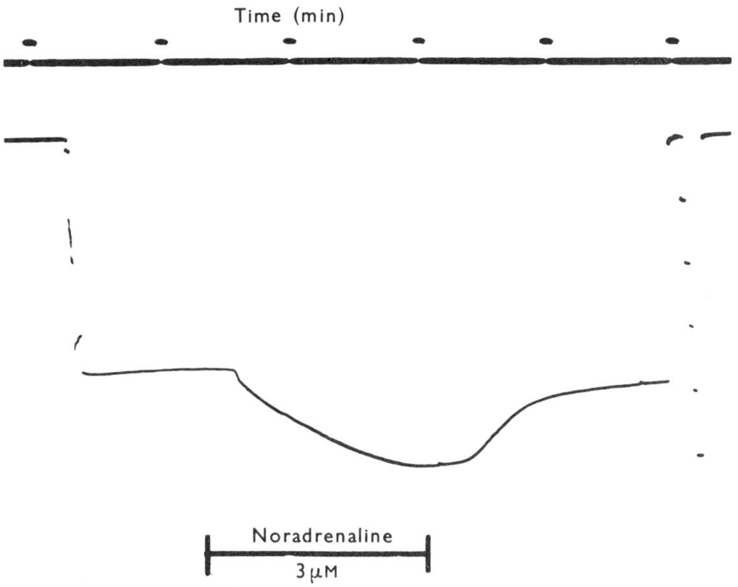


FIG. 2. Effect of (−)-noradrenaline (3 μM), on the membrane potential of a cell in a guinea-pig liver slice. As the record began (left) a microelectrode was lowered towards the slice and inserted in the second cell encountered. Application of noradrenaline (during the bar) caused the membrane potential to increase from −35 to −50 mV. The electrode was then withdrawn, and 10 mV calibration steps applied (right). (From Haylett & Jenkinson, 1972a, with permission.)

Further experiments (Haylett & Jenkinson, 1969, 1972a) showed that the variation of the response with changes in external potassium was in keeping with the idea of an increase in potassium permeability, as was the finding that noradrenaline reduced the amplitude of electrotonic potentials set up by current pulses through a second microelectrode located in a cell some distance (150–350 μm) from the recording site. Nevertheless, although all the evidence obtained was consistent with the hypothesis that has been outlined, it has to be recognized that because of the complex structural arrangement of hepatic tissue, the various tests applied are in general less decisive than the equivalent experiments with excitable tissues (see discussion by Haylett & Jenkinson, 1972a). Thus, certain alternative explanations for the increases in membrane potential and potassium efflux caused by noradrenaline cannot be entirely ruled out. For example, both effects could be accounted for by supposing that noradrenaline activates an active transport mechanism which extrudes potassium ions from the cells, and which can operate electrogenically, although ouabain-insensitive. This seems unlikely, taking the evidence as a whole, although it should be noted that a cation pump with precisely these characteristics may operate in some insect tissues (for references see Keynes, 1969).

## *Classification of receptors in guinea-pig liver*

Further experiments were made to identify the types of receptor concerned in the effect on potassium permeability and glucose release. Since β-receptors have been found to mediate most of the metabolic responses to catecholamines, it was rather surprising to observe that selective α-agonists (methoxamine, phenylephrine and amidephrine*), as well as isoprenaline accelerated the release of glucose. Amidephrine was chosen for more detailed study, and its effect on glucose release was found to be inhibited by phentolamine (10 μM) but not by propranolol (1 μM), whereas the converse held for the action of isoprenaline (Figs. 3 and 4). While these results (see also

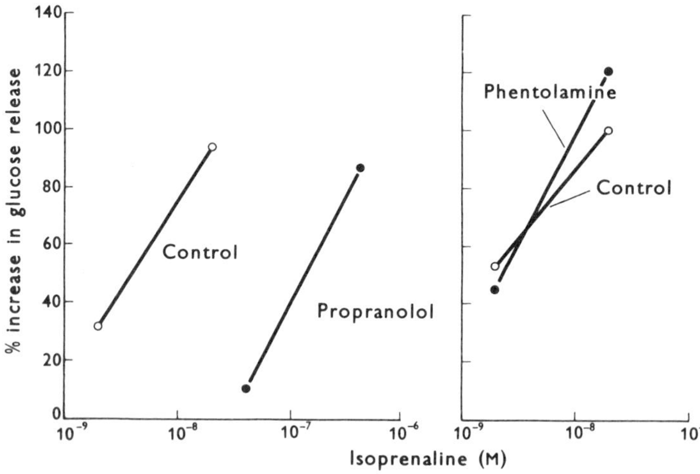


FIG. 3. Inhibition by propranolol (1 μM) but not by phentolamine (10 μM) of the effect of (−)-isoprenaline on glucose release. Both antagonists were included in the bathing fluid from 1 h beforehand. Separate experiments. (From Haylett & Jenkinson, 1972b, with permission.)

* 3(2-methylamino-1-hydroxyethyl)methanesulphonanilide: see Dungan, Stanton & Lish (1965); Buchthal & Jenkinson (1970).

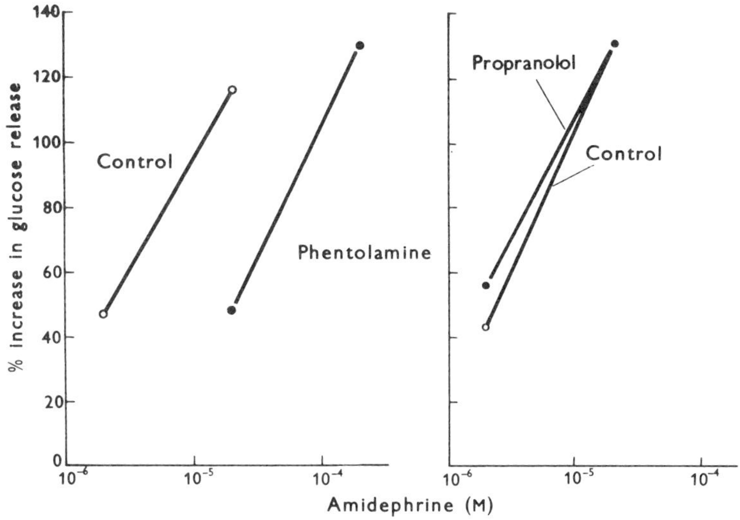


FIG. 4. Inhibition by phentolamine (10 $\mu$M) but not by propranolol (1 $\mu$M) of the effect of ($\pm$)-amidephrine on glucose release. Separate experiments. (From Haylett & Jenkinson, 1972b, with permission.)

Haylett & Jenkinson, 1968, 1972b) strongly suggest that this response can be elicited by activation of either of two distinct adrenergic receptors, it would be premature to conclude that these are identical to the kinds found in other peripheral tissues since the dose ratios (that is, the factor by which the concentration of an agonist has to be increased to restore a given response in the presence of an antagonist) found in the present work were smaller (particularly with phentolamine) than those observed with, for example, vascular and intestinal smooth muscle.

Parallel experiments to classify the receptors concerned in the effect on potassium permeability suggested that under normal circumstances $\alpha$-like receptors were mainly involved (though see later). Thus, amidephrine markedly increased both $^{42}$K efflux and membrane potential, and these effects could be inhibited by phentolamine but not by propranolol, both antagonists being applied at the same concentrations as in the experiments on glucose release. This conclusion is in keeping with the demonstration by Ellis & Beckett (1963) that the hyperkalaemic response in the cat is $\alpha$-mediated.

## *Species variation*

It is well known, mainly from the work of Ellis and his colleagues, that the action of catecholamines on the liver can differ considerably from species to species, the rat being particularly divergent (see reviews by Ellis, 1956, 1967; Hornbrook, 1970). Fig. 5 illustrates an experiment to compare the effects of

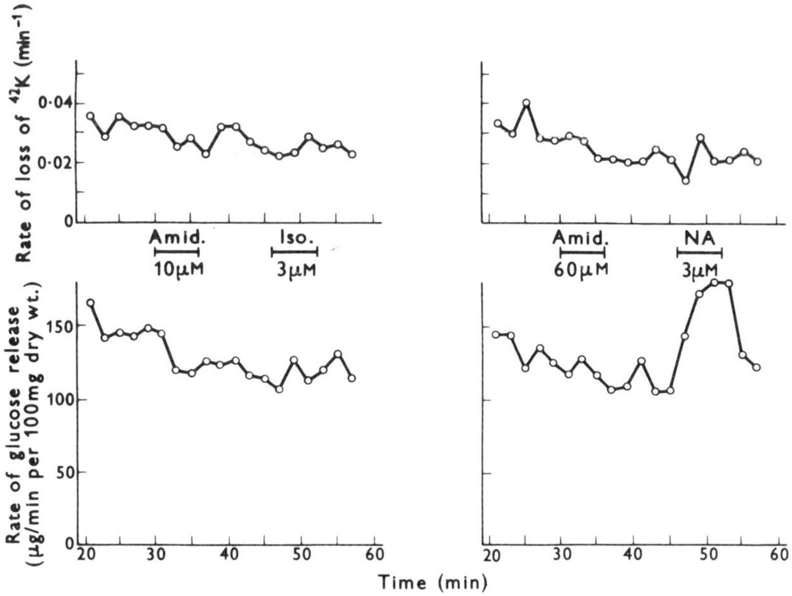


FIG. 5. Effect of (−)-amidephrine (Amid.; 10 μM) and (−)-isoprenaline (Iso.; 3 μM) (left) and of (−)-amidephrine (Amid.; 60 μM) and (−)-noradrenaline (NA; 3 μM) (right) on $^{42}$K efflux (upper) and glucose release (lower) from rat liver slices at 38° C.

amidephrine, noradrenaline and isoprenaline on rat liver slices under conditions identical to those used with the guinea-pig tissue. It can be seen that potassium efflux is little affected by any of these agonists, and only noradrenaline causes any substantial increase in glucose release, in marked contrast to the results obtained with guinea-pig liver. The explanation of this difference is uncertain: it may be that the receptors in rat liver are quite different, or that the agonist concentrations attained in the immediate vicinity of the receptors are much lower than in the bathing fluid, possibly because of the operation of an uptake mechanism for these substances. This remains for further study.

### *Effect of isoprenaline on membrane potential*

Another rather puzzling aspect of the action of catecholamines on the liver was revealed by a study of the effect of isoprenaline on membrane potential. If α-receptors alone were concerned in the action on potassium permeability which has been described, it would be expected that isoprenaline should increase $^{42}$K efflux and cause hyperpolarization only at high concentration, if at all. A first series of experiments with isoprenaline at 1 μM showed that whereas many cells were unaffected, and remained so even when the concentration was increased to 6 μM, others hyperpolarized: in 32 tests in 11 preparations, the membrane potential increased by 4·2 ± 0·9 mV (S.E.) (as compared to 10·1 ± 0·7 mV ($n$=31) in response to the same concentration (1 μM) of noradrenaline).

It was at first thought that this response to isoprenaline could be α-mediated. However, further experiments showed that in responsive preparations much lower concentrations of isoprenaline (10–50 nM), at which little α-receptor activation would be expected, also caused hyperpolarization (see also Somlyo, Somlyo & Friedmann, 1971; Lambotte, 1971). It was also observed that the response to low concentrations of isoprenaline became much larger if tested just after application of the α-agonists amidephrine and methoxamine, as illustrated in Fig. 6.

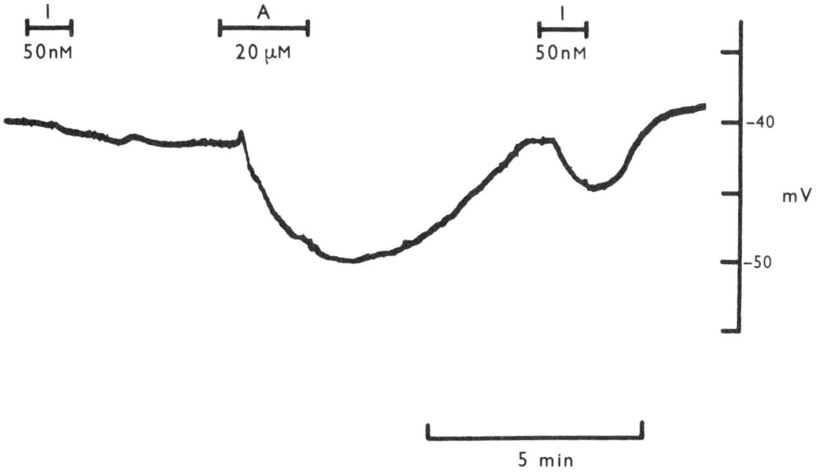


FIG. 6. Potentiation by (±)-amidephrine (20 μM, at 'A') of the hyperpolarization caused by (−)-isoprenaline (50 nM, at 'I').

The mechanism of this facilitation, and indeed of the effect of isoprenaline on membrane potential, is uncertain. Some general possibilities are that isoprenaline may hyperpolarize by increasing the activity of an electrogenic transport mechanism, or by altering membrane permeability. The hypothetical active transport process could be based on movements of either cations or anions. However, further experiments showed that the response to isoprenaline increased rather than diminished on replacing chloride by either isethionate or other large anions such as methylsulphate or pyroglutamate. This suggested that active transport of anions, and certainly of chloride, is unlikely to have been the main factor involved. Considering next cation transport, an important possibility was that isoprenaline hyperpolarized by activating an outwardly-directed sodium pump which, it could be imagined, may become electrogenic when the ratio of sodium to potassium in the tissue rises. Since this occurs as a result of the action of α-agonists such as noradrenaline and amidephrine (Haylett & Jenkinson, 1972a,b), the increased electrogenicity could perhaps account for the facilitation illustrated in Fig. 6. Active transport systems of this kind can often be inhibited by ouabain and by reduction of the external potassium concentration. An experiment to test the effect of these treatments is shown in Fig. 7. It may be seen that the response to isoprenaline still occurs in nominally potassium-free solution, and is little affected by ouabain at a concentration sufficient to abolish the hyperpolarization (presumably electrogenic) which results from reintroduction of potassium to slices bathed in potassium-free solution. It should be mentioned in relation to this that Lambotte (1971) has concluded that the hyperpolarization caused by isoprenaline in perfused dog liver is also ouabain-insensitive.

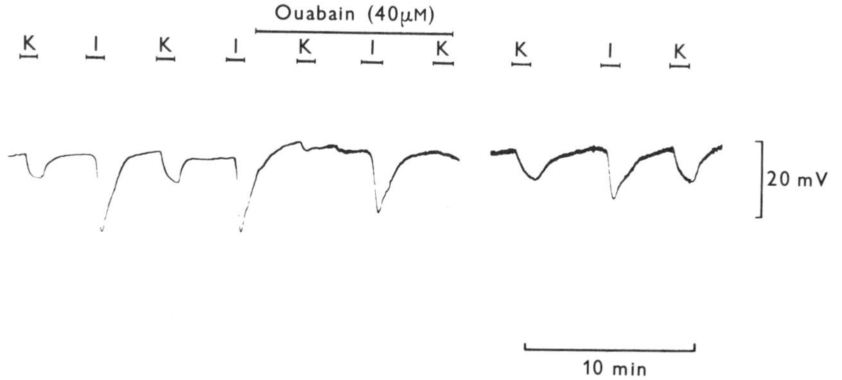


FIG. 7. The effect of ouabain (40 μM) on the hyperpolarizations elicited by applications of isoprenaline (50 nM, at 'I') and brief restoration of the normal external potassium (6 mM, at 'K') to a slice bathed in a potassium-free isethionate solution. The rise in membrane potential which followed the increase in $[K]_o$ is abolished by ouabain, in contrast to the response to isoprenaline. 40 min later the effect of ouabain is largely reversed (right).

Explanations based on changes in membrane permeability may next be considered. The effect of isoprenaline on membrane potential could perhaps be due to a reduction in the ratio of sodium to potassium permeability ($P_{Na}/P_K$). Were a fall in $P_{Na}$ to underly the response, and were $P_K$ to remain unchanged, the efflux of potassium would be expected to decline a little during the action of isoprenaline, as a consequence of the slight increase in membrane potential. An experiment to test this point is shown in Fig. 8 where it is seen that potassium efflux *increases* rather than falls, the effect becoming much more marked after amidephrine (cf. Fig. 6). Thus it would seem that a decline in $P_{Na}$, *per se*, could not explain the effect on membrane potential, although more direct evidence on the point is required.

Another possibility is that isoprenaline influences membrane potential and potassium efflux by increasing potassium permeability. This could certainly account for the observed results and can perhaps provide a better explanation for the findings in preliminary experiments that the effect of isoprenaline on membrane potential, (a) was associated with a fall in the amplitude of the electrotonic potential, as found with noradrenaline, and (b), varied with external potassium in the way which would be expected were $P_K$ to have increased. Thus isoprenaline, like noradrenaline, caused the membrane potential to move toward the potassium equilibrium potential ($E_K$) whether this was smaller or larger than the membrane potential (see Haylett & Jenkinson, 1972a).

Such an hypothesis, however, leaves open the question of why this action of isoprenaline (unlike the effect on glucose release) should become substantial only under some experimental conditions. One possible explanation for the potentiation by amidephrine is that a metaphilic effect (Rang & Ritter, 1969, 1970a,b) may be involved. Thus it was noted that the effect of amidephrine on $^{42}K$ efflux was invariably transient, suggesting that the α-like receptors may have become desensitized; if the change in the receptors was such that they could now be activated by isoprenaline, the facilitation seen in Figs. 6 and 8 could perhaps be accounted for. While further study is clearly needed, some indirect evidence against this tentative hypothesis was provided by the additional findings (1) that the action of glucagon in causing a small increase in potassium efflux also becomes more marked after amidephrine; (2) that the action of isoprenaline both before and after amidephrine could be inhibited by propranolol (see Fig. 9).

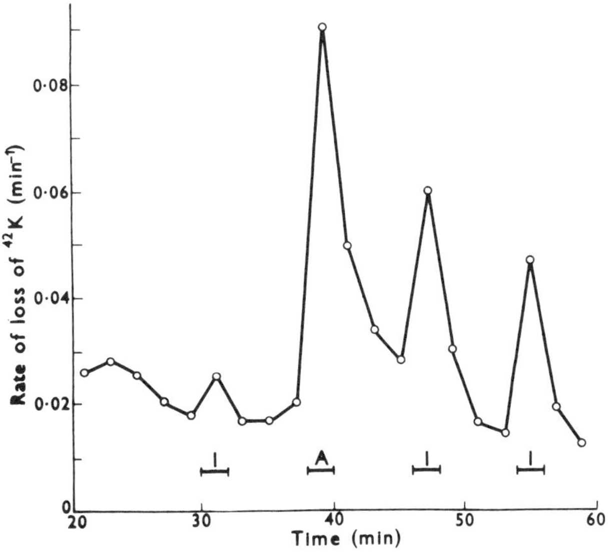


FIG. 8. Potentiation by (±)-amidephrine (20 μM, at 'A') of the effect of (−)-isoprenaline (50 nM, at 'I') on $^{42}K$ efflux.

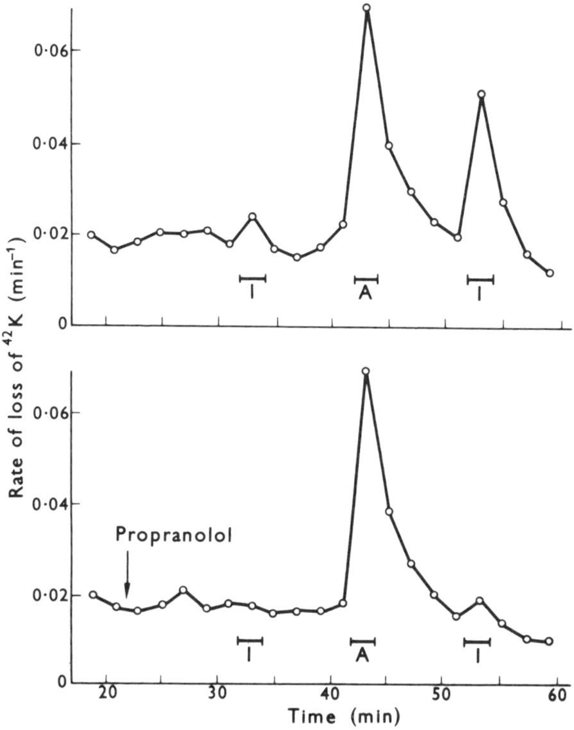


FIG. 9. Upper, as Fig. 8, but from another experiment. Lower, as above, but in the presence of propranolol (1 μM) from arrow onwards. Note the response to isoprenaline is much reduced, in contrast to that to amidephrine.

To summarize, while it has been possible to rule out some explanations for the effect of isoprenaline on membrane properties, the exact mechanism remains uncertain. One possibility is that isoprenaline activates an outwardly-directed, ouabain-insensitive potassium pump that can operate electrogenically. Another is that under certain conditions the β-receptors may, like the α-receptors in normal circumstances, cause an increase in potassium permeability. Taken as a whole, the present evidence tends to favour the second hypothesis which, in common with the first, represents a considerable departure from current views of the mechanisms concerned in the actions of adrenergic receptors.

## *Summary*

Noradrenaline increases glucose release and potassium efflux from guinea-pig liver slices. The latter action can be accounted for as a consequence of an increase in the potassium permeability of the liver cell membrane, and is normally mediated by an α-like receptor, although β-receptor activation may also be effective in some circumstances. Glucose release can be increased by either of two distinct receptors, one α- and the other β-like.

We enjoyed the help of Dr D. W. Littlejohns in some experiments, and our thanks are also due to Mrs J. E. Haylett for unfailing technical assistance. The work was supported in part by the Medical Research Council.

## REFERENCES

Bogach, P. G. & Klevets, M. Yu. (1967). *Biofizika*, **12**, 997.
Buchthal, A. D. & Jenkinson, D. H. (1970). *Eur. J. Pharmac.*, **10**, 293.
Bülbring, E. & Tomita, T. (1968). *J. Physiol., Lond.*, **194**, 74P.
Bülbring, E. & Tomita, T. (1969a). *Proc. Roy. Soc.*, B, **172**, 89.
Bülbring, E. & Tomita, T. (1969b). *Proc. Roy. Soc.*, B, **172**, 103.
D'Silva, J. L. (1934). *J. Physiol., Lond.*, **82**, 393.
D'Silva, J. L. (1937). *J. Physiol., Lond.*, **90**, 303.
Dungan, K. W., Stanton, H. C. & Lish, P. M. (1965). *Int. J. Neuropharmac.*, **4**, 219.
Ellis, S. (1956). *Pharmac. Rev.*, **8**, 485.
Ellis, S. (1967). In: *Physiological Pharmacology*, Vol. 4, ed. Root, W. S. & Hofmann, F. G., p. 179. London: Academic Press.
Ellis, S. & Beckett, S. B. (1963). *J. Pharmac. exp. Ther.*, **142**, 318.
Green, R. D., Dale, M. M. & Haylett, D. G. (1972). *Experientia*, **28**, 1073.
Haylett, D. G. & Jenkinson, D. H. (1968). *Br. J. Pharmac.*, **34**, 694P.
Haylett, D. G. & Jenkinson, D. H. (1969). *Nature, Lond.*, **224**, 80.
Haylett, D. G. & Jenkinson, D. H. (1972a). *J. Physiol., Lond.*, **225**, 721.
Haylett, D. G. & Jenkinson, D. H. (1972b). *J. Physiol., Lond.*, **225**, 751.
Hornbrook, K. R. (1970). *Fedn Proc.*, **29**, 1381.
Jenkinson, D. H. & Morton, I. K. M. (1965). *Nature, Lond.*, **205**, 505.
Jenkinson, D. H. & Morton, I. K. M. (1967a). *J. Physiol., Lond.*, **188**, 373.
Jenkinson, D. H. & Morton, I. K. M. (1967b). *J. Physiol., Lond.*, **188**, 387.
Keynes, R. D. (1969). *Q. Rev. Biophys.*, **2**, 177.
Lambotte, L. (1971). *J. Physiol., Paris*, **63**, 134A.
Ohashi, H. (1971). *J. Physiol., Lond.*, **212**, 561.
Rang, H. P. & Ritter, J. M. (1969). *Mol. Pharmac.*, **5**, 394.
Rang, H. P. & Ritter, J. M. (1970a). *Mol. Pharmac.*, **6**, 357.
Rang, H. P. & Ritter, J. M. (1970b). *Mol. Pharmac.*, **6**, 383.
Somlyo, A. P., Somlyo, A. V. & Friedmann, N. (1971). *Ann. N.Y. Acad. Sci.*, **185**, 108.

## DISCUSSION

*Vrbová (Birmingham)*

Could the different release of glucose in different species be related to the initial levels of liver glycogen, which may vary according to diet?

*Jenkinson (London)*

The variation between species is not so much in the resting release from the slices but rather in the extent to which the rate is increased by different catecholamines. With regard to your interesting suggestion about the possible role of differences in glycogen levels, the only relevant information we have is that the effects of noradrenaline and amidephrine on membrane potential and potassium efflux in guinea-pig liver slices were rather reproducible whereas the amount of glycogen remaining in the incubated slices varied greatly (up to 10-fold). But we have not yet looked at the glycogen content of rat and rabbit liver slices, which would be important. Nor have we gone into the consequences of the well-established diurnal variations in glycogen content (as well as in the activity of certain hepatic enzymes, for example, tyrosine transaminase) although I should perhaps mention in relation to this that the experiments were always made at about the same time of day (between 3 and 6 p.m.).

*Worcel (Paris)*

Perhaps the species differences observed by you and others would be eliminated if experiments were done with high-potassium, depolarizing solution.

*Jenkinson (London)*

Such experiments might serve to eliminate those variations which arise solely from differences in membrane potential; they could also be of value in testing the possibility that the ion specificity of the permeability change caused by catecholamines varies between species. In completely depolarized preparations ion fluxes secondary to alterations in membrane potential are much reduced, or absent, so that effects on permeability can be studied more directly, although of course at the cost of further departure from physiological conditions (see discussion by Jenkinson & Morton 1967, *Ann. N.Y. Acad. Sci.*, **139**, 762).

*Petersen (Copenhagen)*

In the salivary glands adrenaline, like acetylcholine, causes a hyperpolarization of the acinar cell membrane and a release of potassium. The release of potassium is probably coupled to sodium uptake (Petersen 1970, *J. Physiol., Lond.*, **208**, 431). My question to you is: to which other ion movement is the potassium release, following noradrenaline stimulation, of the liver coupled?

*Jenkinson (London)*

Our evidence (Haylett & Jenkinson, 1972) suggests that the net loss of potassium caused by noradrenaline is accompanied by an increase in the sodium content of the slices, although the experiments are not sufficiently precise to show whether there is an exact balance. The rise in tissue sodium could be a consequence of the increase in sodium influx which can be expected to result from the hyperpolarization produced by noradrenaline, although our experiments do not exclude the possibility that a small increase in $P_{Na}$ may accompany the rise in $P_K$.

*Lambotte* (*Paris*)

In isolated dog liver perfused with blood, we have found that adrenaline produces a potassium loss from the liver cell, an equivalent sodium gain and a marked but transient depolarization. These changes persist in the presence of ouabain and have been attributed to an increase in sodium permeability. On the other hand, isoprenaline, or adrenaline in the presence of phenoxybenzamine, produces in 20 min a hyperpolarization without potassium loss. This effect is demonstrable after ouabain administration and could depend on a decrease in $P_{Na}$.

Do you think that the difference between your results and ours depends just on species difference or on methodology since the membrane potential in perfused dog liver is maintained between 45 and 50 mV and is lower in liver slices?

*Jenkinson* (*London*)

I'm afraid that it will not be possible to answer this fully until further work has been done with both dog and guinea-pig liver. We were most interested in your preliminary report (Lambotte, 1971) that adrenaline causes depolarization in dog liver by increasing $P_{Na}$, and this redirected our attention to the problem of whether the permeability change in guinea-pig liver extends to sodium as well as to potassium ions. If this were so, the observation that α-agonists always caused *hyperpolarization* in guinea-pig liver slices could mean that the additional influx of sodium switches on an electrogenic pump so active that one sees an increase in membrane potential rather than the decrease which might be expected to result from a large increase in $P_{Na}$. If this is correct, procedures which should slow the pump (for example, ouabain, dinitrophenol, cooling) might be expected to convert the response to noradrenaline or phenylephrine to *depolarization*. So far we have not been able to demonstrate such a reversal, although this could merely mean that we have not been able to slow the pump sufficiently. It would be of great interest to examine the effect of catecholamines on slices prepared from dog liver as well as on perfused guinea-pig liver, in order to assess the significance both of the differences in membrane potential which you have referred to, and of possible changes in perfusion flow due to the action of catecholamines on hepatic blood vessels.

*Bolton* (*Oxford*)

Would your results support the view that stimulation of α-receptors results in an increase in both chloride and potassium permeability of the liver cell membrane while stimulation of β-receptors increases only potassium permeability? I believe you mentioned some results with chloride deficient solution which would support this. It has probably not escaped you that the effects of adrenergic stimulants on the membrane potential of liver cells are similar to those obtained on certain smooth muscles.

*Jenkinson* (*London*)

We are certainly interested in possible common features in receptor mechanisms in smooth muscle and liver, and indeed several of the present experiments were prompted by the earlier findings that the increase in membrane permeability which catecholamines cause in intestinal muscle is mediated by α- rather than by β-receptors, at least under the conditions so far examined (Jenkinson & Morton, 1967; Bülbring & Tomita, 1969). This seems to apply to the liver as well, except under the special circumstances (chloride-free solutions, prior administration of an α-agonist) discussed in our paper. Under more normal conditions, activation of the β-receptors causes only small and variable increases in membrane potential and potassium efflux in guinea-pig and rabbit liver.

With regard to possible effects on chloride permeability, we observed that the effect of both noradrenaline and isoprenaline on membrane potential became larger in chloride-free solutions. This could be simply a consequence of removal of the shunting effect of the high chloride conductance of the resting membrane. However, an effect on chloride conductance could also be concerned, as you suggest, and it will be important to examine the ion specificity of the effects mediated by both types of receptor.

# RECEPTOR CLASSIFICATION WITH SPECIAL REFERENCE TO β-ADRENERGIC RECEPTORS

H. O. SCHILD

*Department of Pharmacology, University College London, London WC1E 6BT, England*

It may seem somewhat of an anachronism to discuss receptor classification at a symposium mainly devoted to receptor mechanisms and isolation, but to pharmacologists classification remains an important and indeed indispensable tool. Part of its importance lies in the fact that receptor classification may be the first step in the discovery of new drugs.

Methods of receptor classification can generally be reduced to one of three approaches.

### *Classification by desensitization*

Ehrlich, who invented the notion of 'chemoreceptors', proposed an ingenious method of classifying them (Ehrlich, 1960). His method was based on receptor desensitization. He discovered that if a batch of trypanosomes was exposed to increasing doses of an arsenical it eventually became refractory to all arsenicals and he attributed this effect to the loss of chemoreceptors for arsenicals. By applying similar desensitization procedures to other trypanocidal drugs he was able to subdivide them into three classes each acting on a separate chemoreceptor.

Ehrlich also suggested a procedure for discovering new receptors. He argued that if trypanosomes have been desensitized to the three known types of trypanocidal drugs and are then found to be destroyed by a new drug the new drug must be acting on a fourth receptor.

Ehrlich's desensitization method has not been widely employed perhaps because later work showed receptor desensitization to be rather less specific than he believed. Indeed some workers have considered receptor desensitization to be quite unspecific, but Fig. 1 shows that this is not altogether so. It shows that desensitization by excess of either histamine or 5-hydroxytryptamine is partly unspecific and partly specific.

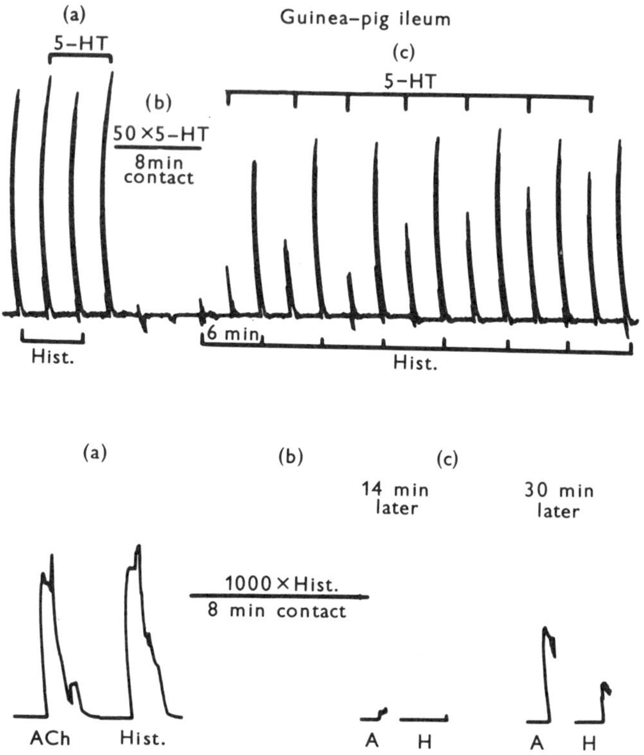


FIG. 1. Receptor desensitization by excess drug. (a), Two drugs administered alternately; (b), period of desensitization (8 min) by applying excess of one drug; (c), drug effects after desensitization. Upper: 5-hydroxytryptamine and histamine. Lower: histamine and acetylcholine.

## *Classification by agonists*

Classification by agonists has been widely employed particularly in relation to adrenergic receptors. Ahlquist's original classification (Ahlquist, 1948) into α- and β-adrenergic receptors and the further classification by Lands, Arnold, McAuliff, Luduena & Brown (1967) into two types of β-receptors have both relied on agonists. In both cases the classification has involved the assumption that agonists acting on similar receptors would show similar activity ratios in different test preparations.

In terms of receptor theory the assumption is not necessarily correct, at least not if it is considered that the effects of agonists are dependent on both their affinity and efficacy (intrinsic activity) (Stephenson, 1956; Ariens, 1964). When the effects of agonists with different efficacies are compared, their activity ratios need not be the same either in different preparations or in the same preparation at different response levels. This could apply even when concentration–effect curves are seemingly parallel since any differences in slope due to different efficacies might be experimentally undetectable. A theoretically sounder procedure would be to determine agonist affinities instead of activities, but this is hardly practicable in view of the complex measurements required to determine the affinity constants of agonists (van Rossum & Ariens, 1962; Arunlakshana & Schild, 1959; Barlow, Scott & Stephenson, 1967; Furchgott, 1966).

In spite of theoretical objections, the classification of receptors on the basis of agonist activity ratios has been highly successful in practice. It has led to the synthesis of new specific agonists with differential effects on adrenergic receptors in different tissues. Examples of results obtained with a specific agonist, salbutamol, are given in Table 1. It shows a clear differentiation of activity ratios in preparations with presumed $\beta_1$ and $\beta_2$ receptors.

TABLE 1. *Differentiation of apparent $\beta_1$ and $\beta_2$ receptors*

| Species | Tissue | Receptor type | R | Reference |
|---|---|---|---|---|
| Guinea-pig | right auricle (rate) | $\beta_1$ | 500 | Black *et al.* (1965) |
| | left auricle (rate) | $\beta_1$ | 2500 | Blinks (1967) |
| Rat | right auricle (rate) | $\beta_1$ | 54 | Black *et al.* (1965) |
| | left auricle (force) | $\beta_1$ | 8000 | Blinks (1967) |
| Rabbit | intestine | $\beta_1$ | 800 | Bowman *et al.* (1970) |
| Guinea-pig | trachea | $\beta_2$ | 6 | Farmer & Coleman (1970) |
| | vas deferens | $\beta_2$ | 1 | Large (1965) |
| Rat | uterus | $\beta_2$ | 3 | Farrant *et al.* (1964) |
| Dog | limb blood flow | $\beta_2$ | 5 | Cullum *et al.* (1969) |
| Chick | colon | $\beta_2$ | 9 | Bartlett & Hassen (1969) |

R = Relative activities isoprenaline/salbutamol. (After Farmer, Levy & Marshall, 1970.)

Fig. 2 shows another example of attempted receptor classification by agonists. Several histamine analogues were tested in two systems, gastric secretion and rat uterine inhibition, both refractory to standard antihistamines. Their activities in the two preparations are correlated (Ash & Schild, 1966) suggesting, if not proving, that a common second histamine receptor may be involved.

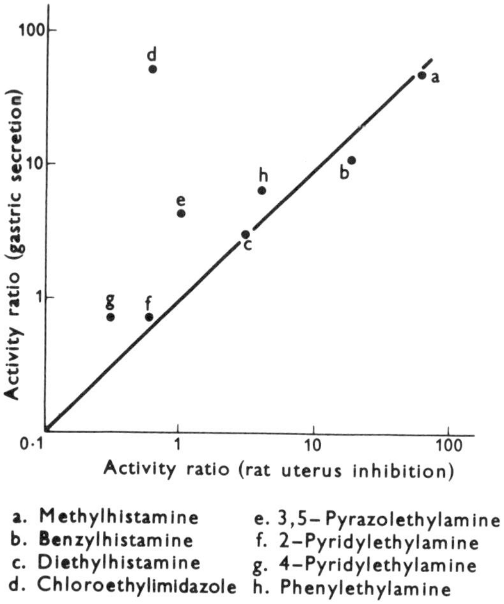


FIG. 2. Correlation between activity ratios of histamine analogues relative to histamine (=100) in two preparations (rat acid secretion; rat uterus inhibition) refractory to standard antihistamines. (After Ash & Schild, 1966.)

## *Classification by antagonists*

Probably the most widely accepted basis of receptor classification is by way of the affinity constants of competitive antagonists, which are readily measurable. Affinity constants of competitive antagonists, can help in the classification of both drugs and receptors. Two simple principles are involved which are a consequence of receptor theory: (1) when different agonists acting on the same receptor are tested with the same competitive antagonist the affinity constants of the latter should be the same, (2) identical receptors in different preparations should produce the same affinity constants with the same competitive antagonists.

When these rules were formulated most of the relevant data had been obtained in terms of $pA_2$ measurements rather than of the affinity constant $K_2$. This could lead to erroneous conclusions unless the antagonism is of a simple competitive kind in which case $pA_2 = \log K_2$. It is preferable, rather than measuring $pA_2$ directly, to determine $K_2$ values from series of parallel log concentration–effect curves. (For a discussion of the significance of parallel curves see Schild, 1969.) It is doubtful whether valid data, suitable for receptor classification, can be derived unless the plot of log $(x-1)$ against $pA_x$ (Arunlakshana & Schild, 1959), referred to henceforth as the A–S plot, is linear with slope = 1.

*β-adrenergic receptors*

The classification by antagonists of β-adrenergic receptors has raised difficult problems partly because of frequently atypical A–S plots with slopes significantly different from 1 and partly due to the apparent heterogeneity of β-adrenergic receptors (Furchgott, 1967). The heterogeneity may be manifested in two ways. The affinity constants of all β-blocking drugs may vary in different test preparations or they may vary according to the particular blocking drug used. Examples of A–S plots for β-blocking drugs are shown in Figs. 3–5 taken from experiments with slope approximately 1. In each case isoprenaline was the agonist.

Fig. 3 shows data (replotted) by Bassett (1971). The affinity constants for propranolol in smooth muscle and heart were similar, whilst methoxy-

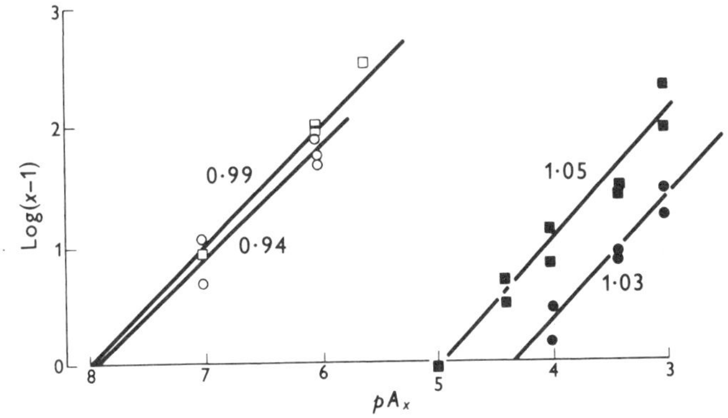


FIG. 3. A–S plots for propranolol (open symbols) and 3-methoxyisoprenaline (closed symbols), with isoprenaline as agonist. $pA_x$ is the negative logarithm of the molar antagonist concentration needed to produce dose ratio $x$ for isoprenaline. Tests were carried out on guinea-pig isolated tracheal chain (○, ●) and on guinea-pig atrial strips (□, ■). Numbers attached to curves indicate the slopes of the lines. (Redrawn after Bassett, 1971.)

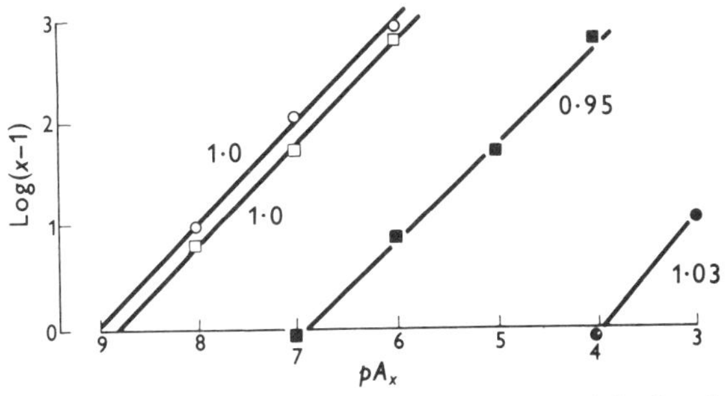


FIG. 4. A–S plots for propranolol (open symbols) and practolol (closed symbols), with isoprenaline as agonist. Tests were carried out on the relaxant effect of isoprenaline on the rabbit aorta (○, ●) and on the increased rate of beating of rabbit atria (□, ■). (Redrawn from Bristow, Sherrod & Green, 1970.)

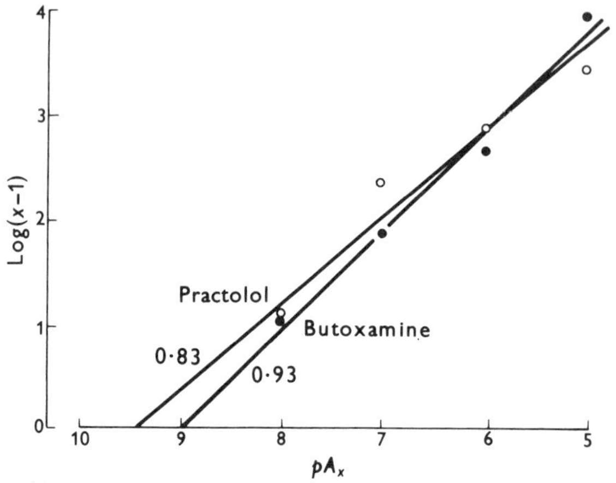


FIG. 5. A–S plots for practolol (○) and butoxamine (●) with isoprenaline as agonist. Tests were carried out on the inhibition by isoprenaline of the anaphylactic histamine release from guinea-pig lung particles. (After Assem & Schild, 1971.)

isoprenaline gave slightly, but significantly, different constants. The receptors thus seemed homogeneous in terms of propranolol but marginally heterogeneous in terms of methoxyisoprenaline.

Fig. 4 (replotted from Bristow, Sherrod & Green, 1970) shows much more pronounced β-receptor differences between heart and smooth muscle revealed by using practolol.

Fig. 5 shows a comparison of practolol, a typical $\beta_1$ blocking agent (Barrett, Crowther, Dunlop, Shanks & Smith, 1968) and butoxamine a $\beta_2$ blocking agent (Parratt & Wadsworth, 1970) in antagonizing the 'anti-anaphylactic' effect of isoprenaline (Assem & Schild, 1971). Both antagonists seemed highly active, suggesting that the anti-anaphylactic effect may not exhibit β-receptor specificity.

It can be concluded from this limited survey that β-adrenergic receptors exhibit considerable heterogeneity. It seems doubtful whether a completely satisfactory classification of β-receptors is possible at present.

## *Atypical plots*

β-Adrenergic blocking drugs frequently exhibit atypical A–S plots. Their slope is sometimes significantly less than 1; in other cases it deviates from linearity. One explanation of these atypical plots is a multimolecular interaction between drugs and receptors (Wenke, Lincova, Cepelik, Cernohorsky & Hynie, 1967).

An entirely different explanation is due to Langer & Trendelenburg (1969) and Waud (1969) and has been further elaborated by Furchgott (1972). This approach is based on two assumptions: (1) that saturable uptake sites for either agonists or antagonists can significantly influence the effective drug concentrations at receptor sites; (2) that the relevant drug concentrations at the receptor site are those occurring in the receptor 'biophase' rather than in the surrounding solution. Calculated theoretical A–S plots based on assumed constants have been published by Furchgott (1972).

It would seem that it is not feasible at present to derive true affinity constants from atypical curves because the necessary constants cannot be independently determined. Nevertheless the new approach underlines the necessity of trying to avoid experimental conditions in which uptake plays an important part. Sometimes this can be achieved by using appropriate drugs not susceptible to uptake. In other cases it may be possible to inactivate the uptake sites by uptake blocking agents such as phenoxybenzamine.

### *Summary*

Three methods of receptor classification are described based on desensitization, activity ratios of agonists and affinity constants of antagonists. The two latter methods have been used to classify β-adrenergic receptors and they agree in showing that these receptors form a heterogeneous group.

### REFERENCES

AHLQUIST, R. P. (1948). *Am. J. Physiol.*, **153**, 586.
ARIENS, E. J. (1964). *Mol. Pharmac.* New York: Academic Press.
ARUNLAKSHANA, O. & SCHILD, H. O. (1959). *Br. J. Pharmac. Chemother.*, **14**, 48.
ASH, A. S. F. & SCHILD, H. O. (1966). *Br. J. Pharmac. Chemother.*, **27**, 427.
ASSEM, E. S. K. & SCHILD, H. O. (1971). *Br. J. Pharmac.*, **42**, 620.
BARLOW, R. B., SCOTT, N. C. & STEPHENSON, R. P. (1967). *Br. J. Pharmac.*, **31**, 188.
BARRETT, A. M., CROWTHER, A. F., DUNLOP, D., SHANKS, R. G. & SMITH, L. H. (1968). *Arch. exp. Path. Pharmak.*, **259**, 152.
BARTLETT, A. L. & HASSEN, T. (1969). *Abst. IVth Int. Congr. Pharmac.*, p. 128.
BASSETT, J. R. (1971). *Br. J. Pharmac.*, **41**, 113.
BLACK, J. W., DUNCAN, W. A. M. & SHANKS, R. G. (1965). *Br. J. Pharmac. Chemother.*, **25**, 577.
BLINKS, J. R. (1967). *Ann. N.Y. Acad. Sci.*, **139**, 673.
BOWMAN, W. C. & HALL, M. T. (1970). *Br. J. Pharmac.*, **38**, 399.
BRISTOW, M., SHERROD, T. R. & GREEN, R. D. (1970). *J. Pharmac. exp. Ther.*, **171**, 52.
CULLUM, V. A., FARMER, J. B., JACK, D. & LEVY, G. P. (1969). *Br. J. Pharmac. Chemother.*, **35**, 141.
EHRLICH, P. (1960). *Collected Papers*, **3**, 183.
FARMER, J. B. & COLEMAN, R. A. (1970). *J. Pharm. Pharmac.*, **22**, 46.
FARMER, J. B., LEVY, G. P. & MARSHALL, R. J. (1970). *J. Pharm. Pharmac.*, **22**, 945.
FARRANT, J., HARVEY, J. A. & PENNEFATHER, J. N. (1964). *Br. J. Pharmac. Chemother.*, **22**, 104.
FURCHGOTT, R. F. (1966). In: *Advances in Drug Research*, Vol. 3, 21.
FURCHGOTT, R. F. (1967). *Ann. N.Y. Acad. Sci.*, **139**, 553.
FURCHGOTT, R. F. (1972). *Handb. exp. Pharmak.*, **33**, 283.
LANDS, A. M., ARNOLD, A., MCAULIFF, J. P., LUDUENA, F. P. & BROWN, T. G. (1967). *Nature, Lond.*, **214**, 597.
LANGER, S. Z. & TRENDELENBURG, U. (1969). *J. Pharmac. exp. Ther.*, **167**, 117.
LARGE, B. J. (1965). *Br. J. Pharmac. Chemother.*, **24**, 194.

PARRATT, J. R. & WADSWORTH, R. M. (1970). *Br. J. Pharmac.*, **39**, 296.
SCHILD, H. O. (1969). *Pharmac. Res. Commun.*, **1**, 1.
STEPHENSON, R. P. (1956). *Br. J. Pharmac.*, **11**, 379.
VAN ROSSUM, J. M. & ARIENS, E. J. (1962). *Arch. int. Pharmacodyn.*, **136**, 385.
WAUD, D. R. (1969). *J. Pharmac. exp. Ther.*, **167**, 140.
WENKE, M., LINCOVA, D., CEPELIK, J., CERNOHORSKY, M. & HYNIE, S. (1967). *Ann. N.Y. Acad. Sci.*, **139**, 860.

## DISCUSSION

*Brittain* (*Ware*)

The ratio of activities of optical isomers of catecholamines has been used to classify β-receptors. On this basis Patil (*J. Pharm. Pharmac.*, **21**, 638, 1969) concluded that the β-receptors in guinea-pig trachea and atria were similar. However, the isomers of salbutamol show the same selectivity of action as (±)-salbutamol between different types of β-receptors, so the isomeric activity ratio is of no help in distinguishing the receptor types. What is your opinion on this method of classifying receptors?

*Schild* (*London*)

Patil suggested that if stereoselective receptors in different tissues are of a single type the activity ratios between (−) and (+) forms (isomeric ratios) of drugs acting on these receptors should be the same. Stated in this form this seems a reasonable proposition particularly when applied to the affinity constants of antagonists but, as mentioned by Patil, isomeric ratios may be obscured by factors such as neuronal uptake and selective degradation of isomers.

*Levy* (*Ware*)

Why does propranolol not distinguish between β-receptors whereas drugs such as practolol do?

*Schild* (*London*)

I do not know; but in my opinion when one antagonist can distinguish between receptors and the other cannot, then the former wins.

# THE ACTION OF ACETYLCHOLINE AND DOPAMINE ON A SPECIFIED SNAIL NEURONE

G. A. KERKUT, J. D. C. LAMBERT AND R. J. WALKER

*Department of Physiology and Biochemistry, University of Southampton, Southampton SO9 3TU, England*

The gastropod central nervous system offers special advantages to the electrophysiologist in that it is often possible to work on a specific nerve cell in the brain from one preparation to another. This is important since there is a pharmacological specificity between neurones. Different nerve cells respond differently to a given drug (Gerschenfeld & Tauc, 1961; Tauc & Gerschenfeld, 1962; Kerkut & Walker, 1961, 1962, 1973; Tauc, 1966, 1967; Kerkut, 1967, 1969; Glaizner, 1967; Gerschenfeld & Chiarandini, 1965; Cottrell, 1967, 1971; Cottrell & Laverack, 1968; Sakharov & Salanki, 1969).

We have mapped the pharmacological and synaptic properties of 150 different nerve cells in the brain of the snail *Helix aspersa* (Kerkut, Lambert, Gayton, Loker & Walker, 1973). The results that will be described here are based on experiments carried out on a specific nerve cell in the right parietal ganglion (Kerkut, Lambert & Walker, 1973).

This nerve cell has a membrane potential of 50–60 mV. If strophanthidin (10 $\mu$g/ml) is applied to the brain, the membrane potential of the neurone falls to 42 mV, that is, a depolarization of 8–10 mV. The response is reversible and when the drug is washed away the membrane potential returns to the original value. The membrane potential of this cell is partially due to the activity of an electrogenic sodium–potassium pump (Kerkut & York, 1971). This view is supported by experiments where the external potassium concentration around the cell is reduced from 4 mM to 0 mM; the membrane potential falls by 8 mV in the 0 mM $K^+$ solution. On restoration back to 4 mM $K^+$, the potential returns to its initial value. Thus a reduction in the membrane potential is brought about by strophanthidin which inhibits the sodium pump, or by removing external potassium ions.

### *Action of acetylcholine and dopamine*

Ionophoretic application of dopamine or acetylcholine on to this nerve cell brought about a hyperpolarization. The cell normally shows action potentials (Fig. 1a). When dopamine was applied ionophoretically there was a 16 mV hyperpolarization, which inhibited the activity of the cell for about 50 s, after which the action potentials reappeared. Ionophoretic application of acetylcholine brought about a hyperpolarization of 15 mV and this effect also lasted for about 50 s.

The solution around the preparation was replaced by control solution containing 10 $\mu$g/ml strophanthidin (Fig. 1b). Application of dopamine still brought about a hyperpolarization of 15 mV, whilst application of acetylcholine brought about a hyperpolarization of only 1 mV. Washing

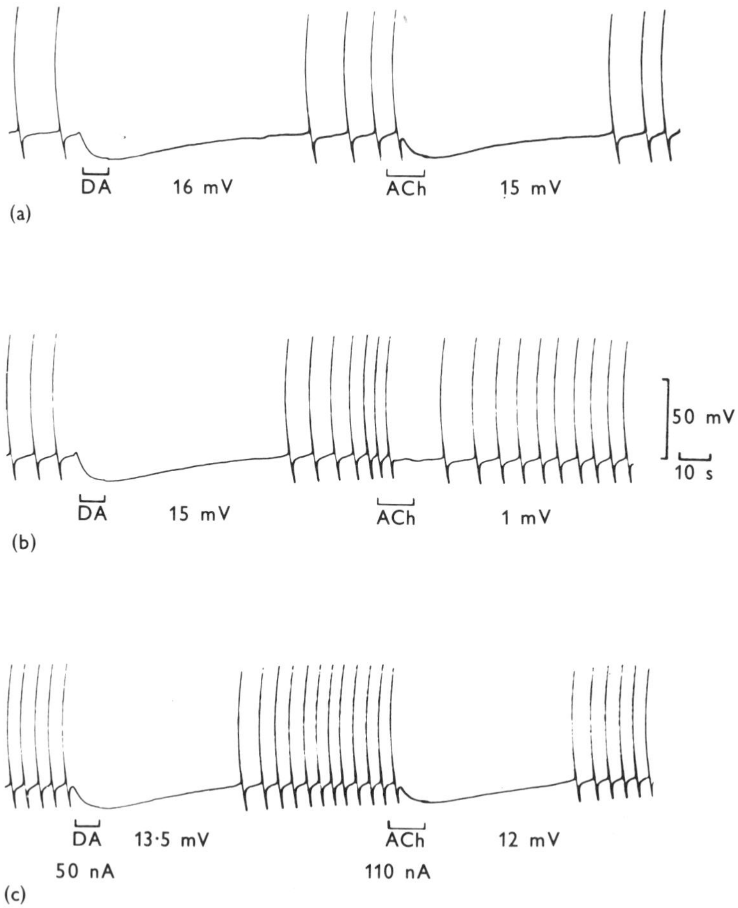


FIG. 1. The effect of ionophoretic application of dopamine and acetylcholine to the nerve cell. The cell membrane potential was initially at $-48$ mV and brought to this value after each change of solution, by passing a current through the electrode. Both dopamine (DA) and acetylcholine (ACh) hyperpolarized the neurone. Under normal conditions (a), ACh and DA caused similar hyperpolarizations in the presence of strophanthidin (10 $\mu$g/ml); (b), the ACh effect was abolished, but recovered after washing (c). Note that the dopamine-induced response had less delay than the ACh-induced response.

away the strophanthidin restored the hyperpolarizing response to acetylcholine (Fig. 1c).

Since we were using microelectrodes filled with 3 M KCl, and since altering the chloride concentration of the bathing solution had little effect on the hyperpolarization induced by dopamine or acetylcholine, chloride ions did not appear to be involved in this case. The effects of the drugs could be due either to an increase in the potassium permeability of the membrane, thus bringing the membrane potential towards $E_K$; or, in the case of acetylcholine, to increased activity of the electrogenic sodium pump, since strophanthidin reduced the effect of acetylcholine.

This was investigated by altering the external potassium ion concentration around the preparation and seeing the effect on the drug-induced hyperpolarization.

Fig. 2 shows the result of such an experiment. Fig. 2b shows the normal preparation in 4 mM K control solution. Dopamine brought about a hyper-

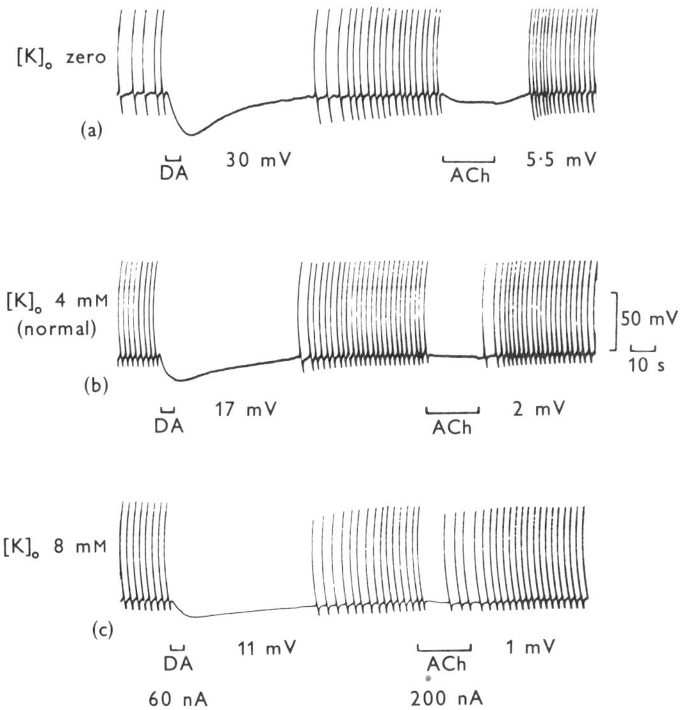


FIG. 2. The effect of changing the external potassium concentration on the ACh- and dopamine-induced hyperpolarization. The cell membrane potential was initially at −41 mV, and brought to this value after each change of solution by passing a current through the electrode. Normal control solution contained 4 mM potassium (b). Decreasing the external potassium concentration to zero (a) increased the hyperpolarization whilst increasing the external potassium concentration to 8 mM (c) decreased the hyperpolarization.

polarization of 17 mV; acetylcholine brought about a hyperpolarization of 2 mV. Reducing the external potassium concentration to 0 mM (Fig. 2a) increased the dopamine hyperpolarization to 30 mV. It also increased the acetylcholine hyperpolarization to 5·5 mV. Increasing the external potassium concentration to 8 mM reduced the dopamine hyperpolarization to 11 mV and the acetylcholine hyperpolarization to 1 mV (Fig. 2c).

Both drugs apparently act by increasing the potassium permeability of the membrane. Acetylcholine was not acting through an electrogenic sodium pump since reduction of the external potassium should in that case reduce the acetylcholine effect. In this cell we saw that reducing $[K]_o$ increased the acetylcholine effect.

We still have to explain why strophanthidin decreased the acetylcholine hyperpolarization from 15 mV to 1 mV whilst the dopamine-induced hyperpolarization was relatively unaffected (16 mV–15 mV).

Kehoe & Ascher (1970) suggested that one effect of strophanthidin is to bring about an increase in the potassium concentration immediately outside the nerve membrane. This increase in $[K]_o$ would reduce the $E_K$ and hence any drug acting by increasing the potassium permeability of the membrane, would have a smaller effect. This could be shown most clearly by studying the potential at which the effect of dopamine or actylcholine became reversed, both in normal control solution and in control solution containing strophanthidin.

Fig. 3 shows the result of experiments in which the membrane potential of the cell was hyperpolarized through an internal electrode, to values between 40 mV and 100 mV. The response to ionophoretic application of dopamine and acetylcholine was measured.

Dopamine (□) applied to a cell in normal control solution whose membrane potential was 40 mV, brought about a hyperpolarization of 20 mV. As the membrane potential of the cell increased, the dopamine effect became reduced until at a membrane potential of 82 mV, the response was zero. When the cell was hyperpolarized beyond 82 mV, dopamine brought about a depolarization of the cell. In solution containing 10 $\mu$g/ml strophanthidin, the dopamine response (■) was similarly studied. The reversal potential was approximately 78 mV, that is, a reduction of about 4 mV from that in normal control solution. Acetylcholine (○) in normal control solution brought about a hyperpolarization of 5 mV and as the membrane potential of the cell became greater so the acetylcholine-induced hyperpolarization decreased to reach zero at about 82 mV. The reversal potential for acetylcholine was approximately the same as that for dopamine. When strophanthidin was present the acetylcholine hyperpolarization was reduced (●) and the reversal potential was now at 55 mV, that is, in the presence of strophanthidin the reversal potential of the acetylcholine-induced response had altered by 27 mV whilst that of the dopamine response had altered by 4 mV.

The fact that both reversal potentials were initially at 82 mV ($\simeq E_K$) is

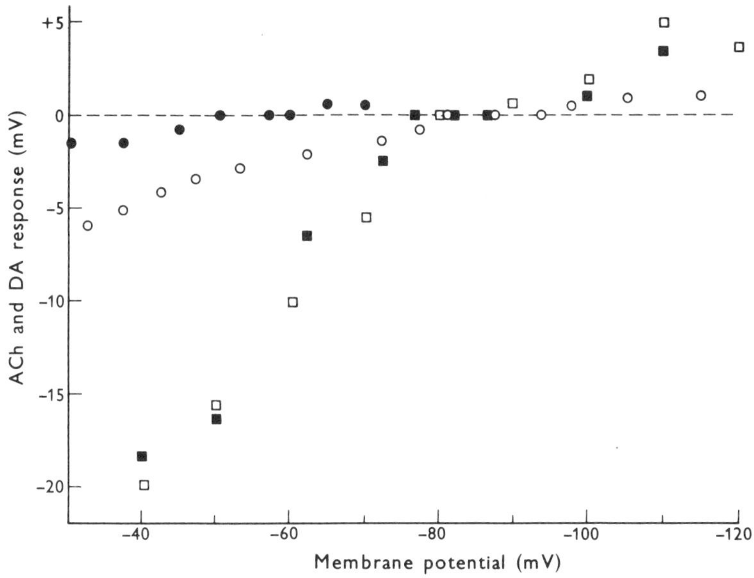


FIG. 3. The reversal potential of the ACh- and dopamine-induced hyperpolarization. The dopamine-induced hyperpolarization had had a reversal potential at −81 mV (□); in strophanthidin solution the reversal potential was −78 mV (■). The ACh-induced hyperpolarization had a reversal potential at −81 mV (○) whilst in strophanthidin solution the reversal potential was approximately −55 mV (●).

indicative that the effect of the drugs is to increase the potassium permeability of the nerve membrane. We have still to explain how the reversal potential for acetylcholine is altered by 27 mV whilst that for dopamine is altered by 4 mV in the presence of strophanthidin.

Gerschenfeld & Stefani (1966, 1968) in analysing the responses of specific neurones of the snail *Crymptomphallus aspersa* to ionophoretically applied acetylcholine and 5-hydroxytryptamine (5-HT) showed that the response to acetylcholine was much more rapid than that to 5-HT. They suggested that the receptors for acetylcholine were mainly over the cell body but that the 5-HT receptors were located close to the axon hillock.

We would like to adapt their answer to our present problem and suggest that the receptors for dopamine are over the surface of the neurone whilst those for acetylcholine are confined to the axon hillock. This would explain why it takes very much longer for acetylcholine to induce a hyperpolarization (2–3 s after onset of ionophoretic pulse) compared with the more immediate hyperpolarization to dopamine (Fig. 1), since the axon hillock region of the neurone is in a more confined space and could form an enclosed microenvironment. It would also explain why strophanthidin has a greater effect on the acetylcholine response than on the dopamine response (Fig. 4).

When strophanthidin stops the sodium–potassium pump, it allows the

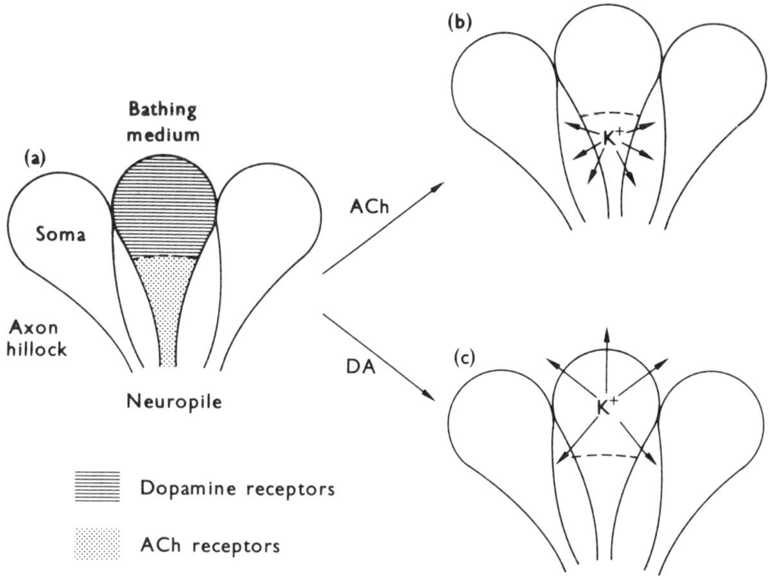


FIG. 4. Diagrammatic representation of suggested location of the dopamine and ACh receptors. It is postulated that the dopamine (DA) receptors are located more over the cell body whilst the ACh receptors are located on the axon hillock. Strophanthidin allows potassium to diffuse out from the cell and the concentration of potassium in the axon hill region could build up and considerably alter the $E_K$ value. The axon hillock region would form a microenvironment when the $[K]_o = 10$ mM, compared to that of 4·3 mM around the cell body and 4 mM in the control solution.

potassium to diffuse out of the cell. In the case of the cell body, the increase in potassium concentration around the cell is small because of the rapid diffusion of potassium into the bathing medium. In the case of the axon hillock, this is a more confined environment surrounded by other axon hillocks and glial cells and the potassium concentration in this microenvironment could build up sufficiently to change the $E_K$ value by 25 mV.

Even though both acetylcholine and dopamine have the same effect on the cell membrane in that they increase the permeability to potassium ions, the difference in the site of the receptors and the microenvironment around the axon hillock could explain the difference in the response to strophanthidin.

It is interesting to speculate whether this situation could have any meaning *in vivo*. It is likely that similar microenvironments occur in the central nervous system and that there could be a difference in the location of receptors over the neuronal surface. In such cases close proximity to a blood capillary would allow some parts of the nerve cell to be more affected than other parts of the cell, and hence critical chemical levels in the blood could alter some synaptic pathways on to a neurone and leave other inputs relatively unaffected. The microenvironments around the nerve cell could be important in the hormonal and chemical modulation of the circuitry within the central nervous system.


## *Summary*

1. A specific nerve cell in the right parietal ganglion of the snail brain has a membrane potential of approximately 55 mV. There is a rapid depolarization of 8 mV in ouabain, attributable to the cessation of an electrogenic sodium pump.
2. The cell is hyperpolarized by the ionophoretic application of dopamine or acetylcholine.
3. The acetylcholine hyperpolarization is markedly reduced by strophanthidin whilst that of dopamine is relatively unaffected.
4. The reversal potentials of the dopamine- and acetylcholine-induced hyperpolarizations are at 82 mV. This is the estimated value of $E_K$, and it would seem that the hyperpolarizations are due to an increased membrane permeability to potassium ions.
5. Strophanthidin reduces the reversal potential for dopamine from 82 mV to 78 mV, namely, a change of 4 mV. It changes the reversal potential for acetylcholine from 82 mV to 55 mV, namely, a change of about 27 mV.
6. Evidence is presented that the dopamine receptors are all over the cell body surface and that the acetylcholine receptors are mainly on the axon hillock.
7. The acetylcholine receptors are in a microenvironment where it would be possible for the external potassium concentration to build up and hence bring about the 27 mV shift in the $E_K$ value.
8. It is possible that differential location of receptors and the development of microenvironments within the central nervous system could play a role in establishing differences in the actions of hormones and chemicals on selected pathways in the nervous system.


We are indebted to a grant from the Medical Research Council to J.D.C.L.

## REFERENCES


COTTRELL, G. A. (1967). *Br. J. Pharmac.*, **29**, 63.

COTTRELL, G. A. (1971). *Comp. gen. Pharmac.*, **2**, 125.

COTTRELL, G. A. & LAVERACK, M. S. (1968). *Ann. Rev. Pharmac.*, **8**, 273.

GERSCHENFELD, H. M. & CHIARANDINI, D. J. (1965). *J. Neurophysiol.*, **28**, 710.

GERSCHENFELD, H. M. & STEFANI, E. (1966). *J. Physiol., Lond.*, **185**, 684.

GERSCHENFELD, H. M. & STEFANI, E. (1968). *Adv. in Pharmacology*, **6A**, 369.

GERSCHENFELD, H. M. & TAUC, L. (1961). *Nature, Lond.*, **189**, 924.

GLAIZNER, B. (1967). In: *Neurobiology of Invertebrates*, ed. Salanki, J., p. 267. New York: Plenum Press.

KEHOE, J. S. & ASCHER, P. (1970). *Nature, Lond.*, **225**, 820.

KERKUT, G. A. (1967). In: *Invertebrate Nervous Systems*, ed. Wiersma, C. A. G., p. 5. Chicago University Press.

KERKUT, G. A. (1969). In: *Handbook of Neurochemistry*, Vol. 2, ed. Lajtha, A., p. 539. Plenum Press.
KERKUT, G. A., LAMBERT, J. D. C., GAYTON, R., LOKER, J. & WALKER, R. J. (1973). *Comp. gen. Pharmac.*, in press.
KERKUT, G. A., LAMBERT, J. D. C. & WALKER, R. J. (1973). *Comp. gen. Pharmac.*, in press.
KERKUT, G. A. & WALKER, R. J. (1961). *Comp. Biochem. Physiol.*, **3**, 143.
KERKUT, G. A. & WALKER, R. J. (1962). *Comp. Biochem. Physiol.*, **7**, 277.
KERKUT, G. A. & WALKER, R. J. (1973). In: *The Biology of the Pulmonates*, ed. Fretter, V. London: Academic Press, in press.
KERKUT, G. A. & YORK, B. (1971). *The Electrogenic Sodium Pump.* Bristol: Scientechnica.
SAKHAROV, D. A. & SALANKI, J. (1969). *Acta physiol. hung.*, **35**, 19.
TAUC, L. (1966). In: *Physiology of the Mollusca*, Vol. 2, ed. Wilbur, H. M. & Yonge, C. M., p. 387. New York: Academic Press.
TAUC, L. (1967). *Physiol. Rev.*, **47**, 521.
TAUC, L. & GERSCHENFELD, H. M. (1962). *J. Neurophysiol.*, **25**, 236.

# ACTIONS OF 5-HYDROXYTRYPTAMINE ON MOLLUSCAN NEURONAL MEMBRANES

H. M. GERSCHENFELD AND DANIELLE PAUPARDIN*

*Laboratoire de Neurobiologie, Ecole Normale Supérieure, 46, rue d'Ulm, Paris 5e, France*

The synaptic transmitter function of 5-hydroxytryptamine (5-HT) has been discussed for many years. However, crucial evidence relating this indoleamine to the function of a specific synapse has not yet been obtained either in vertebrates or in invertebrates.

In a survey of the 5-HT content of invertebrate nervous system, Welsh & Moorhead (1960) found that the molluscan central nervous system is among the richest in 5-HT, the highest content being found in *Venus mercenaria* (40 μg of 5-HT per g of tissue). Central ganglia of gastropods generally contain about 2–6 μg per g of tissue (Welsh & Moorhead, 1960; Cardot & Ripplinger, 1963; Kerkut & Cottrell, 1963; Mirolli & Welsh, 1964; Carpenter, Breese, Schanberg & Kopin, 1971). The Hillarp–Falck histochemical technique (see Falck, 1962) allows the observation in many species of gastropods of yellow fluorescent neurones probably containing 5-HT (see, for instance, Dahl, Falck, von Mecklemburg, Myhrberg & Rosengreen, 1966; Marsden & Kerkut, 1970; Jaeger, Jaeger & Welsh, 1971; Osborne & Cottrell, 1971). However, a localization of 5-HT in synaptic endings has not yet been demonstrated in molluscs. It has been claimed that whole molluscan ganglia (Mirolli, 1968) or identified single neurones isolated from them (Cottrell & Powell, 1971) may synthesize 5-HT from 5-hydroxytryptophan (5-HTP). There is no evidence, however, that molluscan neurones are capable of synthesizing 5-HTP from tryptophan. 5-HT or a related compound may be released from molluscan heart during the stimulation of the cardio-accelerator nerves (Loveland, 1963; S.-Rosza & Perenyi, 1966) and 5-HT was

* Fellow Roussel-Uclaf.

shown to be taken up by nerve endings located in the vicinity of heart muscle fibres (Taxi & Gautron, 1969).

In snail central ganglia, some neurones showing excitatory responses to 5-HT (see below) may also present slow excitatory potentials that could be blocked by 5-HT antagonists (Gerschenfeld & Stefani, 1968). However, it is not certain that the action of these blocking agents is purely postsynaptic (Gerschenfeld & Stefani, 1968). More recently, Cottrell (1970) has described a connection between a giant neurone, presumed to release 5-HT as transmitter, located in each metacerebral ganglion of *Helix* and three other neurones of the ipsilateral buccal ganglion. Proof of the 5-HT-releasing function of these giant metacerebral neurones, of the monosynaptic character of the link between the metacerebral and the buccal neurones and of the involvement of 5-HT as a transmitter at these synapses is still incomplete.

The present paper describes a series of experiments which, together with previous data (Gerschenfeld & Stefani, 1966; Stefani & Gerschenfeld, 1969) demonstrate that 5-HT could at least act as a transmitter on molluscan neurones since it can cause a specific change in the neuronal membrane permeability either to $Cl^-$ or to $K^+$ or to $Na^+$.

### *5-HT effects on membrane potential*

The experiments to be presented here were performed on *in vitro* preparations of the isolated central ganglia of the snail *Helix aspersa*. The ganglia were fixed to the bottom of a small chamber and continuously bathed with a suitable physiological salt solution. The glial-connective envelope of the ganglia was dissected off, and the naked neuronal bodies were impaled with double-barrelled micropipettes filled with a 0·6 M solution of $K_2SO_4$. One of the barrels, connected to a standard d.c. recording set, was used for recording; the other barrel was used for injecting suitable currents through the neuronal membrane to drive the membrane potential to desired levels. 5-HT was applied ionophoretically on the neuronal membranes from micropipettes filled with a saturated solution of a complex of 5-HT and creatine sulphate. The drugs assayed were added to the solution perfusing the preparation. In some experiments the ionic composition of the solution was altered, keeping its tonicity as constant as possible (for technical details see Stefani & Gerschenfeld, 1969).

Application of 5-HT to *Helix* ganglia by perfusion results in the depolarization and excitation of some neurones (Gerschenfeld & Tauc, 1961; Gerschenfeld & Stefani, 1965; Glaizner, 1967), and the hyperpolarization and inhibition of others (Gerschenfeld & Tauc, 1961; Glaizner, 1967). However, since many of these effects could be due to the activation of interneurones, ionophoretic applications of 5-HT were used. These local applications also cause opposite effects on different neurones (Gerschenfeld & Stefani, 1966; Stefani & Gerschenfeld, 1969; Gerschenfeld, 1971).

## Ionic mechanism of 5-HT actions

Ionophoretic applications of 5-HT on some neurones of *Helix aspersa* causes an acceleration of the spontaneous firing frequency (Fig. 1). When the neurone is artificially hyperpolarized and the spontaneous discharge disappears, a depolarization consisting of a relatively rapidly ascending phase and a much slower falling phase can be observed (Fig. 1). The slow decay of the response could probably be explained by a purely diffusional mechanism of removal of 5-HT (Gerschenfeld & Stefani, 1968).

Complete replacement of NaCl in the perfusing solution by Tris-Cl, greatly diminishes the amplitude of the response (Fig. 2), indicating that $Na^+$ ions are very probably involved in the permeability increase caused by 5-HT.

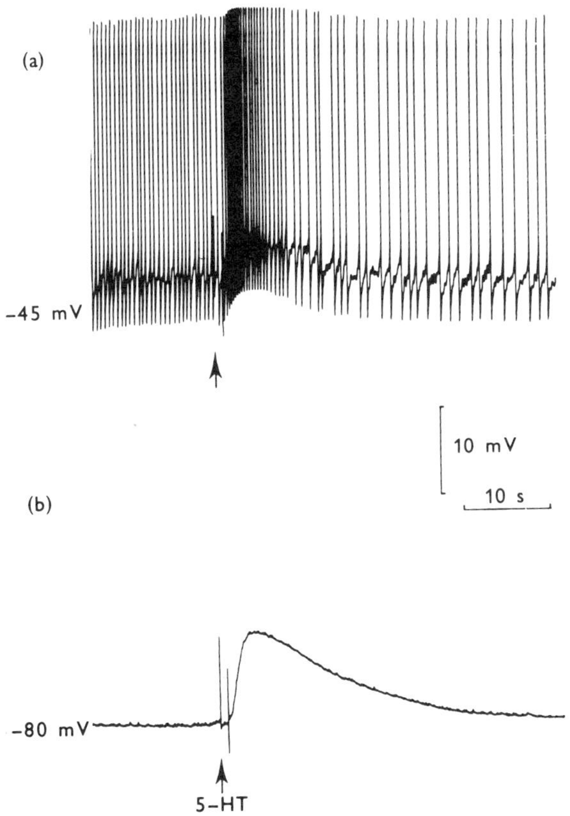


FIG. 1. 5-HT depolarization recorded at two different levels of membrane potential. (a), At the resting level, 5-HT applied ionophoretically causes an increase of the firing frequency. (b), At −80 mV, the time course of the depolarization can be analysed (see text). In all figures, arrows indicate the ionophoretic application of an agonist. All the recordings in this and following figures have been obtained using a Brush-Clevite pen recorder.

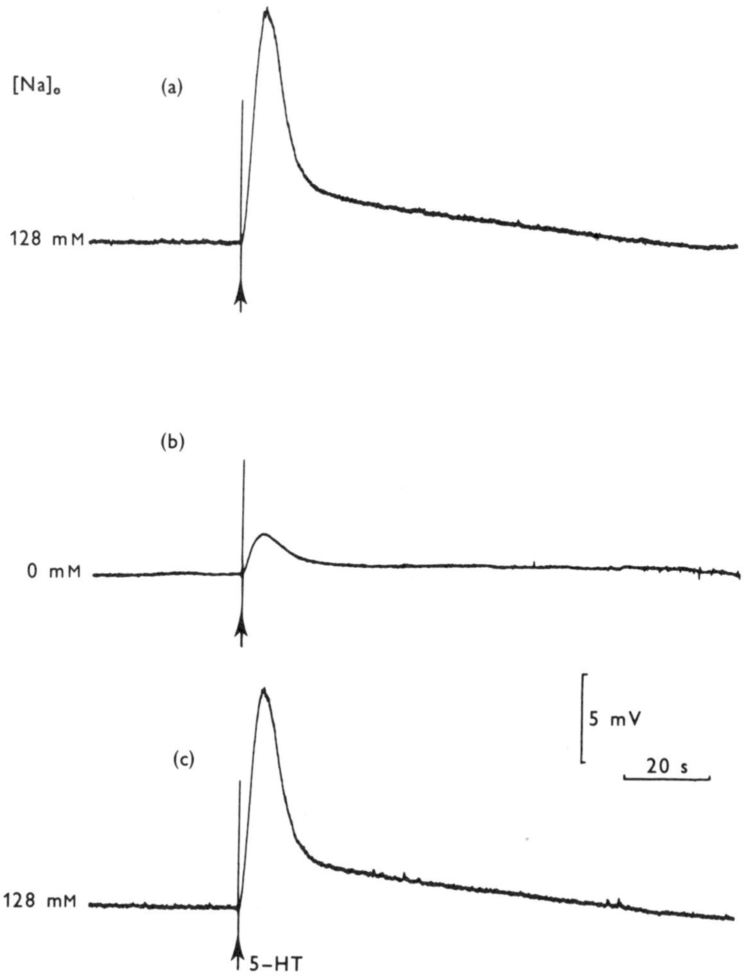


FIG. 2. Dependence of 5-HT depolarization on $Na^+$ ions. (a), Control 5-HT response in control solution. (b), Complete replacement of the NaCl by Tris-Cl greatly diminishes the amplitude of the response. (c), Recovery of the response after washing with control solution.

The receptors involved in this $Na^+$-dependent depolarization will be referred to as A-receptors.

It is not possible to reverse this 5-HT depolarization by artificially depolarizing the neurone, because of delayed rectification of the membrane which typically appears at membrane potentials positive to $-35$ mV. In some cases, the somatic membrane may be driven to apparent potential levels of $+10$ to $+15$ mV without observing any reversal. By plotting the amplitudes of the 5-HT responses against the membrane potential values at which they were recorded, a reversal potential ($E_{5\text{-HT}}$) near the zero level may be calculated by extrapolation. However, the range of membrane potentials at which these responses can be recorded without interference from the nonlinearities of the membrane resistance or the firing of action potentials is very limited (generally between −55 and −70 mV). On the other hand, analysis of the participation of other cations such as $Ca^{2+}$ in the mechanism generating the depolarization is hindered by the direct effects that $Ca^{2+}$ may have on the A-receptors. For instance, the 5-HT depolarizations increase in amplitude when the normal $Ca^{2+}$ content of the salt solution (6·4 mM) is decreased, and their amplitude diminishes when the external $Ca^{2+}$ is increased. A similar effect of the external $Ca^{2+}$ concentration on the responses to ACh of the vertebrate muscle endplate has been attributed to effects of the cation on receptor desensitization (see Nastuk & Parsons, 1970).

On the basis of the available evidence, it may be provisionally concluded that 5-HT depolarizations involve mainly, if not exclusively, an increase in

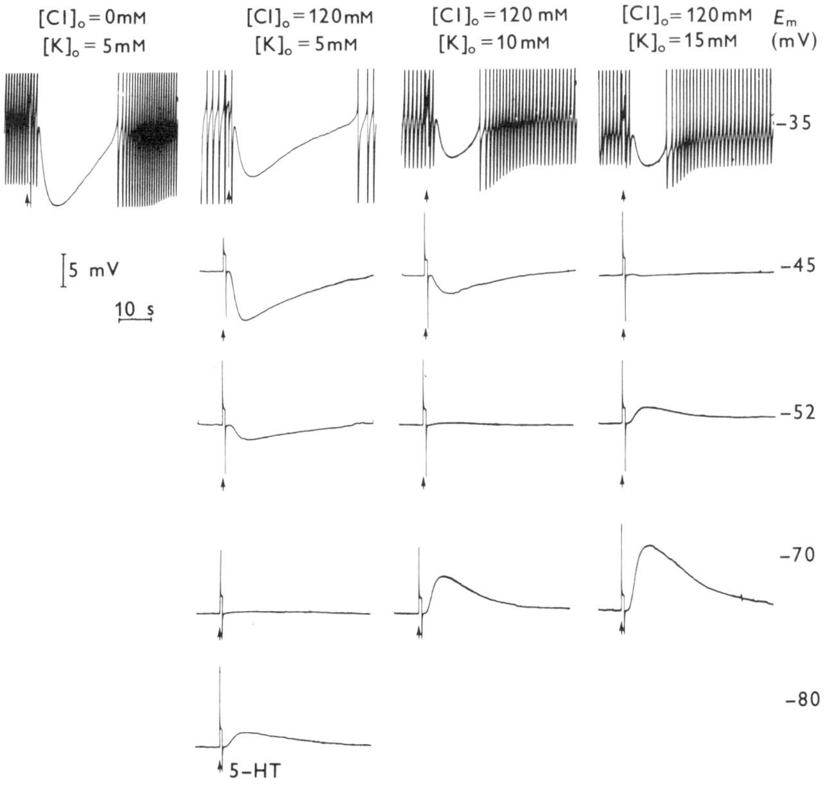


FIG. 3. A 5-HT hyperpolarization reverses at about −70 mV in control solution (second column from the left). A $Cl^-$-free medium depolarizes the cell and slightly increases the response (extreme left column). Increasing two and three times the external potassium concentration (right columns) causes a shift of the reversal potential.

the membrane permeability to $Na^+$ resulting in an influx of this cation. Further work is still necessary to clarify whether $K^+$ or $Ca^{2+}$ fluxes intervene in these 5-HT responses.

Two different mechanisms are responsible for the inhibitory actions of 5-HT. In some neurones of the right pallial ganglion, which are characterized by their rather low resting potential (−35 to −40 mV) and a very regular spontaneous spike discharge, the ionophoretic applications of 5-HT result in a hyperpolarization which becomes reversed when the membrane potential is artificially driven beyond −75 mV (Fig. 3). As will be seen, this first type of hyperpolarization depends on a selective change of the membrane permeability to $K^+$ and the receptors involved will be called B-receptors.

When the $Cl^-$ content of the environment is totally replaced by an impermeant anion such as $SO_4^{2-}$, this first type of 5-HT hyperpolarization is only slightly altered (Fig. 3) and its reversal potential does not change. When the external $K^+$ concentration is increased two or three times (Fig. 3) the 5-HT hyperpolarizations diminish in amplitude and the $E_{5\text{-HT}}$ is shifted. The shift in $E_{5\text{-HT}}$ with the increase in the external $K^+$ concentration in a neurone endowed with B-receptors is showed in Fig. 4. There, the straight

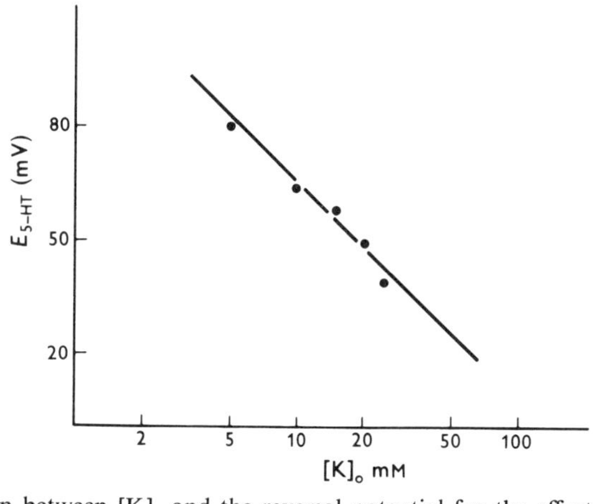


FIG. 4. Relation between $[K]_o$ and the reversal potential for the effect of 5-HT ($E_{5\text{-HT}}$) recorded in a neurone possessing B-receptors. The straight line has been drawn according to the Nernst equation.

line showing a slope of 58 mV for a 10-fold change in $[K]_o$ fits the theoretical values of $E_K$ at 20° C derived from the Nernst equation. It is possible to see that the values of $E_{5\text{-HT}}$ are not far from the theoretical ones for $E_K$. In other cases, such as in the neurone of Fig. 3, the values of $E_{5\text{-HT}}$ fitted a straight line with a slope of 51 mV for a 10-fold change in $[K]_o$. This behaviour is assumed to be due to the activation of more than one 5-HT receptor; that is, apart from the B-receptors involved in the $K^+$ dependent inhibition, some activation of other receptors may cause an increase of the membrane permeability to $Na^+$ or to $Cl^-$ (see below).

In all these cases of B-receptor activation the hyperpolarization is due to a selective increase of the membrane permeability to $K^+$, resulting in a $K^+$ efflux.

In other cases of B-receptor activation, it is not possible to obtain a reversal of the response by hyperpolarizing the neurone by passing inward current through the membrane, even if the soma membrane potential is driven to −110 mV or beyond. In these cases, the hyperpolarization gradually decreases and disappears, but does not reverse. This may be due to a localization of the receptors far from the somatic region and to the anomalous rectification of the membrane which attenuates the signals. Sometimes, by greatly increasing the $[K]_o$, a reversal appears because of the shift of $E_{5\text{-HT}}$ (see Gerschenfeld, 1971).

The second type of inhibition produced by 5-HT is only observed in a small number of neurones of both pallial ganglia. The receptors involved in these responses will be called C-receptors and their activation results in a rather rapid hyperpolarization (specially when compared with the time course of the $K^+$ dependent hyperpolarization) which reverses around −60 mV (Fig. 5). When the entire $Cl^-$ content of the solution is substituted by $SO_4^{2-}$, this 5-HT response reverses polarity (Fig. 6) and its reversal potential

TABLE 1. *Effect of changes in the external concentration of* $Cl^-$ *or* $K^+$ *on the* $E_{5\text{-HT}}$ *(in mV) of the responses to 5-HT of the neurones of the left pallial ganglion group*

| Control | 0 mM $Cl^-$ | 15 mM $K^+$ |
|---|---|---|
| −55 | 0 | −55 |
| −53 | −8 | −53 |
| −54 | −2 | −56 |
| −56 | −2 | −56 |
| −59 | −2 | −54 |
| −58 | 0 | −57 |
| −56 | −6 | −55 |
| −58 | −1 | −52 |
| (−56·1±0·74) | (−2·3±1·0)* | (−54·7±0·59)† |

The values given in parentheses are the means ± the standard errors. * The mean change between this value and the control in physiological salt solution is statistically significant ($P<0·001$). † The mean change between this value and the control in physiological salt solution is not statistically significant ($P>0·05$).

shifts to a value near the zero level (Table 1). Changes in the $[K]_o$ do not affect the $E_{5\text{-HT}}$ values (Table 1). It is evident that this inhibition resulting from the activation of the C-receptors is caused by an increase of the membrane permeability to $Cl^-$, resulting in an influx of this anion.

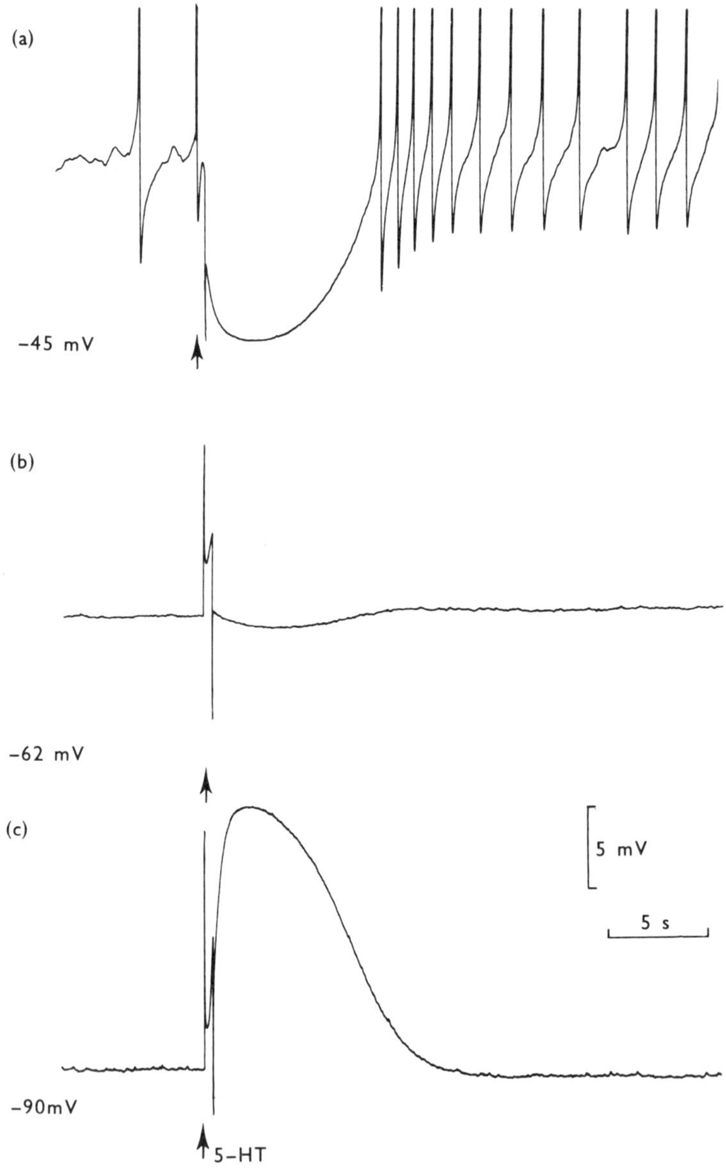


FIG. 5. Reversal potential for the effect of 5-HT produced by activation of C-receptors.

of a series of drugs on the three types of receptor. It may be seen that some 5-HT antagonists like LSD 25 or tryptamine block all three responses to 5-HT. Other 5-HT structural analogues act more specifically. For instance, bufotenine $10^{-5}$ M blocks both the A- and the B-receptors, but potentiates the effect of 5-HT on the C-receptors (Fig. 7). Melatonin or 7-methyltryptamine block the A-receptors without affecting the B-receptors or the C-receptors.

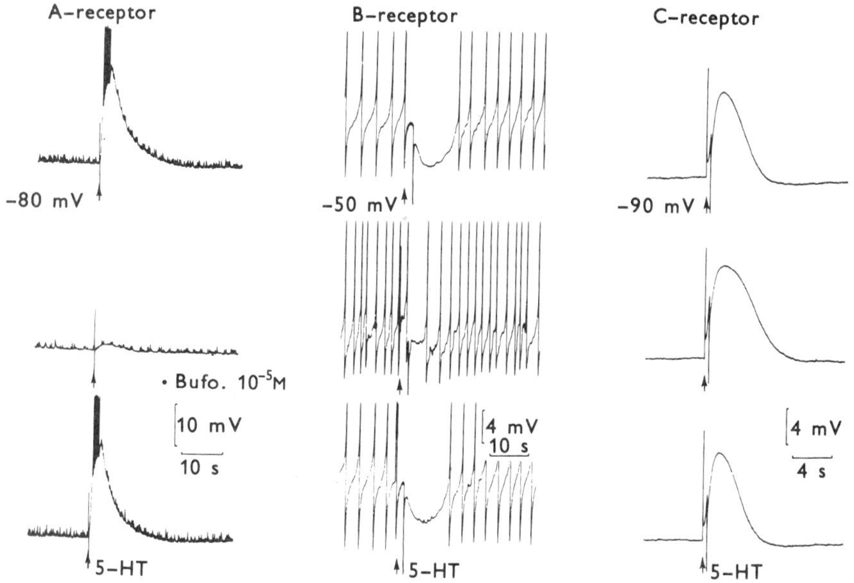


FIG. 7. Effects of bufotenine (Bufo.) on the different types of 5-HT receptors of snail neurones. Each column corresponds to a different neurone, and the receptors involved in each case are indicated above. The upper row of recordings are control 5-HT responses. The middle row are the same responses after perfusion on the preparations of a $10^{-5}$ M solution of bufotenine. The lower row shows the recovering of the responses after washing with control solution. Bufotenine blocks both A- and B-receptors and slightly potentiates the C-receptors.

On the other hand, some drugs active on cholinergic synapses affect the responses to 5-HT. Atropine blocks all the receptors, but (+)-tubocurarine (TC) blocks the responses of the A- and C-receptors without affecting the B-receptors at all. On the other hand, neostigmine blocks the response of C-receptors, without altering those of the A- or the B-receptors. Probably these effects are not totally specific but they are useful for the pharmacological recognition of the receptors.

## *The direct character of 5-HT responses*

There are indications that at least the A-receptors (see Stefani & Gerschenfeld, 1969) and the B-receptors (see above) may be localized on the axon rather

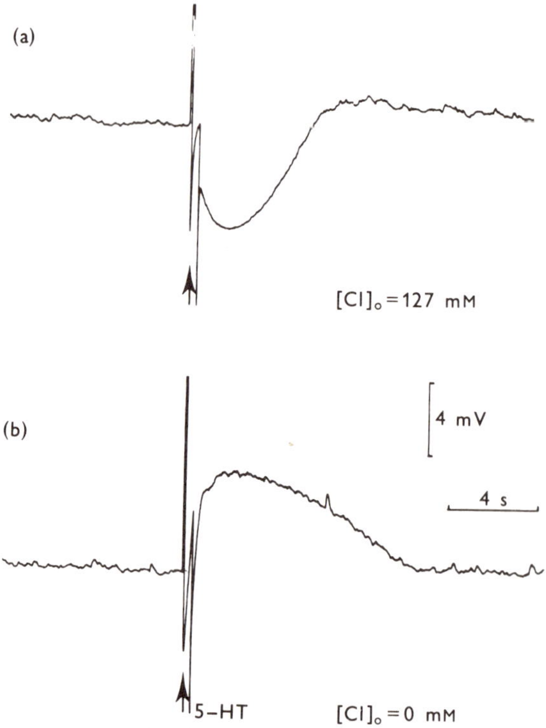


FIG. 6. In the same neurone as in Fig. 5, $Cl^-$-free solution causes a reversal of th
hyperpolarization.

## *Properties of the different 5-HT receptors*

The receptors involved in each of the actions of 5-HT described al appear to be different entities, and each of them may be distinguished fı the others by using pharmacological tools. Table 2 summarizes the eff

TABLE 2. *Pharmacological properties of 5-HT receptors on central neurones of* Helix pomatia

| | A-receptor | B-receptor | C-receptor |
|---|---|---|---|
| LSD 25 | B | B | B |
| Tryptamine | B | B | B |
| Melatonin | B | 0 | 0 |
| Bufotenine | B | B | 0 |
| 7-Methyltryptamine | B | 0 | 0 |
| Atropine | B | B | B |
| (+)-Tubocurarine | B | 0 | B |
| Neostigmine | 0 | 0 | B |

B=Blocks. 0=No blocking effect. Drugs were effective in concentrations between $10^{-5}$ M and $10^{-4}$ M.

than on the soma. This feature, together with the previously mentioned sensitivity of some 5-HT responses to ACh antagonists, may be interpreted as indicating that 5-HT could be acting by exciting interneurones or by producing the release of transmitter from synaptic endings. This hypothesis was discarded on the basis of a series of experiments such as the one in Fig. 8 where a neurone that is depolarized by 5-HT is also depolarized and excited by an ionophoretic application of ACh. The perfusion of neostigmine ($10^{-5}$ M) over the preparation greatly increases both the amplitude and the duration of the ACh response, but does not affect the 5-HT response at all. If 5-HT was causing a release of ACh from cholinergic synapses, a potentiation of the 5-HT response might be expected.

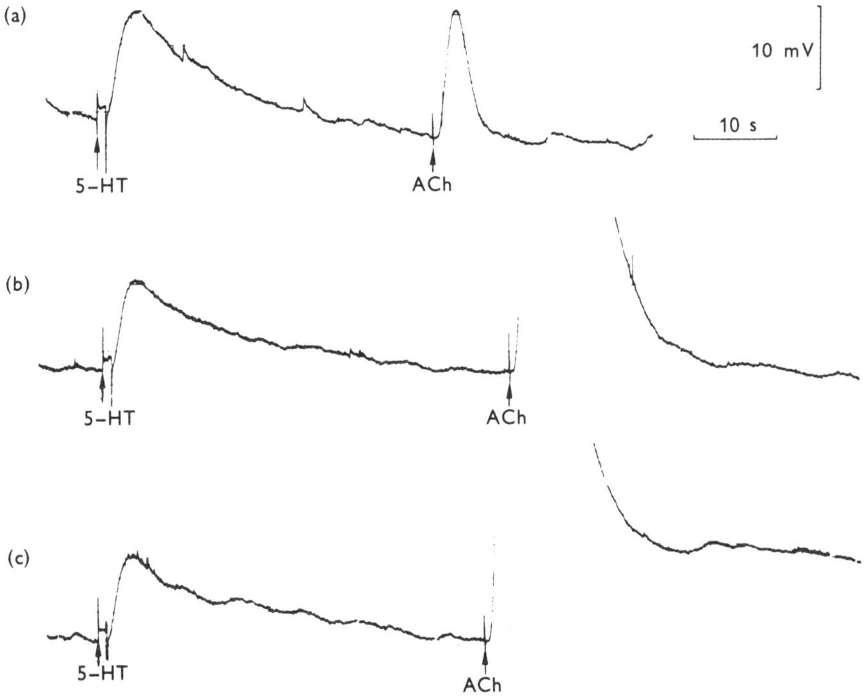


FIG. 8. (a), Control responses to ACh and 5-HT in a neurone possessing A-receptors. (b) and (c), Perfusion of a $10^{-5}$ M solution of neostigmine increases both the amplitude and duration of the ACh response without affecting the 5-HT response.

Other means of demonstrating that the 5-HT effects are exerted directly on the impaled neurone consist of (1) suppressing interneuronal firing or (2) interfering with the transmitter release mechanism at the ganglionic synapses. Figs. 9 and 10 show such experiments in the case of a B-receptor response. The complete removal of both $Na^+$ and $Ca^{2+}$ from the perfusing fluid sup-

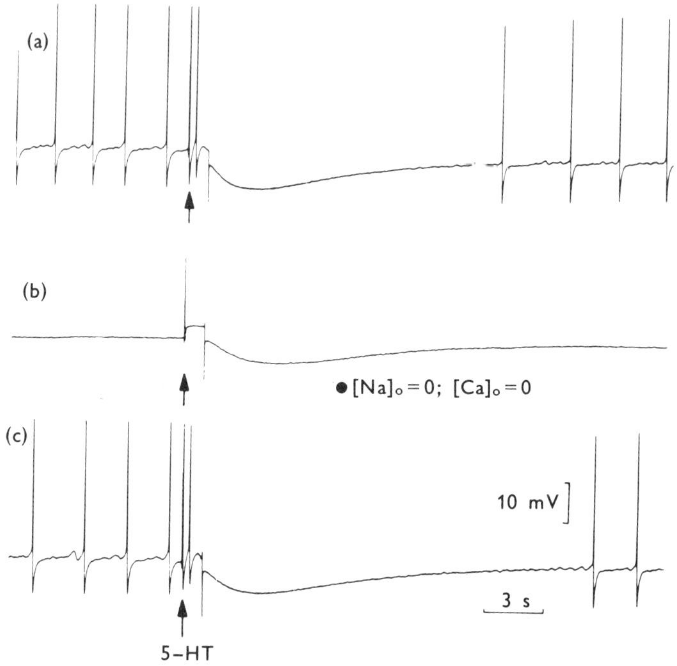


FIG. 9. (a), $K^+$-dependent 5-HT response recorded in control solution. (b), The removal of all $Na^+$ and $Ca^{2+}$ ions from the medium blocks the spike activity of all the neurones of the central nervous system, but the 5-HT response is not altered. (c), Washing with the control solution.

presses all the spike activity in the ganglia, but does not change the 5-HT response. The perfusion of the preparation with iso-osmotic $Mg^{2+}$ also blocks the spikes and blocks the transmitter release at all the ganglionic synapses (Fig. 10). Probably due to an effect of the environmental conditions on the receptors, the response in Fig. 10 is slightly diminished. Again, such drastic procedure shows that the effects of 5-HT are exerted directly on the membrane. In other experiments, the synaptic activity in the CNS was blocked by removing all the $Ca^{2+}$ ions, increasing the $Mg^{2+}$ content five times and adding ethyleneglycol-*bis*(β-aminoethyl ether)-N,N′-tetra-acetic acid (EGTA) 5–10 mM to the bath. Under these conditions, all the 5-HT responses remain unchanged (see Fig. 12).

### *Multireceptor responses*

The membranes of molluscan single neurones may have more than one type of receptor for a given transmitter and polyphasic responses may result from their combined activation (see Kehoe, this symposium). Fig. 11 shows the response of such a multireceptor system combining the activation on a

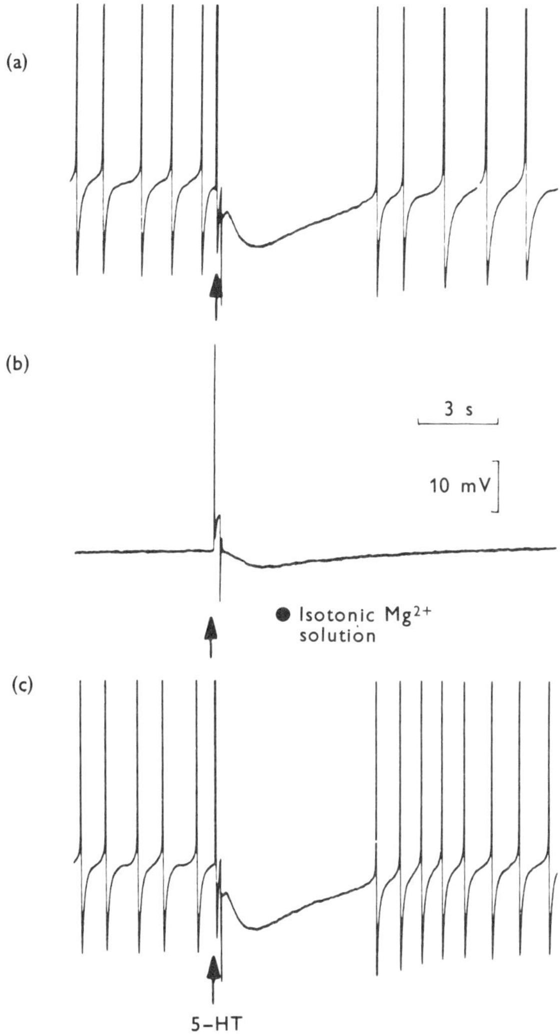


FIG. 10. (a), $K^+$-dependent response to 5-HT recorded in a control solution. (b), Response recorded in isotonic $Mg^{2+}$ solution which suppresses all spike and synaptic activity in the central nervous system. The 5-HT response persists, although somewhat diminished in amplitude. (c), Response recorded after replacement with the control solution.

single cell of A- and B-5-HT receptors, that is, an excitation followed by an inhibition. When the A-receptors involved in the excitation are blocked by TC (Fig. 11), the $K^+$ dependent inhibition remains unaltered. On the other hand, Fig. 12 shows a neurone responding to 5-HT by a combined activation of A- and C-receptors. By replacing all the external $Cl^-$ by $SO_4^{2-}$, the response of the C-receptor is reversed and only a depolarization is then

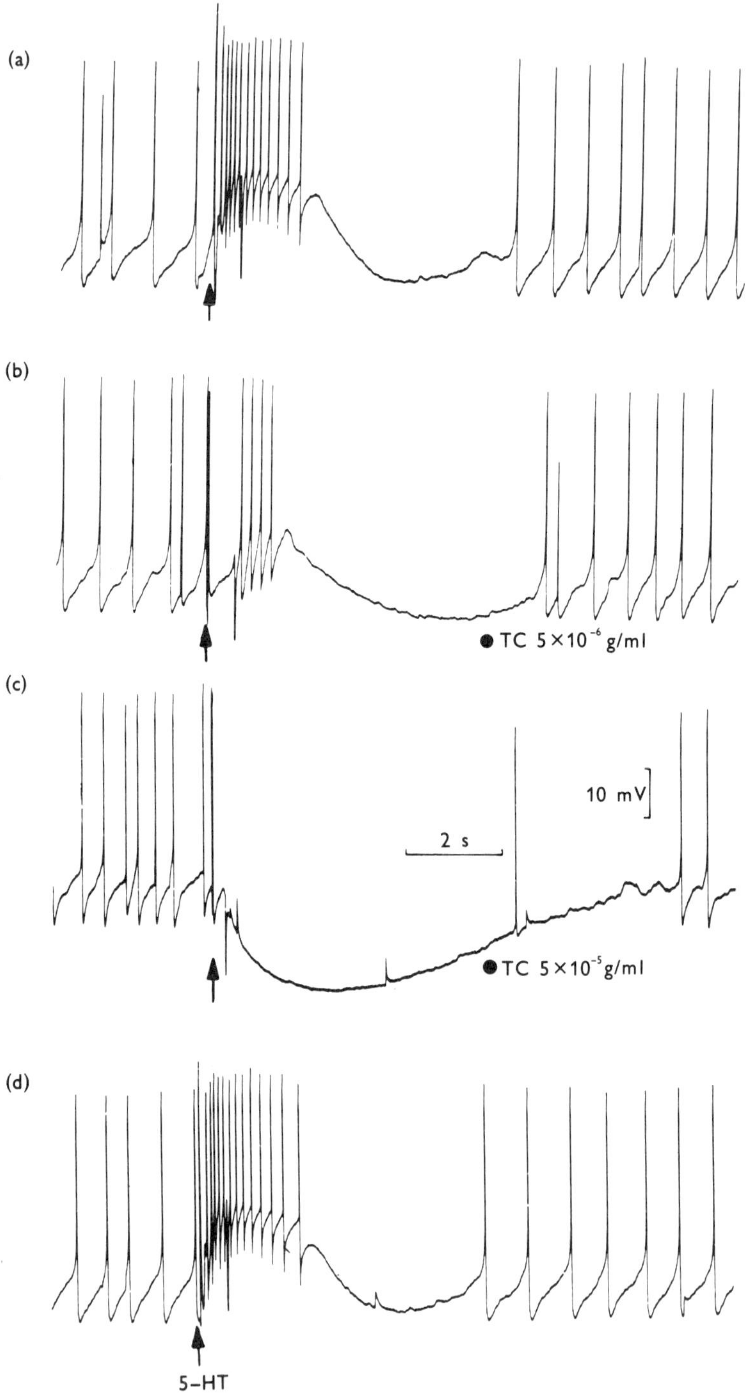


FIG. 11. (a), Biphasic response to ionophoretic application of 5-HT consisting of a depolarization followed by a hyperpolarization. (b) and (c), Two increasing concentrations of TC block the excitatory component. (d), Recovery of the initial response after washing with the control solution.

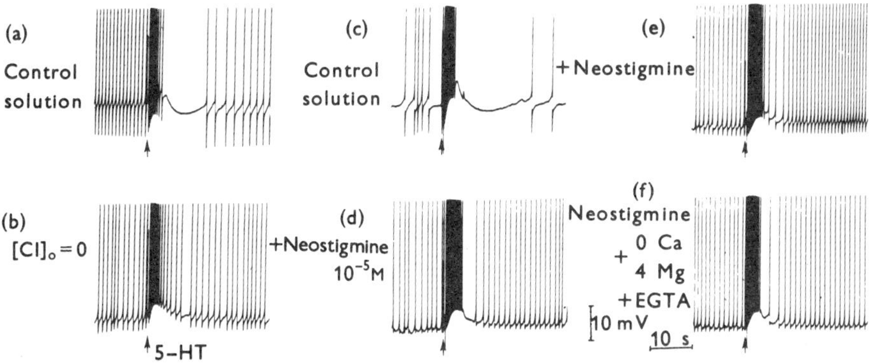


FIG. 12. (a), Biphasic 5-HT response consisting of a depolarization followed by a hyperpolarization, control solution. (b), Disappearance of inhibitory phase in the presence of $Cl^-$-free solution. (c), Recovery in control solution. (d), In presence of $10^{-5}$ M neostigmine, which partly abolishes the inhibitory phase. (e), Complete block of the inhibitory phase by neostigmine. (f), After removal of $Ca^{2+}$ without changing and increase of the $Mg^{2+}$ concentration to 4 mM in the presence of neostigmine.

observed. The effect of neostigmine confirms that the hyperpolarization is due to C-receptor activation, since it blocks the inhibition without affecting the excitation (Fig. 12). The direct character of the depolarization is confirmed by its persistence in a low $Ca^{2+}$, high $Mg^{2+}$ solution containing 5 mM EGTA (Fig. 12).

Other biphasic actions already observed consist of a hyperpolarization mediated by the B-receptors followed by excitation mediated by the A-receptors. In some cases, the multireceptor character of the response is not apparent on first analysis but only when the membrane potential is changed as in Fig. 3 or after the application of specific antagonists which block one of the components.

## *Concluding remarks*

The experiments reported above demonstrate that 5-HT may excite some molluscan neurones by changing their membrane permeability mainly to $Na^+$ ions or may inhibit other neurones by increasing their membrane permeability either to $Cl^-$ or to $K^+$. Each one of these three actions is due to the activation of a different specific receptor, which can be identified by the use of appropriate pharmacological agents. Composite responses involving more than one of the permeability changes described are probably due to the activation of more than one type of receptor. This action of 5-HT on neuronal membranes confirms that 5-HT shares an important property with well-known synaptic transmitters: the ability to produce selective changes in the permeability of the membrane to specific ions.

This work was supported by grants of NIH (grant number 06975 to the Laboratoire de Neurophysiologie Cellulaire, C.E.P.N., C.N.R.S.) and from the Délégation Générale de la Recherche Scientifique et Technique (grants 71-7-3087 and 71-7-3210 to the Laboratoire de Neurobiologie, E.N.S.).

## REFERENCES

CARDOT, J. & RIPPLINGER, J. (1963). *J. Physiol., Paris*, **55**, 217.
CARPENTER, D., BREESE, G., SCHANBERG, S. & KOPIN, I. (1971). *Int. J. Neurosci.*, **2**, 49.
COTTRELL, G. A. (1970). *Nature, Lond.*, **225**, 1060.
COTTRELL, G. A. & POWELL, B. (1971). *J. Neurochem.*, **18**, 1695.
DAHL, E., FALCK, B., VON MECKLEMBURG, C., MYHRBERG, H. & ROSENGREEN, E. (1966). *Z. Zellforsch.*, **71**, 489.
FALCK, B. (1962). *Acta physiol. scand.*, **56**, *suppl.*, 197.
GERSCHENFELD, H. M. (1971). *Science, N.Y.*, **171**, 1252.
GERSCHENFELD, H. M. & STEFANI, E. (1965). *Nature, Lond.*, **205**, 1216.
GERSCHENFELD, H. M. & STEFANI, E. (1966). *J. Physiol., Lond.*, **185**, 684.
GERSCHENFELD, H. M. & STEFANI, E. (1968). *Adv. Pharmac.*, **6A**, 369.
GERSCHENFELD, H. M. & TAUC, L. (1961). *Nature, Lond.*, **189**, 924.
GLAIZNER, B. (1967). In: *Symposium on Neurobiology of Invertebrates*, p. 267. Budapest: Akadémiai Kiadó.
JAEGER, C. P., JAEGER, E. C. & WELSH, J. H. (1971). *Z. Zellforsch.*, **112**, 54.
KERKUT, G. A. & COTTRELL, G. A. (1963). *Comp. Biochem. Physiol.*, **8**, 53.
LOVELAND, R. E. (1963). *Comp. Biochem. Physiol.*, **9**, 95.
MARSDEN, C. & KERKUT, G. A. (1970). *Comp. gen. Pharmac.*, **1**, 101.
MIROLLI, M. (1968). *Comp. Biochem. Physiol.*, **24**, 847.
MIROLLI, M. & WELSH, J. H. (1964). In: *Comparative Neurochemistry*, ed. Richter, D., p. 433. Oxford: Pergamon.
NASTUK, W. L. & PARSONS, R. L. (1970). *J. gen. Physiol.*, **56**, 218.
OSBORNE, N. N. & COTTRELL, G. A. (1971). *Z. Zellforsch.*, **112**, 15.
S.-ROSZA, K. & PERENYI, L. (1966). *Comp. Biochem. Physiol.*, **19**, 105.
STEFANI, E. & GERSCHENFELD, H. M. (1969). *J. Neurophysiol.*, **32**, 64.
TAXI, J. & GAUTRON, J. (1969). *J. Microscopie*, **8**, 627.
WELSH, J. H. & MOORHEAD, M. (1960). *J. Neurochem.*, **6**, 146.

## DISCUSSION

*Walker* (*Southampton*)

Have you any evidence for 5-HT as a transmitter agent at excitatory and inhibitory synapses in the snail?

*Gerschenfeld* (*Paris*)

As has been briefly mentioned in the text, some years ago we reported with Dr E. Stefani (*Adv. Pharmac.*, **6A**, 369, 1968) that neurones endowed with A-5-HT receptors may show two different kinds of excitatory synaptic potentials: (a) fast e.p.s.ps which may be blocked with hexamethonium and other cholinergic agonists and (b) slow e.p.s.ps which are not affected by hexamethonium and may be blocked by LSD 25, tryptamine and 5-HT itself, in the same concentrations as the A-receptors. We considered that the fast e.p.s.ps were probably cholinergic and that the slow e.p.s.ps could possibly involve 5-HT. However, the e.p.s.ps that we studied were unitary and probably not monosynaptic, and we did not know whether the antagonists were not acting at other levels, different from the postsynaptic membrane. Therefore we considered this evidence as incomplete. More recently, Dr Cottrell and his collaborators have identified in snail metacerebral ganglia a pair of giant neurones that probably release 5-HT as transmitter. They also described some connections of these neurones with a series of identified neurones located in the buccal ganglia. The evidence as to whether 5-HT has a role in mediating excitation at these synapses appears to me still incomplete.

*Cottrell* (*St Andrews*)

I would like to comment on Dr Gerschenfeld's reference to our work. First, we now have extra evidence that the yellow, 5-HT-like, fluorescence in the giant metacerebral cell of *Helix pomatia* brain is indeed due to the presence of this amine. This evidence comes from bioassay, from electrophoresis and, most significantly, from microchromatography using dansyl chloride of extracts of individually dissected neurones. Thus, there can be little doubt that these giant neurones do contain 5-HT. Secondly, we have observed that 10 h after injecting TEA into this cell, there is a dramatic increase in the size of the excitatory postsynaptic potential seen in the 'middle buccal cell' hitherto presumed to be directly innervated by the giant serotonin-containing neurone (GSN) on the basis of constant latency and response to GSN stimulation. These data provide extra valuable evidence for a monosynaptic connection. Applied 5-HT activates the 'middle buccal cell'. Thirdly, Mr V. Pentreath and I have observed that tritium-labelled 5-HT is specifically taken up by axon terminals in the region of the buccal ganglia where the synapses onto the 'middle buccal cell' are thought to be made. Electron microscope autoradiograms show that these endings contain small dense cored vesicles of the same appearance as those observed in the soma of the GSN. Imipramine blocks 5-HT uptake and markedly potentiates transmission at the synapse.

Our results then do indeed argue for a transmitter role for 5-HT in the central nervous system of gastropod molluscs and fit well with Dr Gerschenfeld's pharmacological observations on the excitatory effects of 5-HT on different snail neurones.

# ACETYLCHOLINE RECEPTORS IN *APLYSIA* NEURONES

JACSUE KEHOE

*Laboratoire de Neurobiologie, Ecole Normale Supérieure, 46, rue d'Ulm, Paris 5e, France*

In 1962, Tauc and Gerschenfeld reported that an ionophoretic injection of acetylcholine (ACh) causes a depolarizing response in some *Aplysia* neurones and a hyperpolarizing response in others. Both of these responses could be blocked by (+)-tubocurarine. The additional finding that the depolarizing responses could be selectively eliminated by hexamethonium showed that the two effects were mediated by different receptor types. Moreover, certain spontaneous i.p.s.ps in the ACh-hyperpolarized cells were, like the ACh response, blocked by (+)-tubocurarine, suggesting that at least one of the two receptor types plays a physiological role.

Further investigation of the transmitter role of ACh in *Aplysia* has been facilitated by the identification of apparently cholinergic neurones and their follower cells (Kandel, Frazier, Waziri & Coggeshall, 1967; Kehoe, 1969, 1972b; Gardner, 1971) in the central ganglia. In the experiments described below, one of these cholinergic neurones was used to show that:

1. A single cholinergic neurone—like an ionophoretic injection of ACh—can cause three different types of elementary postsynaptic potentials (an e.p.s.p., a 'rapid i.p.s.p.', and a 'slow i.p.s.p.') (see also Strumwasser, 1962; Kandel *et al.*, 1967; Kehoe, 1972c; Gardner, 1971) which are due to the activation of three pharmacologically distinct receptors.
2. The response of a given cell to the presynaptic neurone can be single- or multicomponent (see also Pinsker & Kandel, 1969; Wachtel & Kandel, 1971) depending upon how many of the three receptor types it possesses.
3. Whereas the receptors mediating the rapid potentials (e.p.s.p. and rapid i.p.s.p.) correspond to those already described by Tauc & Gerschenfeld (1962), the receptor mediating the slow i.p.s.p. bears no resemblance to previously described vertebrate or invertebrate receptors.
4. Each of the three receptors controls a selective change in membrane permeability. The excitatory response has been shown by Blankenship, Wachtel & Kandel (1971) to be due, at least in part, to a permeability change to sodium ions. It is shown below that the rapid i.p.s.p. (see also

Blankenship *et al.*, 1971) and slow i.p.s.p. are due to selective changes in permeability to $Cl^-$ and $K^+$ ions, respectively.

5. The potassium-dependent slow i.p.s.p. (mediated by the 'new' receptor type) is affected in such a way by the conditions known to block the Na–K pump that this potential could be misinterpreted as an activation of that pump (see Pinsker & Kandel, 1969; Kehoe & Ascher, 1970).

The methods employed in these experiments have been reported elsewhere in detail (Kehoe, 1972a–c). The identifiable, presumably cholinergic neurone of the pleural ganglion (presynaptic neurone I) was used in conjunction with three groups of postsynaptic cells with which it makes monosynaptic contact: 'anterior', 'medial', and 'unidentified' cells of the pleural ganglion (Kehoe, 1972b,c). When the synaptic responses were studied, both the pre- and postsynaptic cells were impaled with double-barrelled microelectrodes filled with 0·6 M $K_2SO_4$, permitting independent recording and polarizing barrels for each cell of the pair. These electrodes were sometimes filled with other solutions to permit the intracellular injection of other ions (for example, tetraethylammonium, chloride) into either of the cells. When ACh was applied electrophoretically, only the postsynaptic cell was impaled, and an electrode filled with ACh was brought close to the surface of the somatic membrane where the ionophoretic application of ACh was made.

### *A single presynaptic neurone can cause three different types of elementary postsynaptic potentials which are due to the activation of three pharmacologically distinct receptors*

As can be seen in Fig. 1, an action potential in presynaptic neurone I provokes an e.p.s.p. in the *anterior* cells of the pleural ganglion, a rapid i.p.s.p. in a group of *unidentified* cells, and a slowly-developing, long-lasting inhibitory response (slow i.p.s.p.) in the *medial* cells (Fig. 1). An electrophoretic injection of ACh imitates, in each case, the synaptic potential observed in a given cell (Fig. 1).

Whereas the response seen in the anterior and unidentified cells resembles those already observed by Tauc & Gerschenfeld (1962) and by Kandel *et al.* (1967) in the visceral ganglion, the third potential type (medial cell response) has a considerably slower time course (see also, Pinsker & Kandel, 1969).

A brief pharmacological analysis of these three response types shows that each is mediated by a pharmacologically distinct receptor. The first two synaptic responses appear to be mediated by the two receptor types already distinguished by Tauc & Gerschenfeld (1962), since both can be blocked by (+)-tubocurarine (TC), whereas only the depolarizing one (the e.p.s.p.) is affected by hexamethonium (C6) (see Fig. 2).

The slow i.p.s.p., on the other hand, does not appear to be mediated by either of the previously described receptor types since it is unaffected by both

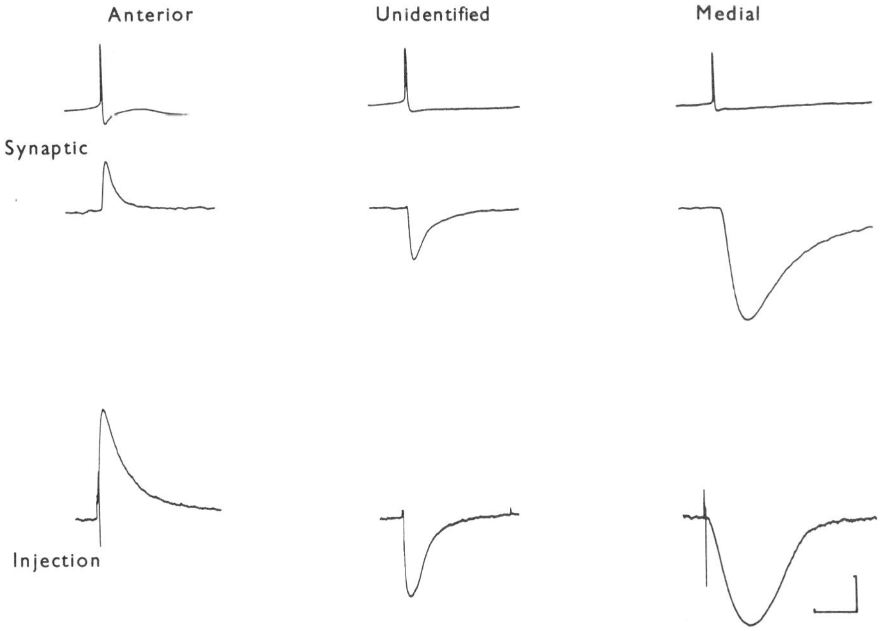


FIG. 1. Synaptic: firing of presynaptic neurone I (see action potentials in the upper trace) causes different types of potentials (lower trace) in different pleural neurones: an e.p.s.p. in the anterior cell; a rapid i.p.s.p. in the unidentified cell; and a slow i.p.s.p. in the medial cell. Calibration: 0·5 s, 5 mV. No amplitude calibration is given for the presynaptic action potential. Injection: responses of the same three types of pleural neurones to an ionophoretic injection of ACh: a rapid depolarizing response in the anterior cell; a rapid hyperpolarization in the unidentified cell; and a slow hyperpolarization in the medial cell. In all cases the postsynaptic neuronal membranes were preset at −45 mV. Under normal conditions, the slow i.p.s.p. of the medial cells is accompanied by a rapid i.p.s.p. like that seen in the 'unidentified' cell. To permit the presentation of the slow i.p.s.p. in isolation, the records of the medial cell responses were made in preparations in the presence of (+)-tubocurarine. Furthermore, all synaptic responses shown in this figure are atypically large in amplitude due to experimental treatment of the presynaptic neurone (see text). Calibration: Anterior cell: 3 s, 5 mV; Unidentified and Medial cells: 10 s, 5 mV.

(+)-tubocurarine and hexamethonium (see TC and C6 of Fig. 2). However, the slow i.p.s.p. and its imitative ACh potential can be blocked by methylxylocholine (see β TM10, Fig. 2), showing that they are mediated by a third type of acetylcholine receptor. Thus, three different ACh receptor types can be pharmacologically distinguished in *Aplysia* neurones, and all three can be activated by the firing of a single presynaptic neurone.

*The response of a given cell to the presynaptic neurone can be single- or multi-component, depending upon how many of the three receptor types it bears*

The synaptic response in the pharmacologically untreated preparation is often complex, made up of a combination of superimposed excitatory and inhibitory elements due to the juxtaposition of more than one type of

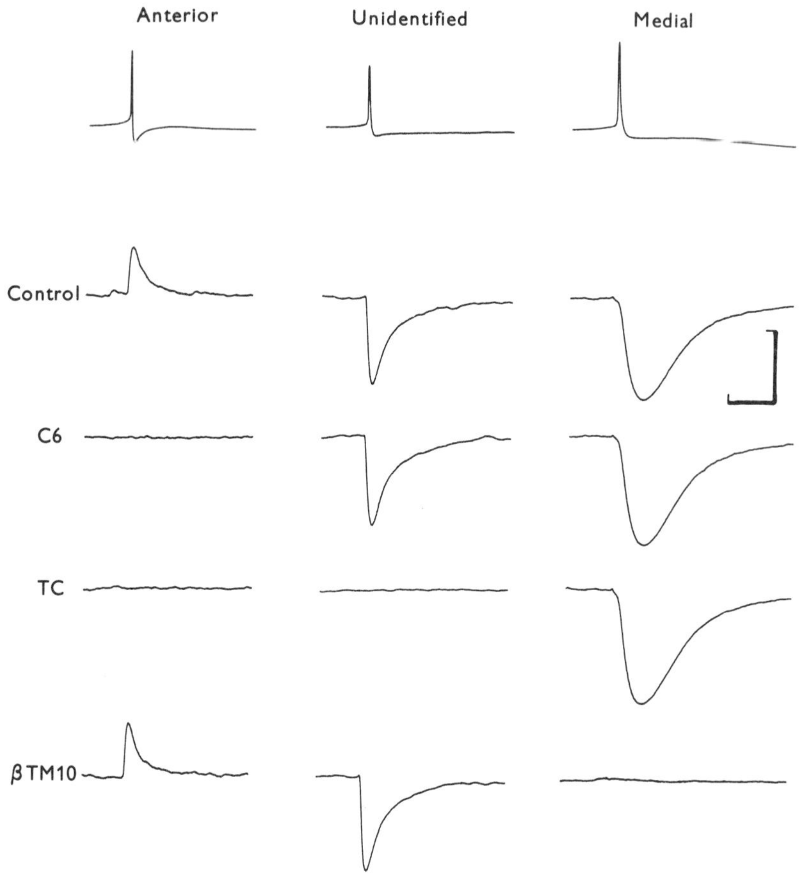


FIG. 2. Effects of hexamethonium (C6), (+)-tubocurarine (TC) and methylxylocholine (βTM10) on the three types of postsynaptic potentials (e.p.s.p., rapid i.p.s.p. and slow i.p.s.p.) evoked by presynaptic neurone I in three different types of pleural ganglion cells (anterior, unidentified and medial cells, respectively). Each of the postsynaptic potentials is a response to a single presynaptic action potential. The action potentials presented in the upper trace are those associated with the control responses; for the sake of simplicity, the action potentials causing the other responses were not included. In all cases, the postsynaptic neuronal membranes were preset at −45 mV. It can be seen that C6 selectively blocks the e.p.s.p.; TC, the e.p.s.p. and rapid i.p.s.p.; and βTM10, the slow i.p.s.p. Under normal conditions, the slow i.p.s.p. of the medial cells is accompanied by a rapid i.p.s.p. like that seen in the unidentified cell (see for example, Figs. 3 and 4). To permit the presentation of the slow i.p.s.p. in isolation, the records of the medial cell responses were made in preparations in the presence of (+)-tubocurarine. Furthermore, all synaptic responses shown in this figure are atypically large due to experimental treatment of the presynaptic neurone (see text). Calibration: 0·5 s, 5 mV. No amplitude calibration is presented for the action potentials.

cholinergic receptor on the postsynaptic cell. In fact, in the normal preparation, it has not as yet been possible to observe the slow i.p.s.p. unaccompanied by one of the other two potential types. For this reason, in order to obtain the records of the isolated slow i.p.s.p. shown in Figs. 1 and 2, preparations were used in the presence of (+)-tubocurarine.

Also, in most preparations the postsynaptic potential changes caused by a single presynaptic spike are not of sufficient amplitude for experimental use. In particular, the slow i.p.s.p. is only barely measurable following a single presynaptic spike. Consequently, for the 'simplified' presentation given above, transmitter liberation from the presynaptic neurone was artificially increased by an intracellular injection of tetraethylammonium (Kehoe, 1969, 1972c; see also Katz & Miledi, 1967; Kusano, Livengood & Werman, 1967) thus permitting an evaluation of the response to a single presynaptic action potential rather than to the series of action potentials that is necessary in the normal preparation.

The records of Fig. 3, in contrast, are typical responses recorded under

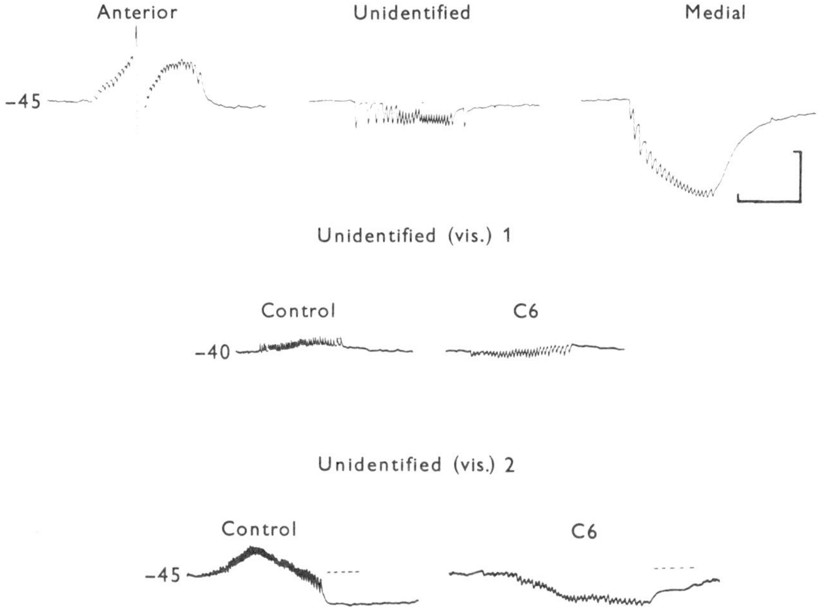


FIG. 3. Upper trace: responses of three pleural neurones (anterior, unidentified and medial) to repetitive firing of presynaptic neurone I. Excitatory potentials are elicited in the anterior cells; rapid i.p.s.ps in the unidentified cell; and a composite inhibitory response, consisting of rapid i.p.s.ps superimposed upon a slow hyperpolarizing wave, is seen in the medial cells. Calibration: 2 s, 5 mV. Lower traces: responses of two unidentified cells in the visceral ganglion to repetitive firing of cholinergic neurone L10. Unidentified (vis.) 1: under control conditions, the response appears to consist of a series of 'simple' e.p.s.ps. However, when hexamethonium is added to the bathing medium, blocking the excitatory potential, underlying rapid i.p.s.ps are revealed. Unidentified (vis.) 2: under control conditions, the response in this neurone appears to consist of rapid e.p.s.ps superimposed upon a slow hyperpolarizing wave. When the excitatory responses are blocked by hexamethonium, it is seen that these two response types (excitatory and slow inhibitory) are accompanied by rapid i.p.s.ps. Calibration: 3 s, 7 mV.

normal conditions (that is, without pharmacological isolation of any of the postsynaptic responses and without an increase in transmitter release from the presynaptic neurone) in the same cell groups as those used in Figs. 1 and 2. Repetitive firing of presynaptic neurone I causes a series of e.p.s.ps in the *anterior* cell; a series of rapid i.p.s.ps in an *unidentified* pleural cell, and a composite inhibitory response in the *medial* cell. This composite response consists of rapid i.p.s.ps superimposed upon the slowly-developing, long-lasting hyperpolarizing wave—the slow i.p.s.p.

Other combinations of the three response types have been observed in the visceral ganglion in response to activation of another cholinergic neurone (L10, see Kandel *et al.*, 1967). These complex responses have likewise been shown to be due to the simultaneous activation of two or three of the cholinergic receptors (see Kehoe, 1972c). As can be seen in Fig. 3 (Unidentified (vis.) 1 and 2) it is often not possible to detect, in the pharmacologically untreated preparations (Controls), all components of the response. For example, in *Unidentified (vis.) 1*, the response in normal conditions appears to be a simple excitatory potential, whereas it is found, following a block of the e.p.s.p. with hexamethonium (C6) to be a complex response, consisting of superimposed e.p.s.ps and rapid i.p.s.ps. Likewise, in *Unidentified (vis) 2*, what appears to be a two-component response (consisting of e.p.s.ps superimposed upon a slow i.p.s.p.) in the pharmacologically untreated condition is in fact a three-component response in which the rapid i.p.s.ps are masked by the e.p.s.ps. Adding hexamethonium (C6) to the bathing medium eliminates the e.p.s.ps, and the two-component inhibition is revealed.

*Whereas the two receptors mediating the rapid responses (e.p.s.p. and rapid i.p.s.p.) resemble previously described receptors, the receptor underlying the slow i.p.s.p. appears to have unique pharmacological characteristics*

Since the two receptors mediating the rapid responses correspond to those previously described by Tauc & Gerschenfeld (1962) (see Fig. 2) the experiments presented below deal primarily with the 'new' receptor type which mediates the slow i.p.s.p. Moreover, as the slow i.p.s.p. is never found in isolation but is always accompanied by one of the two rapid response elements, it has been studied as a component of the two-component inhibition seen in the medial cells. Thus, the pharmacological characteristics of the receptor mediating the slow i.p.s.p. are constantly compared to those of the receptor mediating the rapid i.p.s.p.

Even without pharmacological manipulation, it is possible to 'separate' the two components of the two-component inhibition by observing the response at a variety of membrane potential levels, as is done in Fig. 4. A hyperpolarization of the postsynaptic cell beyond the resting level progressively reduces the size of the rapid i.p.s.p. as it approaches its 'equilibrium potential' at $-60$ mV. At this level, the rapid i.p.s.p. is no longer visible, and one can

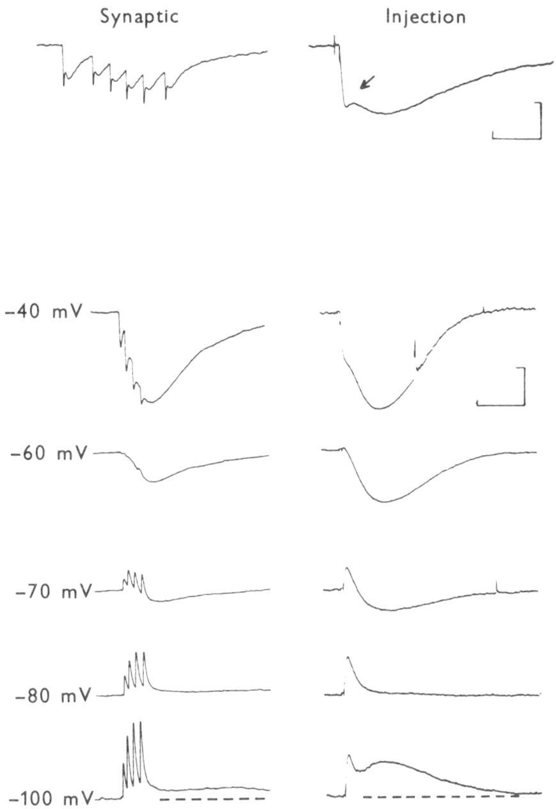


FIG. 4. Response of medial pleural neurones to firing of presynaptic neurone I (Synaptic) and to an ionophoretic injection of ACh (Injection). Upper trace: responses, at resting level, to 6 successive presynaptic action potentials (not shown) (Synaptic) and to an ionophoretic injection of ACh (Injection). Note the biphasic nature of each p.s.p. and of the response to ACh injection (arrow indicating break between rapid and slow components). Calibration: Synaptic and Injection: 2 s, 5 mV. Lower traces: response to 4 presynaptic spikes (Synaptic) and an ionophoretic injection of ACh (Injection) as a function of preset membrane potentials. Note that the rapid component of both the synaptic and ACh potentials (indicated in this and subsequent figures by values on the left) reverses at $-60$ mV, whereas the slow component reverses at $-80$ mV. The response to stimulation of presynaptic neurone I in the lower traces had been experimentally increased by an intracellular injection of TEA in the presynaptic neurone. Calibration: Synaptic: 2 s, 5 mV; Injection: 10 s, 5 mV.

observe the slow i.p.s.p. with minimal interference from the rapid one. However, since the slow i.p.s.p. is not as yet in equilibrium at $-60$ mV, it hyperpolarizes the cell further, and thus the membrane crosses the reversal potential of the rapid response, which reappears as a rapid depolarizing potential superimposed upon the slow, still-hyperpolarizing wave. The slow i.p.s.p. is 'in equilibrium' at $-80$ mV. At this potential one can observe the rapid i.p.s.p. with the least interference from the slow component of the response. The reversal of the slow i.p.s.p. can be detected (at −100 mV) as a slow return of the membrane to the preset potential following the last (reversed) rapid i.p.s.p. (see broken line indicating preset potential). Note that the rapid phase of the ACh potential, like the rapid i.p.s.p., reverses at −60 mV; the slow phase of the ACh potential, like the slow i.p.s.p., at −80 mV (see Fig. 4, Injection).

That the rapid i.p.s.p. is selectively eliminated by (+)-tubocurarine, and the slow i.p.s.p. untouched by that drug, is shown in Fig. 5 (Synaptic). Fig. 5 (Injection) gives a comparable picture of the effect of (+)-tubocurarine on the two components of the ACh response in the same cells. Since almost all previously described tubocurarine-resistant cholinergic responses have been shown to be blocked by atropine (see Koelle, 1970 for review; see Levitan & Tauc, 1972 for an exception), this drug was of course tested. However, atropine—even at concentrations of $10^{-3}$ g/ml, has no blocking effect on either component of the inhibitory response (see Kehoe, 1972b). (In some experiments, atropine affected the conduction of the spike in the presynaptic neurone, and by this indirect means caused a reduction in both components of the inhibitory response.)

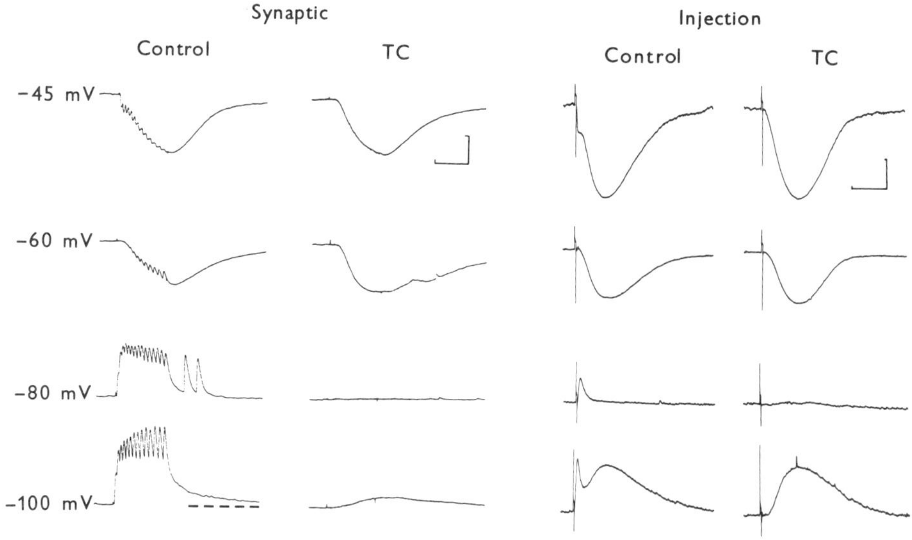


FIG. 5. Effects of (+)-tubocurarine (TC) on the two-component inhibitory response of a medial pleural neurone to a series of approximately 14 action potentials in presynaptic neurone I (Synaptic) and to an ionophoretic injection of ACh (Injection). Note that in the presence of (+)-tubocurarine ($10^{-4}$ M) the rapid i.p.s.p. of the synaptic response and the early component of the injection potential are completely eliminated, whereas the slow i.p.s.p. and the slow injection potential are unaffected. The elimination of the rapid responses by (+)-tubocurarine can best be observed at −80 mV (the reversal potential of the slow response). The persistence in the presence of (+)-tubocurarine of the slow responses is best observed at −60 mV (the reversal potential of the rapid response). Calibration: Synaptic: 1 s, 5 mV; Injection: 10 s, 5 mV. (From Kehoe, 1972b, modified.)

Although both (+)-tubocurarine and atropine are without effect on the slow i.p.s.p., it is possible to eliminate that response selectively with a variety of different compounds. As was shown in Fig. 2, the slow i.p.s.p. can be blocked by methylxylocholine—a drug better known for its adrenergic neurone blocking properties (McLean, Geus, Mohrbacher, Mattis & Ullyot, 1960). Fig. 6 shows a similarly selective block of the slow i.p.s.p. which was obtained with tetraethylammonium (TEA). Although tetraethylammonium is known as a cholinolytic, its blocking action has previously been demonstrated at tubocurarine-sensitive rather than tubocurarine-resistant synapses (Volle & Koelle, 1970).* Finally, the slow i.p.s.p. can also be blocked by phenyltrimethylammonium. This drug, known for its cholinomimetic (Koelle, 1970) and anticholinesterasic actions (see Nachmansohn,

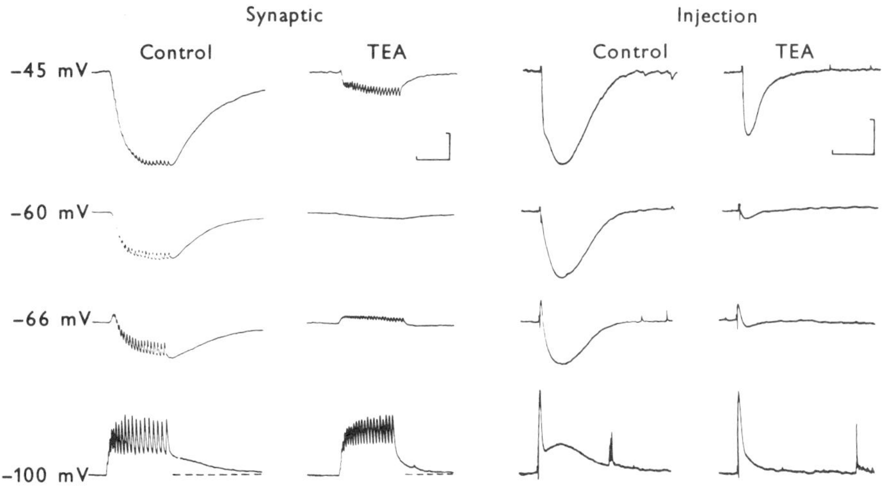


FIG. 6. Effect of tetraethylammonium (TEA) $10^{-4}$ M on the two-component inhibitory response of the medial pleural neurones elicited by stimulation of presynaptic neurone I (Synaptic) or by an ionophoretic injection of ACh (Injection). Note that under TEA the slow i.p.s.p. of the synaptic response and the slow component of the injection potential are eliminated, whereas the rapid i.p.s.p. and the early component of the injection potential are unaffected. The elimination of the slow responses by TEA can best be observed at −60 mV (the reversal potential of the rapid responses). The retention, in TEA, of the rapid responses is best observed at −100 mV. Calibration: Synaptic: 2 s, 5 mV; Injection: 10 s, 5 mV.

* TEA has been shown to block potassium permeability in many preparations. The fact, shown below, that the slow i.p.s.p. is due to a change in potassium permeability raises the possibility that the block observed in Fig. 5 could be due to a general interference with potassium permeability rather than to a specific cholinergic receptor block. However, it has been shown (Kehoe, 1972a,c) that although TEA, applied intracellularly, can greatly reduce potassium permeability in *Aplysia* neurones (acting on the potassium currents of the action potential as well as on those of the synaptic potentials) the block observed at low concentrations with external application cannot be attributed to a general effect on potassium permeability since neither the action potential nor a potassium-dependent dopamine potential in these neurones is affected.

1959) at other junctions, blocks the receptor mediating the slow i.p.s.p. without an antecedent stimulation of that receptor.

Thus, the receptor for the slow i.p.s.p. (and the slow component of the ACh potential) is unaffected by both (+)-tubocurarine and atropine, but can be blocked by methylxylocholine, tetraethylammonium, and phenyltrimethylammonium—drugs not typically grouped together in the pharmacological literature. This atypical pharmacological profile constructed from the study of cholinolytic effects at this synapse is paralleled by the atypical character of the sensitivity of the underlying receptor to cholinomimetics. Whereas the rapid (tubocurarine-sensitive) i.p.s.p. is imitated by all nicotinic agents tested (nicotine, tetramethylammonium, decamethonium, suxamethonium, and dimethyl-4-phenylpiperazinium) none of these agents is capable of imitating the slow i.p.s.p. Furthermore, muscarine and most muscarine-like drugs (methacholine, oxotremorine and pilocarpine) are essentially without effect on the receptor which mediates the slow i.p.s.p. Other than ACh and carbachol (which mimics all three actions of ACh) the only cholinomimetic tested which elicits the slow inhibitory response is arecoline. Moreover, arecoline acts selectively on the receptor mediating that response. The selectivity of its action can be seen in Fig. 7, which compares the effects of bath-applied ACh, tetramethylammonium (TMA), and arecoline (Arec.) on the medial pleural neurones. The membrane was preset at −70 mV in these experiments, from which level activation of the receptor mediating the rapid response causes a depolarization (towards −60 mV); of that mediating the slow i.p.s.p., a hyperpolarization (towards

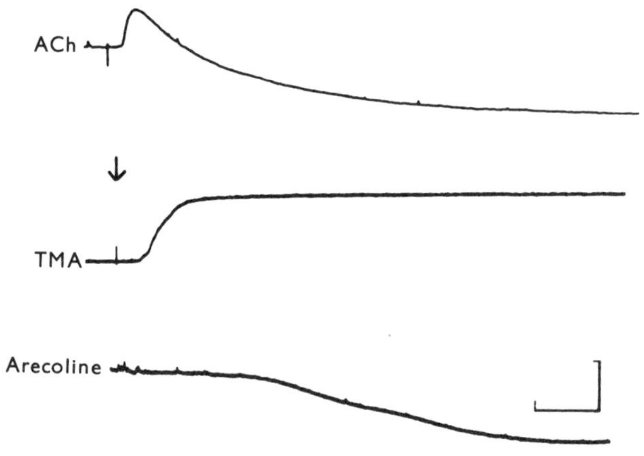


FIG. 7. Effects of bath application of ACh ($2 \times 10^{-4}$ M), TMA ($5 \times 10^{-5}$ M), and arecoline ($10^{-4}$ M) on medial cells of the pleural ganglion. The neuronal membranes are preset at −70 mV in all cases. Arrow indicates application of the drugs. Calibration: ACh: 10 s, 10 mV; TMA: 2 s, 5 mV; Arecoline: 10 s, 5 mV. (Modified presentation of data from Kehoe, 1972b.)

– 80 mV). ACh, which stimulates both receptors, causes a biphasic response (depolarization followed by hyperpolarization). Tetramethylammonium, acting on the tubocurarine-sensitive 'inhibitory' receptor, depolarizes the cell towards – 60 mV. The fact that the response to arecoline application has no depolarizing phase strongly suggests that it acts only on the tubocurarine-resistant receptor. This impression was confirmed by the finding that cells which appear to bear only the tubocurarine-sensitive receptors are unaffected by arecoline (Kehoe, 1972b).

The selective action of arecoline is further shown by its secondary blocking effects. Whereas nicotine selectively blocks the tubocurarine-sensitive receptor (thus eliminating the rapid i.p.s.p. of the two-component inhibition while leaving the slow i.p.s.p. intact) arecoline selectively blocks the receptor mediating the slow i.p.s.p. (see Fig. 8).

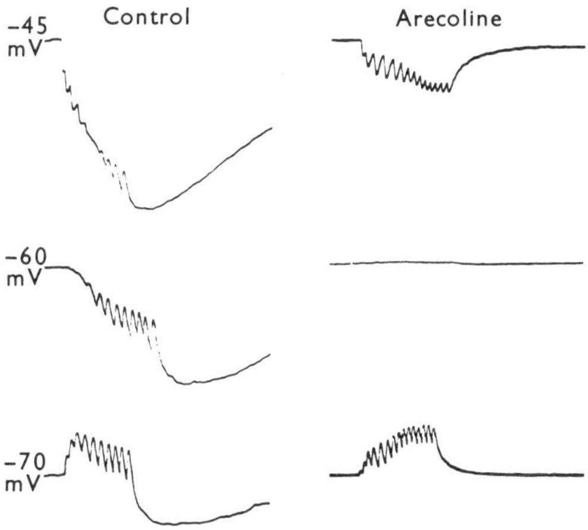


FIG. 8. Effect of arecoline ($5 \times 10^{-6}$ M) on the response of a medial pleural neurone to repeated firing of presynaptic neurone I. Arecoline completely blocked the slow i.p.s.p. without affecting the amplitude of the rapid i.p.s.p.

A résumé of the drugs capable of blocking the three different response types is presented in Table 1 (see Kehoe, 1972b for further details). In many respects, the two receptors mediating rapid responses resemble vertebrate nicotinic receptors. The receptor mediating the slow i.p.s.p., on the other hand, seems to have no known counterpart in the vertebrate system. It is insensitive to both nicotine and muscarine, and is unaffected by both (+)-tubocurarine and atropine. The fact that it can be selectively blocked by such diverse agents as tetraethylammonium, methylxylocholine and phenyltrimethylammonium, and selectively stimulated by arecoline, does not facilitate its incorporation into standard classification schemes.

TABLE 1. *Blocking effects of cholinolytics and cholinomimetics on cholinergic synaptic responses of anterior and medial pleural neurones*

| Drug | e.p.s.p. | Rapid i.p.s.p. | Slow i.p.s.p. |
|---|---|---|---|
| Hexamethonium<br>Atropine | C | N | N |
| (+)-Tubocurarine<br>Dihydro-β-erythroidine<br>Strychnine<br>Brucine<br>Nicotinic agents | C | C | N |
| Methylxylocholine<br>Tetraethylammonium | P | N | C |
| Phenyltrimethylammonium<br>Arecoline | N | N | C |

C: complete block; N: no effect; P: partial block.

Almost all the effects listed in this table can be obtained with drug concentrations of $10^{-4}$ M. Exceptions are atropine (for which a dose of $10^{-3}$ M or greater is required), and the nicotinic agents (for which the effective doses are unknown since a test for a block of the synaptic response can be made only after washing). Not all the nicotinic agents were tested on the synaptic inputs to either the anterior or medial pleural cells; however, the tests performed strongly suggest that they block completely and selectively the two rapid synaptic responses, as they do the corresponding ACh potentials. The nicotinic agents and arecoline cause a fall in membrane resistance due to their cholinomimetic action which can sometimes cause a 'shunting' of the 'unaffected' response in the medial pleural neurones. (From Kehoe, 1972b.)

## *Each of the receptors mediating inhibition controls a selective change in membrane permeability*

Blankenship *et al.* (1971) have shown that sodium ions contribute in large part if not exclusively to the development of the excitatory cholinergic response in *Aplysia* neurones.

The inhibitory responses, on the other hand, obviously depend on the movement of other ions. Moreover, the fact that the rapid and slow inhibitory responses reverse at different levels suggests that the two inhibitory potentials are the result of different ionic permeability changes. This has been confirmed by manipulation of the external (or internal) concentrations of chloride and potassium ions.

As can be seen in Fig. 9, replacement of half of the external chloride by sodium sulphate (or methylsulphate) causes a 17 mV shift in the reversal potential of the rapid phase (from −60 mV to −43 mV) (see Kehoe, 1972a for methodological details). Such a shift would be predicted by the Nernst equation if chloride is the only ion causing the rapid potential, and if the synaptic membrane is impermeable to sulphate ions. A comparison of the shifts in the rapid i.p.s.p. and the rapid component of the ACh response as a

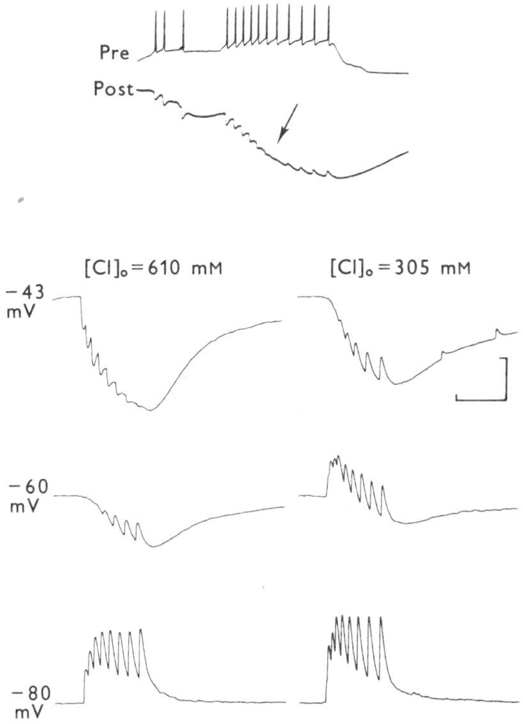


FIG. 9. Upper two traces: the postsynaptic response (Post) of a medial neurone to a series of presynaptic (Pre) action potentials recorded in a cell whose membrane was preset at approximately −50 mV. These records are included to facilitate the recognition of the reversal potential of the rapid phase of the two-component synaptic inhibitory response. With repetitive firing of the presynaptic neurone, the initially hyperpolarizing i.p.s.p. associated with each presynaptic spike is reduced in amplitude, becomes imperceptible (see arrow) and eventually reverses as the summating slow i.p.s.p. pulls the postsynaptic membrane beyond the reversal potential of the rapid i.p.s.p. The reversal potential of the rapid i.p.s.p. is defined as the polarization level at which the rapid i.p.s.p. becomes imperceptible. Calibration: 1 s, 5 mV. Lower three traces: effect of a reduction by half of the extracellular chloride concentration on the reversal potentials of the two components of the synaptic inhibitory potential. Both in normal sea water (610 mM) and after half of the chloride had been replaced by sulphate the reversal potential of the slow i.p.s.p. was approximately −80 mV. The reversal potential of the rapid i.p.s.p., on the other hand, moved from −60 mV (its value in normal chloride concentration) to −43 mV when external chloride was halved. Calibration: 2 s, 5 mV. (From Kehoe, 1972a, modified.)

function of external chloride concentration is shown in Fig. 10, where the straight line represents the changes in reversal potential predicted by the Nernst equation for a chloride electrode.

In contrast, alterations in chloride concentration had no effect on the reversal potential of the slow i.p.s.p. or on that of the corresponding ACh response. Although this conclusion is qualitatively evident in Fig. 9, in the

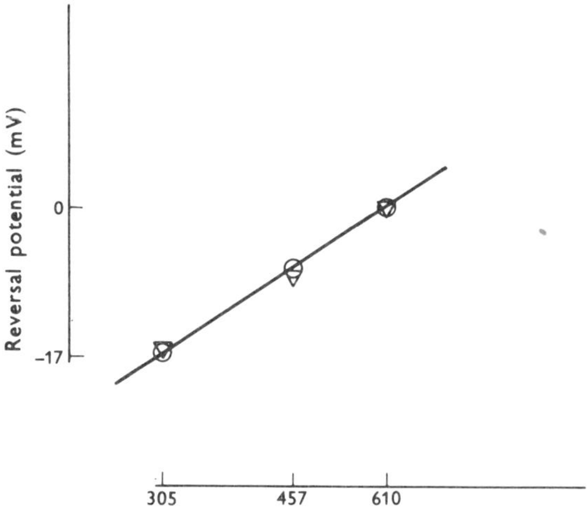


FIG. 10. Mean change in reversal potential of the rapid component of the cholinergic two-component inhibition caused by reducing $[Cl]_o$. Circles represent the mean of 5–9 values at each $Cl^-$ concentration obtained for the rapid response to ACh injection. Triangles represent one or the mean of two values for the rapid synaptic response. The range never exceeded $\pm 1$ mV around the mean value. The line represents the changes in $E_{Cl}$ anticipated by the Nernst equation. The reversal potential in the control solution ($-60$ mV) is represented by 0 mV on the ordinate scale. The line describing the theoretical behaviour of $E_{Cl}$ was drawn through this reference point. In approximately half of the experiments, chloride was replaced by methylsulphate; in the other half, by sulphate. (From Kehoe, 1972a.)

presence of the 'dominating' rapid component of the response, it was quantitatively confirmed by experiments in the presence of (+)-tubocurarine where the reversal potential of the slow i.p.s.p. could be measured more precisely.

On the other hand, when the external *potassium* concentration was altered, the reversal potential of the *slow* component of the inhibition was selectively affected. In Fig. 11, the slow i.p.s.p. (studied in a preparation in the presence of (+)-tubocurarine) is shown to be in equilibrium at $-80$ mV in normal external potassium concentration (10 mM), at $-96$ mV when $[K]_o$ is halved, and at $-63$ mV when $[K]_o$ is doubled. A similar change was observed in the slow component of the ACh response. These experimentally determined shifts in the reversal potential of the slow i.p.s.p. and the slow ACh potential are practically identical with those predicted by the Nernst equation for a potassium electrode (see lower half of Fig. 11). The reversal potential of the rapid response is unaffected by alterations of external potassium concentrations (at least within the limits tested: 5–20 mM).

The data thus far presented show that the cholinergic inhibitory response of the medial cells of the pleural ganglion consists of two descriptively distinct components (one rapid, one slow) which are mediated by pharmacologically distinct receptors. It is now also evident that each component is due to the

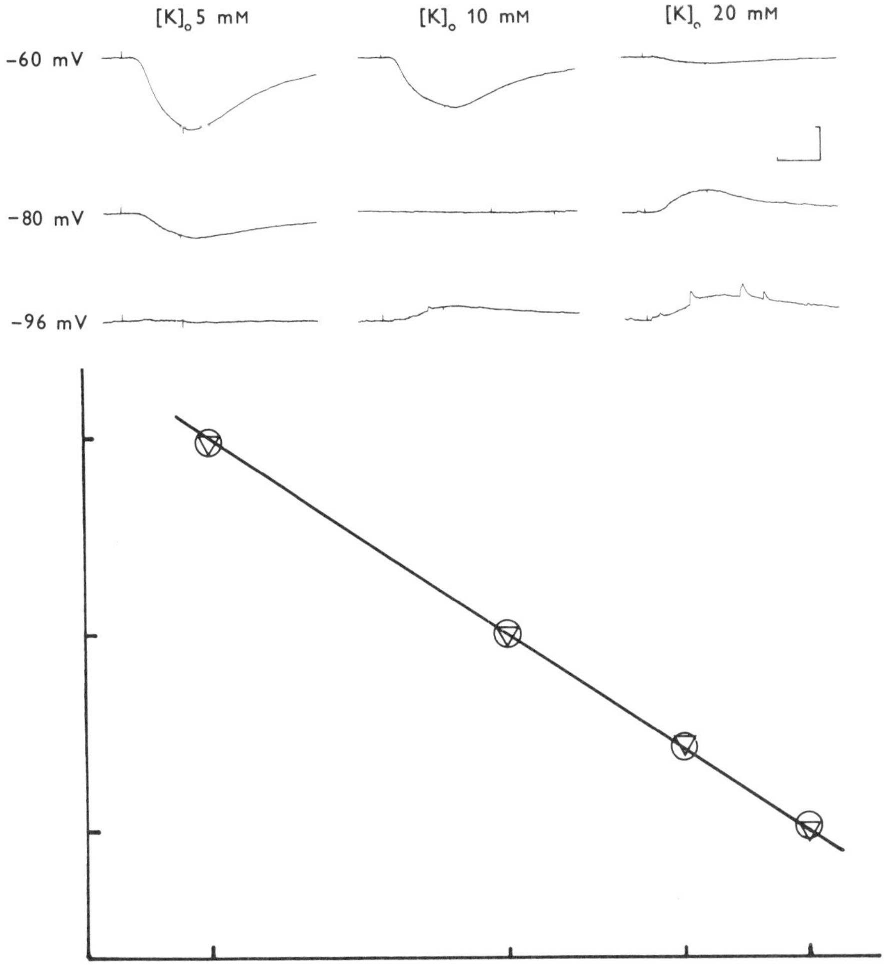


FIG. 11. Upper half: effect of alteration in the external potassium concentration on the reversal potential of the slow i.p.s.p. in a preparation in the presence of (+)-tubocurarine. The reversal potential was found to be at −96 mV in 5 mM potassium, at −80 mV in 10 mM potassium, and at −63 mV in 20 mM potassium. Calibration: 1 s, 5 mV. Lower half: mean change in reversal potential of the slow component of the cholinergic potential as a function of external potassium concentration. Circles represent the mean of 6–8 values at each potassium concentration obtained for the slow response to ACh injection. Triangles represent one or the mean of two values of the slow synaptic response. The range never exceeded ±1 mV around the mean value. The line represents the changes in $E_K$ predicted by the Nernst equation. The reversal potentials measured under 10 mM potassium, which varied only slightly around −80 mV, were arbitrarily assigned the 0 value from which all changes in reversal potentials were estimated. The line describing the anticipated changes in $E_K$ was drawn through this zero point. All the experiments dealing with the synaptic response, and half of those concerned with the ACh potential, were performed on preparations in which the rapid phase had been pharmacologically eliminated. (From Kehoe, 1972a.)

movement of a different ion. It becomes clear from such data that the fact that a synaptic potential (or the response of a cell to artificial application of a supposed transmitter) is altered by changes in the concentrations of more than one ion does not necessarily imply a lack of selectivity in permeability change caused by a transmitter–receptor interaction. It is possible that certain potentials previously considered to be 'bi-ionic' should be reconsidered in light of such findings.

*Under what conditions can a potassium-dependent synaptic potential appear to be due to the activation of an electrogenic sodium pump?*

The data presented above call attention to the atypical time course and peculiar pharmacological characteristics of the slow i.p.s.p. One other aspect of this response which deserves particular consideration is the change it undergoes when exposed to conditions known to affect the Na–K pump; for example, cooling and ouabain. An evaluation of these changes is particularly appropriate since a comparable, potassium-dependent, cholinergic synaptic potential in the visceral ganglion of *Aplysia* was in fact assumed to be due to the synaptic activation of an electrogenic pump (Pinsker & Kandel, 1969; see also Kerkut, Brown & Walker, 1969). The following data (see also Kehoe & Ascher, 1970; Kehoe, 1972a; and Kerkut, Lambert & Walker, this symposium) show how such a misinterpretation might develop.

Firstly, the potassium-dependent cholinergic potential (whether elicited synaptically or by ACh injection) is very sensitive to cooling. As can be seen in Fig. 12, cooling the ganglion to approximately 4° C practically eliminates the potassium-dependent component of both the synaptic and ACh two-component inhibition. A similar reduction in a potassium-dependent potential elicited in *Aplysia* neurones by an ionophoretic injection of dopamine was observed by Ascher (1972). Although cooling also slows down the chloride-dependent response, this slowing is minor compared to that shown by the potassium-dependent component.*

Ouabain, likewise known to block the Na–K pump, causes an apparent reduction in the potassium-dependent response which could be misinterpreted if the response were observed over a limited range of membrane potentials. For example, Fig. 13 shows the effect of ouabain on the synaptic response of the medial cells. Comparing the records before and after ouabain ($10^{-4}$ M) at $-60$ mV (the reversal potential of the rapid i.p.s.p.) could lead to the conclusion that ouabain had almost completely eliminated the slow component of the inhibitory response. The mechanism underlying this apparent reduction, however, is better understood by comparing the response measured after ouabain (Fig. 13) to that observed (in the absence of ouabain) when the

* Since cooling also prolongs the presynaptic action potential—thereby increasing transmitter liberation—the chloride-dependent synaptic response (which is not blocked by the temperature reduction) is greatly enlarged and prolonged (see Fig. 11).

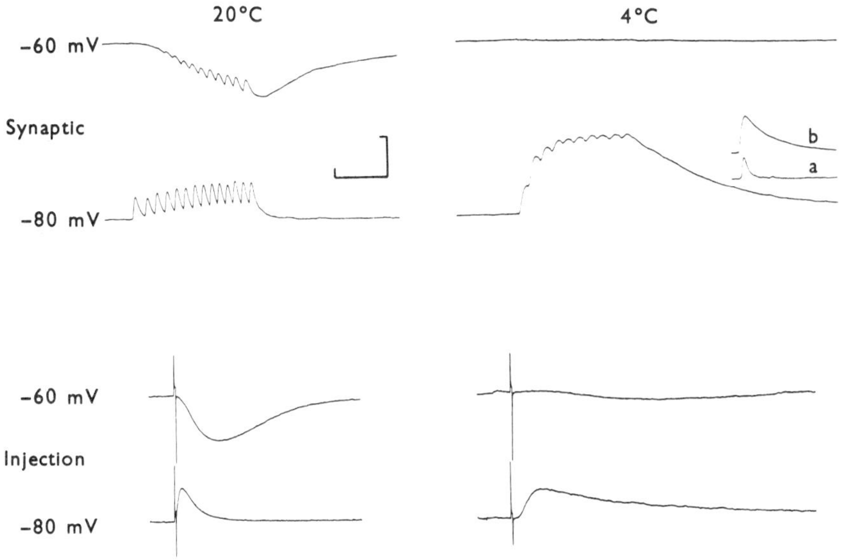


FIG. 12. Effect of cooling on the two-component cholinergic response in medial pleural neurones. Synaptic: response to firing of presynaptic neurone I. Injection: response to an ionophoretic injection of ACh. Cooling the preparation from 20° to 4° C eliminates the slow component (see −60 mV) of both the synaptic and ACh responses. The rapid component of the synaptic response is markedly increased and prolonged, causing a fusion of the reversed i.p.s.ps (measured at −80 mV) in response to repetitive firing of the presynaptic neurone. The change in the rapid synaptic potential can best be seen in the individual records of the reversed i.p.s.ps shown between the upper two traces. 'a' is the i.p.s.p. recorded at 20° C; 'b', that recorded at 4° C. The rapid component of the ACh response is relatively unaffected by cooling. Calibration: Synaptic: 1 s, 5 mV; Injection: 10 s, 5 mV.

external potassium concentration is doubled (to 20 mM) (Fig. 13). In both cases (under ouabain and in 20 mM $[K]_o$), whereas the slow i.p.s.p. measured at −60 mV is diminished, there is an appearance, at −80 mV, of a reversed slow potential (note slow return to the preset baseline). Under normal conditions, no slow i.p.s.p. is evident at this level since the slow response is normally 'in equilibrium' at −80 mV (see controls). This ouabain-induced shift in reversal potential is more clearly seen in Fig. 14, where the rapid i.p.s.p. of the response has been eliminated by (+)-tubocurarine. A similar ouabain-induced change was seen by Ascher (1972) in the potassium-dependent dopamine inhibitory potential.

The fact that there is no change in intracellular potassium concentration during such a short exposure to ouabain (see Kunze & Brown, 1971) and that there is no shift in the reversal potential of the potassium-dependent ACh potential (which is evoked by an injection of ACh on the well-dissected somatic region) suggests that the shift in the reversal of the slow i.p.s.p. is due to an accumulation of potassium in the extrasynaptic space due to the

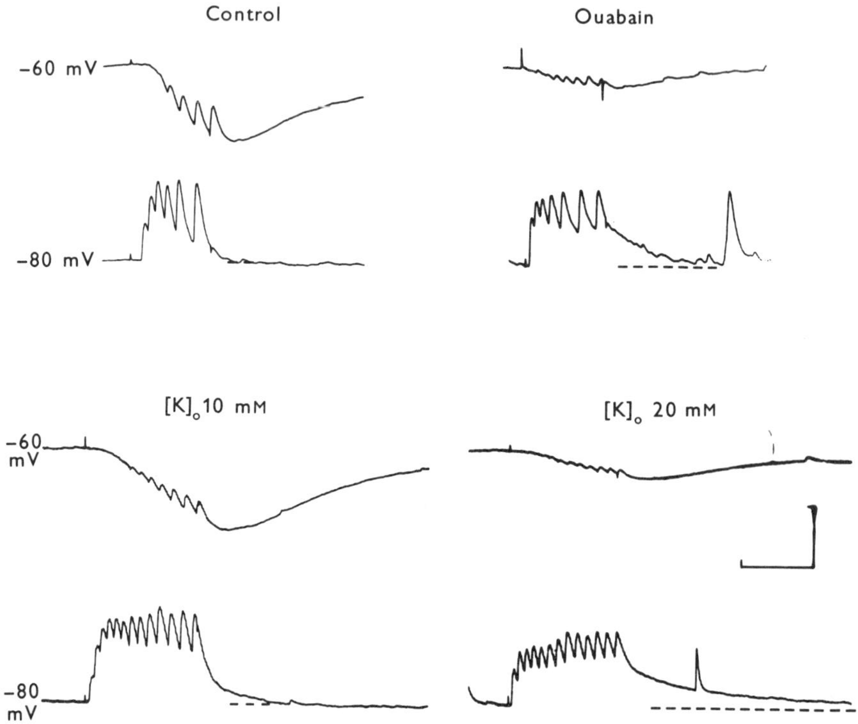


FIG. 13. Upper two traces: effect of ouabain ($5 \times 10^{-4}$ M) on the two-component inhibitory response. Note that the slow component of the inhibitory response (seen at −60 mV) appears to be abolished by ouabain. However, a comparison of the records at −80 mV shows that the slow component, in equilibrium in control conditions at −80 mV, has become a slow depolarizing response under ouabain (note slow return to baseline following the final rapid, reversed i.p.s.p.). Lower two traces: effect of doubling external potassium concentration on the two-component synaptic inhibition. Whereas the rapid i.p.s.p reverses at −60 mV in both normal and twice-normal external potassium, the reversal potential of the slow i.p.s.p. is markedly lowered by doubling external potassium. The change in reversal potential can be seen by the reduction in the slow hyperpolarization measured at −60 mV, and the slow return of the membrane to the preset baseline at −80 mV in twice-normal potassium. Calibration: 1 s, 5 mV.

blocking of the Na–K pump. A similar interpretation was given by Frankenhaeuser & Hodgkin (1956) to explain changes in the undershoot of the action potential during successive impulses in squid axons, and by Orkand, Nicholls & Kuffler (1966) to explain a depolarization in the glial cells following action potentials in amphibian optic nerves.

A shift in reversal potential of the slow i.p.s.p. similar to that caused by ouabain is also seen when sodium is replaced by lithium in the seawater bathing the ganglion. Unlike the change caused by ouabain, however, the effects of sodium replacement by lithium are reversible, and are proportional to the percentage of sodium removed (see Kehoe, 1972a and Ascher, 1972).

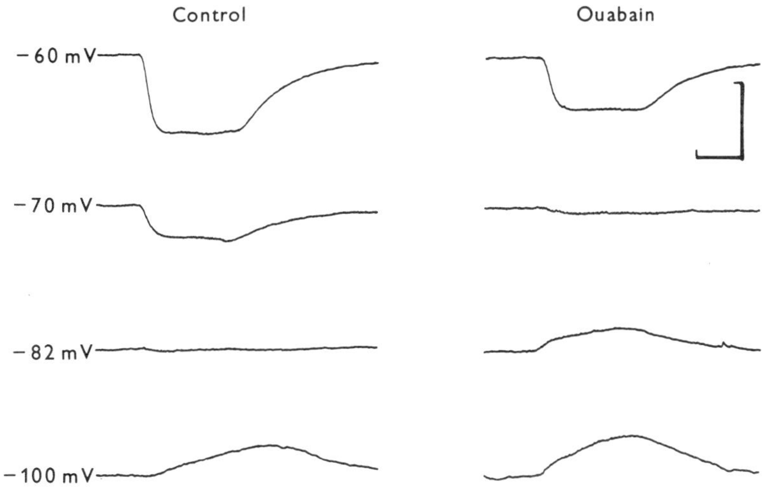


FIG. 14. Effect of ouabain ($5 \times 10^{-4}$ M) on the reversal potential of the slow i.s.p.a. in a preparation in the presence of (+)-tubocurarine (medial pleural neurone). Note that after 10 min exposure to ouabain, the reversal potential has shifted from −80 mV to approximately −71 mV. Calibration: 2 s, 5 mV.

Finally, when such potassium-dependent synaptic potentials are observed in certain of the large *Aplysia* cells (which are more easily damaged by dissection and show more prominent anomalous rectification) it is often difficult to reverse the potassium-dependent synaptic potential or to observe a conductance change during the course of that response. For example, in Fig. 15 are records taken of responses of a medial pleural neurone (Medial) and of the left giant cell (Giant) to activation of the same presynaptic neurone. In both experiments, the recording and polarizing electrodes were placed in the soma of the postsynaptic cell. The slow i.p.s.p. in the smaller of the two cells (Medial) reverses at −80 mV, as does the slow ACh potential. In contrast, the slow component of the response in the giant cell diminishes markedly with polarization of the postsynaptic cell (presumably because of the marked anomalous rectification shown by that cell) and is reversed only when the soma is polarized beyond −100 mV. (It should also be noted that the rapid i.p.s.ps in this preparation of the giant cell were almost invisible; compare with recording from the medial cell.) The reversal potential of the slow i.p.s.p. in the giant cell was moved to approximately −80 mV in the presence of ouabain (Giant, ouabain, Fig. 15). The slow component of the response of such large cells to an ionophoretic injection of ACh on the soma reverses at the same potential (−80 mV) as the synaptic and ACh slow responses in the medial cells.

That the change in reversal potentials as a function of cell 'size' is due to the failure of the somatic electrode to polarize the synaptic region effectively is

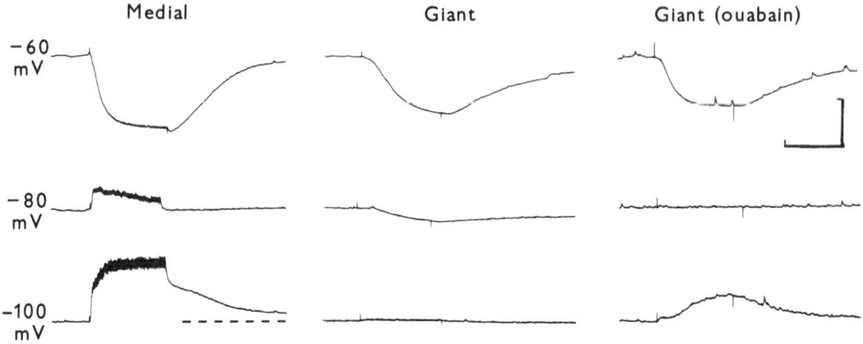


FIG. 15. Response of a medial pleural neurone and of the left giant cell (Giant) to repetitive firing of presynaptic neurone I. Note that the rapid i.p.s.p. is much more evident in the medial cell than in the giant, and that whereas the reversal potential of the slow component is −80 mV in the medial cell, it is beyond −100 mV in the giant cell. (Under normal conditions, the hyperpolarization disappears around −100 mV, but it is often, though not always, difficult to obtain a clear reversal with further hyperpolarization—in part due to the extremely low resistance of the membrane at these polarization levels.) In the presence of ouabain, the reversal potential was moved by at least 20 mV. The same duration and frequency of firing of the presynaptic neurone were used to elicit both series of responses. Calibration: 4 s, 5 mV.

suggested by an experiment in which simultaneous records were taken from the soma and from the assumed synaptic region of the axon (see Kandel *et al.*, 1967) of one of the large cells of the visceral ganglion which registers a similarly distorted potassium-dependent synaptic response. Fig. 16, which presents these data, shows that polarization of the soma to −80 mV polarizes the presumed synaptic region of the axon to only approximately −60 mV; conversely, the hyperpolarization of the distant axonal region is registered as an attenuated potential change in the soma. Since such 'distant' junctions can impede the reversal of a synaptic response and prevent the recording 'in the soma' of concomitant conductance changes, it is clear how these distortions—combined with the effects shown above of cooling and ouabain—can facilitate the misinterpretation of a potassium-dependent potential as an activation of an electrogenic pump.

## *Summary and Conclusions*

It is appropriate to summarize at this point the data which permit the conclusion that presynaptic neurone I is indeed cholinergic. (1) The type of postsynaptic potential caused in a given postsynaptic cell by presynaptic neurone I is invariably mimicked by an ionophoretic injection of ACh, as seen in the relative rapidity of the response and its underlying ionic mechanism. (2) All drugs capable of selectively eliminating any one of the three synaptic responses have similarly selective actions on the corresponding

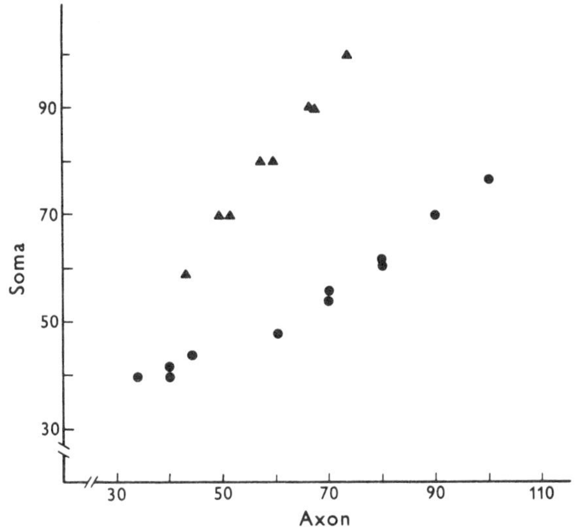


FIG. 16. Differences between axonic and somatic membrane potentials. Data from a visceral cell of Group L1–L6 in which double-barrelled microelectrodes had been inserted in both the soma and in the presumed synaptic region of the axon (see Kandel *et al.*, 1967). Somatic and axonic membrane potentials were compared when current was passed through either one barrel of the somatic electrode (▲) or through one barrel on the axonic electrode (●). Note that if there was no decrement with distance in the potential changes caused by such polarization, all points would fall on the 45° angle. (From Kehoe, 1972c.)

ACh potential. (3) Finally, all three synaptic responses, like the responses to ACh injection, are increased in the presence of neostigmine (unpublished observations).

Thus, it can be concluded that three types of cholinergic receptors can be distinguished in *Aplysia* neurones; each one mediates a different response type by controlling a selective change in permeability; and all three can be activated by a single presynaptic neurone with which it makes monosynaptic contact (see Kehoe, 1972c).

It is clear from the data of Ascher (1972), Gerschenfeld & Paupardin (see this symposium) and Gerschenfeld & Lasansky (1964) that dopamine, 5-hydroxytryptamine and glutamic acid, respectively, have similar multireceptor systems in molluscs. Furthermore, many identifiable neurones liberating as yet unknown transmitters show similarly complex responses (see, for example, Kehoe, 1971) and cause different responses in different cells (unpublished observations), suggesting that these transmitters too work with more than one type of postsynaptic receptor in the same nervous system. In fact, it appears that, in molluscs, a single-receptor system is the exception rather than the rule.

REFERENCES

ASCHER, P. (1972). *J. Physiol., Lond.*, **225**, 173.
BLANKENSHIP, J. E., WACHTEL, H. & KANDEL, E. R. (1971). *J. Neurophysiol.*, **34**, 76.
FRANKENHAEUSER, B. & HODGKIN, A. L. (1956). *J. Physiol., Lond.*, **131**, 341.
GARDNER, A. (1971). *Science, N.Y.*, **173**, 550.
GERSCHENFELD, H. M. & LASANSKY, A. (1964). *Intern. J. Neuropharmac.*, **3**, 301.
GERSCHENFELD, H. M. & PAUPARDIN, D. (1973). This symposium.
KANDEL, E. R., FRAZIER, W. T., WAZIRI, R. & COGGESHALL, R. E. (1967). *J. Neurophysiol.*, **30**, 1352.
KATZ, B. & MILEDI, R. (1967). *J. Physiol., Lond.*, **192**, 407.
KEHOE, J. S. (1969). *Nature, Lond.*, **221**, 866.
KEHOE, J. S. (1971). *Proc. XXV Int. Congr. Physiol. Sci.*, Munich, **9**, 877.
KEHOE, J. S. (1972a). *J. Physiol., Lond.*, **225**, 85.
KEHOE, J. S. (1972b). *J. Physiol., Lond.*, **225**, 115.
KEHOE, J. S. (1972c). *J. Physiol., Lond.*, **225**, 147.
KEHOE, J. S. & ASCHER, P. (1970). *Nature, Lond.*, **225**, 820.
KERKUT, G. A., BROWN, L. & WALKER, R. J. (1969). *Nature, Lond.*, **223**, 864.
KERKUT, G. A., LAMBERT, J. D. C. & WALKER, R. J. (1973). This symposium.
KOELLE, G. B. (1970). In: *The Pharmacological Basis of Therapeutics*, 4th Ed., ed. Goodman, L. S. & Gilman, A., p. 402. London: Macmillan.
KUNZE, D. L. & BROWN, A. M. (1971). *Nature, New Biol., Lond.*, **229**, 229.
KUSANO, K., LIVENGOOD, D. R. & WERMAN, R. (1967). *J. gen. Physiol.*, **50**, 2579.
LEVITAN, H. & TAUC, L. (1972). *J. Physiol., Lond.*, **222**, 537.
MCLEAN, R. A., GEUS, R. J., MOHRBACHER, R. J., MATTIS, P. A. & ULLYOT, G. E. (1960). *J. Pharmac. exp. Ther.*, **129**, 11.
NACHMANSOHN, D. (1959). *Chemical and Molecular Basis of Nerve Activity*. New York: Academic Press.
ORKAND, R. K., NICHOLLS, J. G. & KUFFLER, S. W. (1966). *J. Neurophysiol.*, **29**, 788.
PINSKER, H. & KANDEL, E. R. (1969). *Science, N.Y.*, **163**, 931.
STRUMWASSER, F. (1962). *Proc. XXII Int. Congr. Physiol. Sci.*, Leyden, **2**, 801.
TAUC, L. & GERSCHENFELD, H. M. (1962). *J. Neurophysiol.*, **25**, 236.
VOLLE, R. L. & KOELLE, G. B. (1970). In: *The Pharmacological Basis of Therapeutics*, 4th Ed., ed. Goodman, L. S. & Gilman, A., p. 585. London: Macmillan.
WACHTEL, H. & KANDEL, E. R. (1971). *J. Neurophysiol.*, **34**, 56.

## DISCUSSION

*Stefani* (*Paris*)

Is the synaptic delay affected by the blocking agents that you have used?

*Kehoe* (*Paris*)

Measuring the synaptic delay of the slow i.p.s.p. is quite difficult, since the response (under normal conditions) is very slow and develops very gradually. Consequently, I would not like to say that there is never a change in latency of that response since I find its latency difficult to define. As for changes in latency of the rapid responses (e.p.s.p. and rapid i.p.s.p.), I have never seen a change in latency in the presence of the blocking drugs cited here, but I have not studied the problem systematically. Certain drugs capable of blocking one or two of the cholinergic responses (for example, atropine and strychnine) cause changes in the form of the presynaptic action potential when they are applied in high doses. Under these conditions I would not be surprised to see changes in latency of the postsynaptic responses.

*Stefani* (*Paris*)

How long does it take for recovery from the effect of ouabain on the shift of the equilibrium potential to the ACh response? This could give some information on the diffusion of potassium ions in the space close to the neuronal membrane.

*Kehoe* (*Paris*)

During the 45-min period in which I examined the effects of ouabain on the response to ACh injection, I saw no shift in the reversal potential of the slow component of that response. This ionophoretic injection is made on the dissected somatic region. The 'ouabain effect' of which you are speaking refers to the shift in the slow *synaptic* i.p.s.p., which is generated in the non-dissected neuropile. I have never seen a return to the normal reversal level following the ouabain treatment, but I have perhaps not persisted long enough.

# THE PERMEABILITY CHANGE PRODUCED BY ACETYLCHOLINE IN SMOOTH MUSCLE

T. B. BOLTON

*Department of Pharmacology, University of Oxford, Oxford OX1 3QT, England*

It is well known that acetylcholine depolarizes the membrane of visceral smooth muscle (Bülbring, 1954, 1955, 1957; Burnstock, 1958; Bülbring & Burnstock, 1960; Bülbring & Kuriyama, 1963; Hidaka & Kuriyama, 1969; Bolton, 1971, 1972), but much less is known about the way in which it does this. The main objective of this paper is to discuss the applicability to the action of acetylcholine on the smooth muscle membrane of a simple model of transmitter action which has been developed from studies on other excitable membranes (Fatt & Katz, 1951; Coombs, Eccles & Fatt, 1955; Takeuchi & Takeuchi, 1960; Takeuchi, 1963a,b; Ginsborg, 1967). Of particular interest will be the permeability to various ion species of the channels which are opened in the membrane when the muscarinic receptor is stimulated. All results were obtained by intracellular recording of membrane potential from the longitudinal muscle of the guinea-pig terminal ileum which was separated from the underlying circular muscle. More details of the method are given elsewhere (Bolton, 1972).

### *Characteristics and distribution of muscarinic receptors*

There are a number of uncertainties concerning the muscarinic receptor which may affect the interpretation of the results that follow. In other situations it is known that the acetylcholine receptor is located on the outer surface of the cell membrane (del Castillo & Katz, 1955). This is likely to be the case in smooth muscle also; muscarinic antagonists are bound to sites that are found mainly in the microsomal fraction of homogenates (Fewtrell & Rang, 1971, 1972). It may be that there is more than one type of muscarinic receptor as defined by pharmacological criteria—Burgen & Spero (1968) produced evidence that supports this view. Another possibility is the existence in visceral smooth muscle of pharmacologically identical receptors operating ion channels that are heterogeneous in their ion selectivities as in frog skeletal muscle (Feltz & Mallart, 1970, 1971). Responses to carbachol recorded from different cells of the same preparation of longitudinal ileal muscle show little variation. As the potential set up by injecting current intracellularly declines to half its value within 30 μm (Sperelakis & Tarr, 1965; Kobayashi, Prosser & Nagai, 1967) this suggests that appreciable discontinuities in the distribution of receptors do not exist. Beyond this, however, nothing is known about the distribution of muscarinic receptors on the smooth muscle cell or throughout the tissue as a whole.

*Effects of muscarinic stimulants on the movements of radioactive ions*

As it is intended to draw inferences concerning the fluxes of various ions from measurements of membrane potential and changes in conductance, it is necessary first to consider briefly the results of studies by others where ion fluxes have been measured directly (Born & Bülbring, 1956; Lembeck & Strobach, 1956; Hurwitz, 1960, 1965; Robertson, 1960; Durbin & Jenkinson, 1961a; Schatzmann, 1961, 1964a,b; Weiss, Coalson & Hurwitz, 1961; Banerjee & Lewis, 1963, 1964; Breeman, Daniel & Breeman, 1966; Herrlinger, Lüllmann & Schuh, 1967; Burgen & Spero, 1968; Brading, 1971b). Unfortunately, in such studies it is not possible to measure the exchange of ions across the smooth muscle membrane, but only their exchange between a piece of tissue and the bathing fluid. This very considerably complicates their interpretation (for example, see Brading, 1971a). Such investigations, and some electrophysiological experiments, have led various reviewers to conclude that the increase in permeability of the smooth muscle membrane, produced by stimulation of the muscarinic receptor, is nonspecific, that is, the channels operated by the muscarinic receptor allow both cations and anions to pass (Burnstock, 1958; Durbin & Jenkinson, 1961a; Bülbring & Kuriyama, 1963; Burnstock & Holman, 1963, 1966; Burnstock, Holman & Prosser, 1963; Ginsborg, 1967; Setekleiv, 1970), although others have suggested, by analogy with the frog endplate, that the increase in permeability is restricted to cations (Holman, 1970; Kuriyama, 1970).

*Action of carbachol on the membrane potential and conductance*

The action of acetylcholine is illustrated in Fig. 1. In most experiments carbachol was used because of its greater stability. The relationship between the concentration of carbachol and its depolarizing action on the longitudinal muscle of the guinea-pig ileum is shown in Fig. 2. It will be noted that depolarization increases very little when the concentration of carbachol is increased beyond $10^{-6}$ M. The same is true for acetylcholine (Fig. 1). A number of lines of evidence indicate that it is not the availability of unoccupied receptors which limits depolarization (Bolton, 1972). Calculations of receptor occupancy show that less than 10% of receptors are expected to be occupied

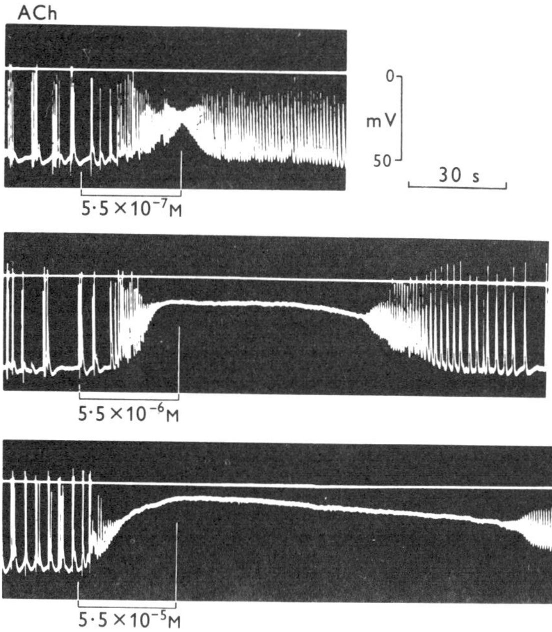


FIG. 1. Action of three concentrations of acetylcholine on the electrical activity of the longitudinal muscle of the guinea-pig ileum. Acetylcholine was introduced to the tissue by changing the solution bathing the tissue to one which contained it. All records are from the same tissue, the upper two from the same cell. The upper line in this and subsequent records is at zero potential.

by carbachol at $10^{-6}$ M (Fig. 2) and the effect of carbachol on $^{86}$Rb efflux was found to increase sharply above $10^{-6}$ M (Burgen & Spero, 1968, see Fig. 2). Furthermore, the effect of carbachol on conductance increases steeply over the range $1{\cdot}4 \times 10^{-6}$ M to $5{\cdot}5 \times 10^{-5}$ M (Bolton, 1972, Fig. 2). Thus it appears that increasing the concentration of carbachol beyond $10^{-6}$ M results in a substantial increase in receptor occupancy and that the occupation of these additional receptors opens further ion channels in the smooth muscle membrane.

A satisfactory explanation for the results summarized in Fig. 2 could be provided by a simple electrical model (Fig. 3a) which has been developed by others from studies of the actions of transmitters on other excitable membranes (see review by Ginsborg, 1967). Activation of the muscarinic receptor is seen as opening additional channels or pores in the membrane which allow ions to pass. The conductance and permeability of the membrane are thereby increased. According to this model, the ion channels opened by stimulation of the muscarinic receptor have an equilibrium potential, $\mathscr{E}$ volts, at which the inward and outward ionic currents they pass are equal (that is, there is no net current flow through them when

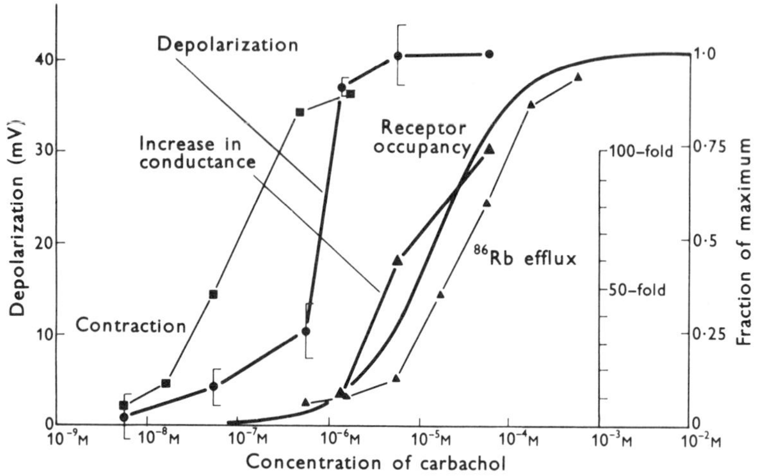


FIG. 2. The action of carbachol on the membrane potential (means ± S.E.) and membrane conductance of longitudinal ileal muscle (data from Bolton, 1972, reproduced by permission of the Editors of the *Journal of Physiology*). Also shown are the action of carbachol on the contraction of this tissue and on the efflux of $^{86}$Rb (data from Burgen & Spero, 1968, reproduced by permission of the Editors of the *British Journal of Pharmacology*) and the fractional receptor occupancy. The latter is calculated from the value of the dissociation constant for carbachol given by Furchgott (1966) and Furchgott & Bursztyn (1967). Scaled depolarization on the left-hand ordinate, contraction, $^{86}$Rb efflux, and receptor occupancy as a fraction of maximum on extreme right-hand ordinate, and increase in conductance ($\Delta G/G$) on the remaining ordinate. For further details see text and Bolton (1972).

$V = \mathscr{E}$); their conductance is $\Delta G$ mho cm$^{-2}$. The potential across the system, $V$ volts, during the action of carbachol is given by

$$V = E - \frac{\Delta G}{\Delta G + G}(E - \mathscr{E}) \qquad (1)$$

where $E$ and $G$ are the resting membrane potential (in volts) and resting membrane conductance (in mho cm$^{-2}$) respectively.

The behaviour of this model (Fig. 3a) as described by equation (1), predicts that concentrations of carbachol that increase the membrane conductance more than 10-fold ($> 10^{-6}$ M) should shift the membrane potential to within a few millivolts of the equilibrium potential for the receptor-operated channels. Thus, the extent of depolarization in this smooth muscle is limited by the position of the equilibrium potential and not by the availability of receptors (Bolton, 1972). A similar situation apparently occurs at the endplate (Koester & Nastuk, 1970). For the moment the effects on the distribution of ions of opening large conductances in the membrane will be ignored.

The data summarized in Fig. 2 from several authors suggests that the maximal increase in conductance produced by carbachol in this tissue would

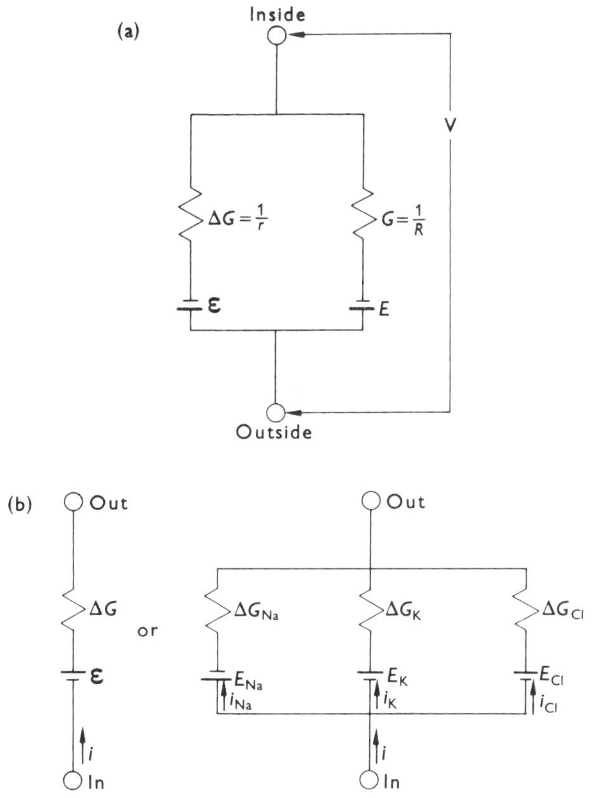


FIG. 3. (a), Suggested electrical model for the action of muscarinic stimulants on the smooth muscle membrane. Stimulation of muscarinic receptors is envisaged as opening additional channels in the membrane which allow ions to pass. These channels have an equilibrium potential ($\mathcal{E}$) at which the net current through them is zero. (b), The facility with which each ion species passes through these channels may be represented by a separate conductance. The equilibrium potential for each ion species is given by the Nernst equation. For further explanation see text. (The results suggest that $\Delta G_{Cl}$ is very small or zero, that is, very little chloride current can pass through these channels.)

be somewhere between 100 and 1000 times the resting membrane conductance of $2 \times 10^{-5}$ mho cm$^{-2}$ (Tomita, 1970), that is, between $2 \times 10^{-3}$ and $2 \times 10^{-2}$ mho cm$^{-2}$.

However, it is possible that an action on permeability is not the only primary mechanism by which carbachol contracts smooth muscle. The line relating contraction to concentration of carbachol lies to the left of that for depolarization (Fig. 2), and is probably coincident with that for the effect of carbachol on spike frequency (Kuriyama, 1970). It has been noted that muscarinic stimulants increase spike frequency at concentrations that have no effect on the resting membrane potential (Kuriyama, 1970; Bolton, 1972) and not all the effects of muscarinic stimulants on the activity of longitudinal ileal muscle can be easily explained by the assumption that they introduce an additional, voltage-independent conductance into the membrane (Bolton, 1971).

### *Ability of various ions to move through the channels opened by stimulation of the muscarinic receptor*

The electrophysiological investigation of the permeability or conductance change produced by stimulation of the muscarinic receptor in this tissue has special problems. In many excitable membranes it is possible to examine the effects of a fixed amount of transmitter or drug at different membrane potentials, by passing constant currents of various strengths. This technique reveals a null point, the equilibrium potential, at which there is no net transfer of charge across the membrane when the receptor-operated channels are opened. Sometimes this point can be obtained by extrapolation (for example, Takeuchi & Takeuchi, 1960). The value of the equilibrium potential may immediately give a clue concerning the identity of the ions that move through the channels opened by stimulation of the receptor. However, as the membrane potential and conductance of a spontaneously active smooth muscle are continuously varying, it is difficult to measure with accuracy the effects of transmitter on either of these parameters, although the technique has been used (Hidaka & Kuriyama, 1969).

In the face of these difficulties a much simpler technique is sometimes adopted. This involves examining the effects of varying the concentrations of ions in the external solution on the response to a fixed, *submaximal*, concentration of transmitter or drug at the resting membrane potential. In such circumstances, however, misleading results may be obtained if the reaction of the receptor with the agonist molecule is altered by the ionic environment (Jenkinson, 1960), or if the current–voltage relationships of the ion channels which determine the membrane potential during spontaneous activity are altered. In either case, such interactions may obscure any effect an ion change may have on the ionic current passing through the receptor-activated channel.

The additional conductance introduced into the membrane by stimulation of the muscarinic receptor (Fig. 3a) may be defined as

$$\Delta G = i/(\mathscr{E} - V) \tag{2}$$

where $i$ is the net current (in A cm$^{-2}$) passing through the receptor-operated channels. When only sodium, potassium, and chloride ions can carry significant currents (designated $i_{\mathrm{Na}}$, $i_{\mathrm{K}}$, and $i_{\mathrm{Cl}}$) through these channels we may similarly write

$$\Delta G_{\mathrm{Na}} = i_{\mathrm{Na}}/(E_{\mathrm{Na}} - V) \tag{3}$$

$$\Delta G_{\mathrm{K}} = i_{\mathrm{K}}/(E_{\mathrm{K}} - V) \tag{4}$$

$$\Delta G_{\mathrm{Cl}} = i_{\mathrm{Cl}}/(E_{\mathrm{Cl}} - V) \tag{5}$$

The simple element which is the left-hand branch of the circuit in Fig. 3a, is now elaborated into three elements shown in Fig. 3b, which represent the behaviour of currents carried by individual ion species. It is not intended to imply that stimulation of the muscarinic receptor opens separate channels for each ion species; the model represents equally well the facility with which different ion species might pass through the same channel. Equating $i$ to $i_{Na}+i_K+i_{Cl}$ gives from equations (2)–(5)

$$\mathscr{E}=\frac{\Delta G_K \,.\, E_K+\Delta G_{Na} \,.\, E_{Na}+\Delta G_{Cl} \,.\, E_{Cl}}{\Delta G} \tag{6}$$

(Takeuchi & Takeuchi, 1960; Takeuchi, 1963b; Ginsborg, 1967).

Equation (6) indicates that if an ion species moves through the channel opened by stimulation of the muscarinic receptor, then varying the concentration of that ion in the external solution should alter the equilibrium potential, $\mathscr{E}$, as the equilibrium potentials for the various ions ($E_{Na}$, $E_K$, $E_{Cl}$) are related to their concentration outside the cell by the Nernst equation (for example, $E_{Na}=RT/F \ln [Na^+]_o/[Na^+]_i$). If the conductances do not depend on either the membrane potential or the ionic concentrations in the bathing solution, as appears to be true (to a limited extent) at the neuromuscular junction (Takeuchi, 1960), and if there is no interaction between ion species, $\mathscr{E}$ will vary linearly with the equilibrium potential of any ion which passes through the channel. Conversely, if an ion species does not pass through a channel then $\mathscr{E}$ will be independent of changes in its concentration.

Thus, the problem of identifying the ion species moving through a particular channel is reduced to one of detecting changes in the equilibrium potential when the concentrations of ions in the external solution are varied.

If it is assumed that the membrane potential in the presence of large concentrations of carbachol ($>10^{-6}$ M) is close to the equilibrium potential, it may be used to detect changes in the latter. This will be possible only if the increase in conductance continues to be large ($>$10-fold) in solutions of modified ionic composition. This method of detecting changes in the carbachol equilibrium potential involves a number of other assumptions, some of which will be examined in due course.

### *Effects of variations in the external sodium concentration*

As muscarinic stimulants depolarize smooth muscle (Fig. 1), it seems likely that they increase sodium permeability. Thus, we would expect that changes in the external sodium concentration would shift the level of peak depolarization produced by large concentrations of carbachol ($>10^{-6}$ M). Fig. 4 shows that this is the case: reducing the sodium concentration in the bathing solution from 137 mM to 17 mM produced a large negative shift in the level of peak depolarization (which is the term that will be used to refer to the most positive membrane potential attained in the presence of the depolar-

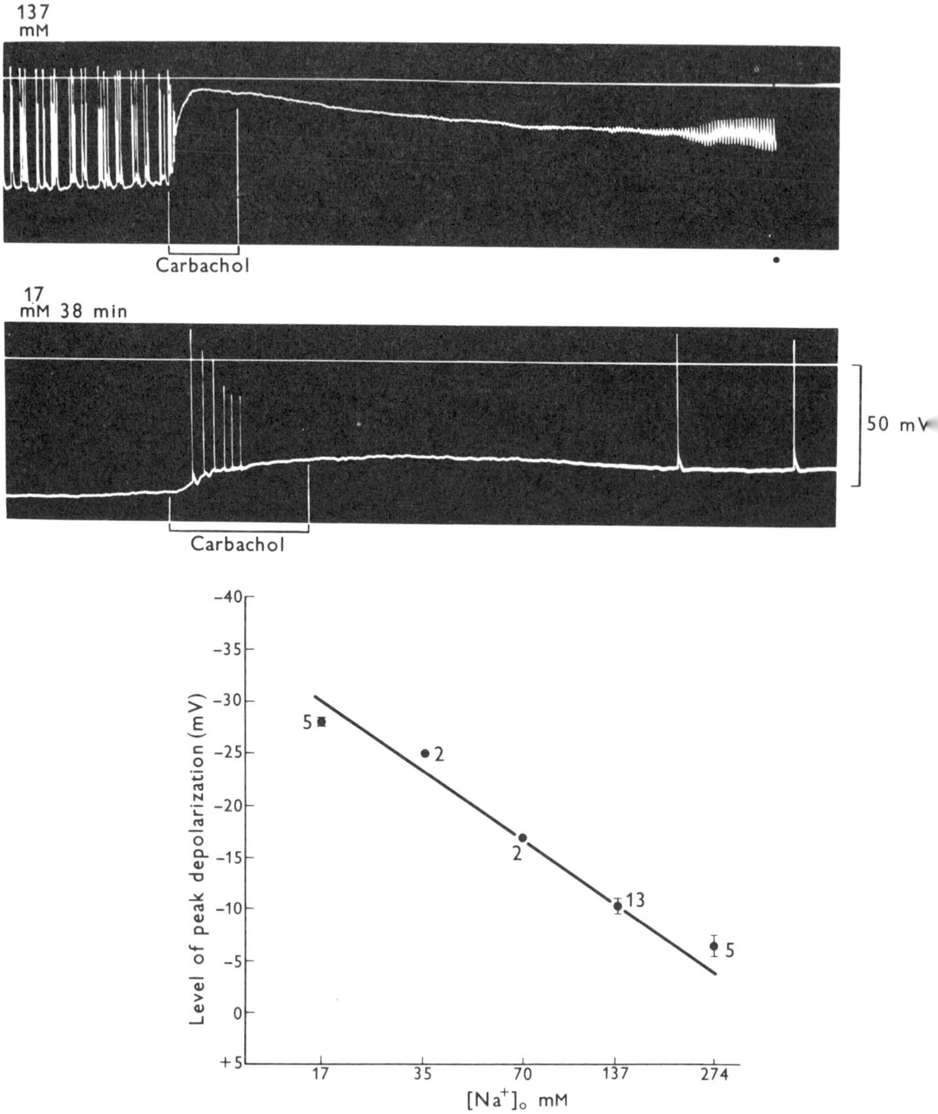


FIG. 4. The effects on the level of peak depolarization of varying the sodium concentration of the bathing solution. The records show that reducing the sodium concentration from 137 mM to 17 mM shifted the level of peak depolarization produced by $5 \cdot 5 \times 10^{-5}$ M carbachol negatively. In this experiment the sodium chloride was replaced by sucrose, so that the chloride concentration was also reduced. At ● the electrode was withdrawn to check the zero level. The graph (from Bolton, 1972, reproduced by permission of the Editors of the *Journal of Physiology*) shows the effects of varying the sodium concentration on the level of peak depolarization (means ± S.E.). In these experiments sodium chloride was replaced by Tris chloride (the chloride concentration remaining unchanged), or the sodium concentration was increased by adding solid sodium benzenesulphonate to Krebs solution making it hypertonic.

izing agent). In this experiment the sodium chloride of Krebs solution was replaced by sucrose; consequently the external chloride concentration was also reduced. In another series of experiments, sodium chloride was replaced with Tris chloride (so that the chloride concentration was unchanged) or the concentration of sodium increased by adding solid sodium benzenesulphonate to Krebs solution, making it hypertonic. Reducing the sodium concentration from 137 to 17 mM shifted the level of peak depolarization from −10 mV to −28 mV, while increasing it to 274 mM shifted it positively by a few millivolts (Fig. 4) even though hypertonicity (produced by sucrose) normally shifts it in a negative direction. Carbachol still produced a large increase in membrane conductance in sodium deficient solution so that we would expect the level of peak depolarization to be close to the equilibrium potential (Bolton, 1972). These results indicate that activation of the muscarinic receptor causes the opening of channels which allow sodium ions to pass. Others have found that carbachol increases the influx of $^{24}$Na into smooth muscle (Durbin & Jenkinson, 1961a), although surprisingly it has little or no effect on the efflux of $^{24}$Na (Durbin & Jenkinson, 1961a; Brading, 1971b). This requires investigation. It is possible that the efflux of sodium is affected by ions outside the membrane (Kasai & Changeux, 1971).

### *Effects of variations in the external chloride concentration*

Because $E_{Cl}$ is probably more negative than −10 mV, chloride should show a net movement into the cell in normal solution if carbachol opens ion channels that allow it to pass. This will be true whether chloride is passively distributed ($E_{Cl} \approx -50$ mV) or actively accumulated by the smooth muscle cells as Casteels (1966, 1969) asserts. In chloride-free solution, and also probably in chloride-deficient solutions, chloride shows a net outward movement (Casteels, 1971). Depolarization will decrease the tendency for chloride to leave the cells but it is likely that it continues to show a net outward movement ($E_{Cl}$ still more positive than −10 mV, Fig. 5). Thus in the presence of carbachol the direction of any chloride flux which might occur when carbachol is applied is probably reversed upon going into chloride-free or -deficient solution.

In two series of experiments the chloride concentration was reduced from its level in normal Krebs solution (134 mM) to 7 mM or zero, and responses to carbachol obtained before, and within the first 5 min of switching to chloride-deficient (or free) solution; it is at this time that $E_{Cl}$ would be expected to show its greatest change. A shift in the level of peak depolarization was found in one series (Fig. 5) but it was small and could well have been due to factors other than a change in chloride flux across the membrane (Bolton, 1972). This result was not confirmed when similar experiments were done in which isethionate instead of benzenesulphonate was used as the major replacement for the chloride ion (Fig. 5)

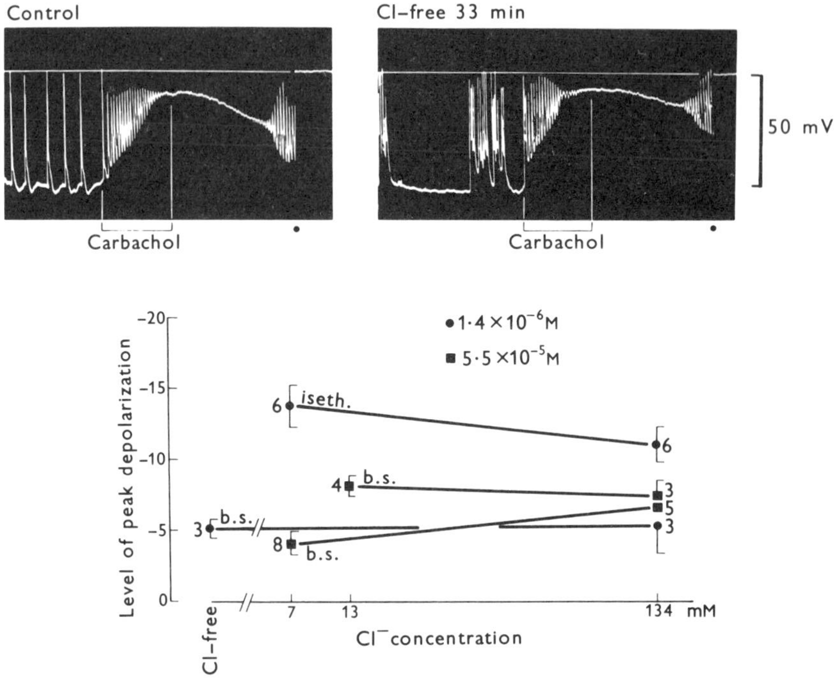


FIG. 5. Lack of effect of varying the chloride concentration on the level of peak depolarization. The control response to $5 \cdot 5 \times 10^{-6}$ M carbachol was obtained in 134 mM chloride and the other after 33 min in chloride-free solution. The levels of peak depolarization do not vary more than consecutive records from the same tissue in normal solution. At ● the electrode was withdrawn to check the zero level. The graph summarizes the results of four series of experiments: in two series the chloride concentration was reduced to 7 mM and responses obtained within 5 min of changing to chloride-deficient solution. In one series chloride was replaced by isethionate (iseth.), in the other by benzenesulphonate (b.s.). In two other series chloride was reduced to 13 mM (responses in the first h averaged) or to zero (responses in the first 90 min averaged). Only one series (134 mM → 7 mM, b.s. replacement) showed a significant ($P < 0 \cdot 025$) shift.

Responses to carbachol were also obtained after periods up to $2\frac{1}{2}$ h in chloride-free, and up to 1 h in chloride-deficient solutions, at which times very little chloride can be present at either side of the membrane (Casteels, 1971). Although it sometimes appeared that there was a slight positive shift in the level of peak depolarization (Fig. 5) in the few responses obtained after periods in excess of 1 h in chloride-deficient (or free) solution, when the results obtained in the first 90 min (chloride-free) or 60 min (chloride-deficient) were averaged, no shift was apparent (Fig. 5). Doubling the external chloride concentration or reducing it from 122 mM to 7 mM was also without effect on the depolarization produced by submaximal concentrations of carbachol in sucrose-hypertonic solution (Bolton, unpublished). These results have been confirmed in guinea-pig uterus (Bülbring & Szurszewski,

1971). In some experiments chloride was replaced by isethionate, in most, by benzenesulphonate, which has a volume of distribution in smooth muscle approximately equal to the extracellular space (Casteels, 1971). It seems very unlikely that this ion moves freely through the channels operated by the muscarinic receptor. It must be concluded that the electrophysiological evidence does not support the hypothesis that chloride ions move readily through the channels that are opened when the muscarinic receptor is stimulated.

However, Durbin & Jenkinson (1961a) found that carbachol increased both the inward and outward fluxes of $^{36}Cl$ in potassium-depolarized taenia. A similar apparent contradiction between electrophysiological and flux data exists for the nicotinic receptor of skeletal muscle (cf. Jenkinson & Nicholls, 1961, with Takeuchi & Takeuchi, 1960; Takeuchi, 1963a) although the effects of carbachol on $^{36}Cl$ fluxes are relatively smaller in skeletal muscle compared with its effects on the fluxes of $^{42}K$. The factors that affect the rate of movement of ions through portions of smooth muscle are not by any means understood (see Brading, 1971a). It is possible for example that the contraction that still occurs in potassium-depolarized smooth muscle when carbachol is applied (Durbin & Jenkinson, 1961a) can accelerate the exchange of ions between the tissue and the bathing fluid. On the other hand, several lines of evidence indicate that the efflux $^{42}K$ is not dependent on contraction although influenced by it (Hurwitz, Tinsley & Battle, 1960; Durbin & Jenkinson, 1961b; Burgen & Spero, 1968; Spero, quoted by Setekleiv, 1970).

It seems very unlikely that chloride moves through the channels opened by stimulation of the muscarinic receptor to any appreciable extent. However, it is not possible at present to decide whether chloride permeability is increased by carbachol to a *small extent*, or whether the increased fluxes of $^{36}Cl$ which it causes have some explanation other than an increase in chloride permeability of the membrane.

### *Effects of variations in the external potassium concentration*

If the equilibrium potential for the receptor-operated channels is less positive than $E_{Na}$, an ion species other than sodium must move through them and carry outward current. Apparently chloride is not involved. The only other ion present in appreciable amounts and with a negative equilibrium potential, is potassium. Carbachol is known to increase both its inward and outward fluxes in potassium-depolarized taenia (Durbin & Jenkinson, 1961a, and others).

When the external potassium concentration was increased to 20 or 50 mM, the level of peak depolarization moved positively (significance $P<0{\cdot}001$) as expected (Fig. 6). However, the shift was much less than that predicted by the model shown in Fig. 3b, from which it is possible to calculate, using the data obtained upon altering the external sodium and chloride concentrations,

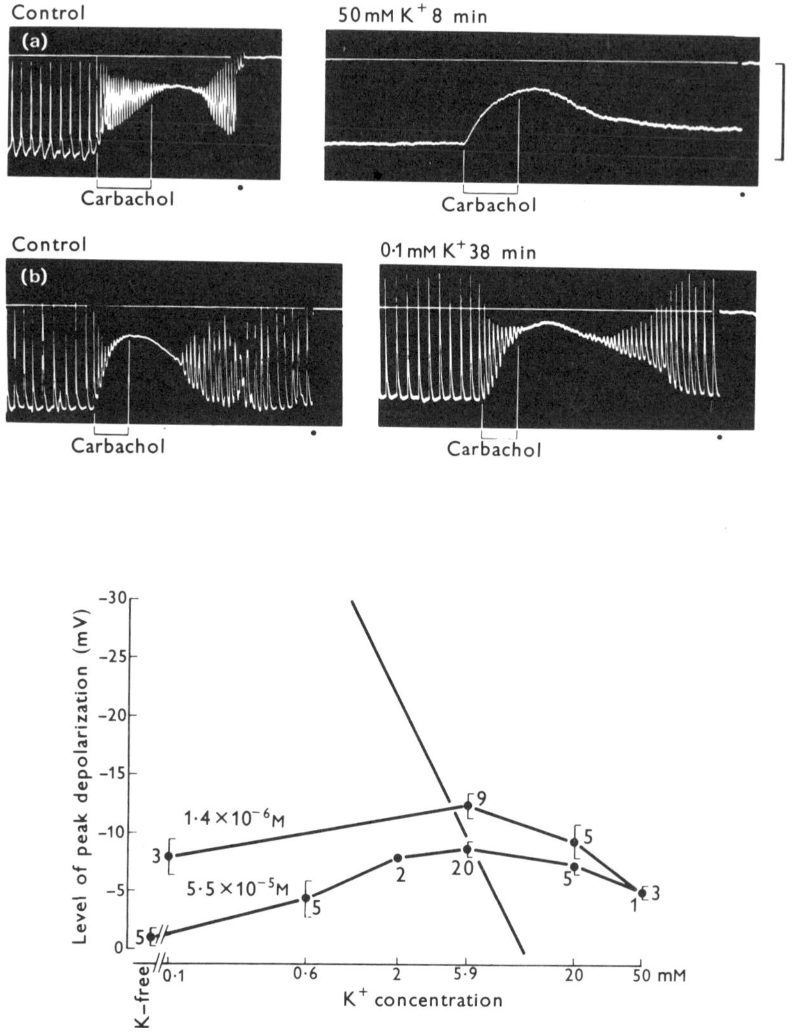


FIG. 6. The effects on the level of peak depolarization of varying the potassium concentration of the bathing solution. The records show the effects on the response to carbachol ($1 \cdot 4 \times 10^{-6}$ M) of (a), 50 mM; (b), 0·1 mM potassium. The vertical calibration represents 20 mV in 50 mM potassium and 50 mV in the other records. In 50 mM potassium the membrane was depolarized and spontaneous activity stopped. At ● the electrode was withdrawn to check the zero level. The graph summarizes the effects of varying the potassium concentration on the level of peak depolarization obtained in two series of experiments using $1 \cdot 4 \times 10^{-6}$ M and $5 \cdot 5 \times 10^{-5}$ M potassium. The straight line is calculated from the model shown in Fig. 3b and equation (6), using the data obtained by varying the sodium and chloride in the external solution (details in Bolton, 1972). It is assumed in the calculation of this line that the relative conductances to various ion species of the channels opened by stimulation of the muscarinic receptor do not change when external ion concentrations are varied. For further details see text.

the expected shifts in the level of peak depolarization if this follows the equilibrium potential closely (Bolton, 1972). The calculated line is shown in Fig. 6.

When the external potassium concentration was reduced, the level of peak depolarization moved positively, in the opposite direction to the one predicted by the model (Fig. 6).

In potassium-free solution the internal potassium concentration falls (Casteels, Droogmans & Hendrickx, 1971) and this is also probably true in potassium-deficient solutions. However, the potassium concentration immediately adjacent to the outside of the membrane may be determined mainly by the rate at which potassium leaves the cell, because potassium might escape relatively slowly from the vicinity of the cell membrane. For example, calculations based on the value of the membrane conductance (Tomita, 1970), the measured increase in conductance produced by carbachol, and an estimate of the ratio $\Delta G_K/\Delta G_{Na}$ (Bolton, 1972) indicate that, *in the absence of ion pumping*, $1{\cdot}4\times10^{-6}$ M carbachol might increase the extracellular potassium concentration at a rate of 0·5 mM/s, if escape of potassium to the bathing solution is negligibly slow. A 10 s exposure would double the extracellular potassium concentration under these conditions. Larger concentrations would have an even greater effect. Suppose in normal solution $E_K$ is $-84$ mV when the external potassium concentration is 6 mM and that in potassium-free solution the internal concentration is halved (to 70 mM) while the external potassium concentration close to the membrane is reduced to a quarter (1·5 mM). Then $E_K$ will be $-102$ mV. When carbachol is applied (assuming equation (4) is applicable) the potassium current will be initially greater in potassium-free than in normal solution. Let us imagine that in normal solution this current increases the external potassium concentration by 10 mM while reducing the internal potassium concentration by 5 mM (intracellular space twice extracellular space); $E_K$ will become $-56$ mV (see Table 1). A similar 10 mM increase in the extracellular potassium concentration when carbachol is applied in potassium-free solution will change $E_K$ from $-102$ to $-45$ mV (Table 1) that is, in potassium-free or -deficient solution upon the application of carbachol $E_K$ may be shifted in the opposite direction to the one anticipated. These considerations illustrate that conditions can be envisaged in which the actual shift in the potassium equilibrium potential when carbachol is applied after reducing the potassium concentration of the bathing solution might be in a positive direction, and not negatively as expected.

There are a number of possible explanations for the apparently small shift in the equilibrium potential in high potassium solutions. It seems unlikely that increasing the external potassium concentration seriously reduces the increase in conductance produced by carbachol (although this has not been tested) so that the level of peak depolarization and the equilibrium potential are still probably close. Calcium current may become

TABLE 1. *Possible effect of carbachol on the potassium equilibrium potential in normal and potassium-free solution*

| | Before carbachol | | In presence of carbachol | |
|---|---|---|---|---|
| Normal solution 6 mM K | $[K]_i$ | 140 mM | $[K]_i$ | 135 mM |
| | $[K]_o$ | 6 mM | $[K]_o$ | 16 mM |
| | $E_K$ | −84 mV | $E_K$ | −56 mV |
| Potassium-free solution | $[K]_i$ | 70 mM | $[K]_i$ | 65 mM |
| | $[K]_o$ | 1·5 mM | $[K]_o$ | 11·5 mM |
| | $E_K$ | −102 mV | $E_K$ | −45 mV |

$[K]_o$ represents the immediate pericellular potassium concentration, which is assumed to be affected by loss of potassium from the cells when carbachol is applied. Note that $E_K$ in the presence of carbachol can be *less* negative in potassium-free than in normal solution.

important when the external sodium is reduced in which case the line relating $\mathscr{E}$ to $E_{Na}$ (Fig. 4) would overestimate the effects of varying $E_K$ on the equilibrium potential. It is also possible that Tris is not completely impermeable as bigger shifts in the level of peak depolarization were observed in the few experiments where sucrose was used instead of Tris chloride to replace sodium chloride (Fig. 4). This would also result in an overestimate of the effects of varying $E_K$. Another likely explanation is that the ratio $\Delta G_K/\Delta G_{Na}$, which has been assumed to be constant in calculating this line, increases when the external potassium concentration is increased. An effect of this type is important at the frog endplate when the external potassium concentration exceeds 8 mM (Takeuchi & Takeuchi, 1960; Takeuchi, 1963a). It is not possible at present to say which of these possibilities might be involved.

It must be admitted that the electrophysiological evidence for an involvement of potassium is not overwhelming. It rests on a small but very significant positive movement of the level of peak depolarization in high potassium concentrations, and on the presumed position of the equilibrium potential about midway between $E_K$ and $E_{Na}$.

## *Summary*

The electrophysiological evidence indicates that stimulation of the muscarinic receptor of the longitudinal muscle of the guinea-pig terminal ileum results in depolarization and an increase in the conductance of the cell membrane. The conductance continues to increase when depolarization has reached a maximum. The limitation of depolarization can be explained if the ion channels opened in the cell membrane by stimulation of the muscarinic receptor have an equilibrium potential of about −10 mV. Depolarization is apparently not limited by the availability of receptors.

The results suggest that the channels operated by the muscarinic receptor allow sodium ions to pass, but probably do not allow chloride ions to pass to any appreciable extent. A *small increase* in chloride permeability would be sufficient to explain the increased fluxes of $^{36}Cl$ which carbachol produces in smooth muscle, but it is possible that these have some other explanation.

The electrophysiological evidence that potassium moves through the channels operated by the muscarinic receptor rests on the presumed position of their equilibrium potential (and insignificant involvement of chloride) and on a small but very significant effect of high potassium concentrations. It is known that muscarinic stimulants produce large increases in $^{42}K$ influx and efflux. However, to explain fully the electrophysiological results it was necessary to postulate special mechanisms and it will require further work before these can be substantiated.

Work described in this paper was supported by the Medical Research Council. I am grateful to Professor E. Bülbring for her interest and encouragement and to Professor W. D. M. Paton for granting me the facilities of his department.

## REFERENCES

Banerjee, A. K. & Lewis, J. J. (1963). *J. Pharm. Pharmac.*, **15**, 409.
Banerjee, A. K. & Lewis, J. J. (1964). *J. Pharm. Pharmac.*, **16**, 134.
Bolton, T. B. (1971). *J. Physiol., Lond.*, **216**, 403.
Bolton, T. B. (1972). *J. Physiol., Lond.*, **220**, 647.
Born, G. V. R. & Bülbring, E. (1956). *J. Physiol., Lond.*, **131**, 690.
Brading, A. F. (1971a). *J. Physiol., Lond.*, **214**, 393.
Brading, A. F. (1971b). *J. Physiol., Lond.*, **215**, 46P.
Breeman, van C., Daniel, E. E. & Breeman, van D. (1966). *J. gen. Physiol.*, **49**, 1265.
Bülbring, E. (1954). *J. Physiol., Lond.*, **125**, 302.
Bülbring, E. (1955). *J. Physiol., Lond.*, **128**, 200.
Bülbring, E. (1957). *J. Physiol., Lond.*, **135**, 412.
Bülbring, E. & Burnstock, G. (1960). *Br. J. Pharmac.*, **15**, 611.
Bülbring, E., Casteels, R. & Kuriyama, H. (1968). *Br. J. Pharmac.*, **34**, 388.
Bülbring, E. & Kuriyama, H. (1963). *J. Physiol., Lond.*, **166**, 59.
Bülbring, E. & Szurszewski, J. H. (1971). *J. Physiol., Lond.*, **217**, 39P.
Burgen, A. S. V. & Spero, L. (1968). *Br. J. Pharmac.*, **34**, 99.
Burnstock, G. (1958). *J. Physiol., Lond.*, **143**, 165.
Burnstock, G. & Holman, M. E. (1963). *A. Rev. Physiol.*, **25**, 61.
Burnstock, G., Holman, M. E. & Prosser, C. L. (1963). *Physiol. Rev.*, **43**, 482.
Burnstock, G. & Holman, M. E. (1966). *A. Rev. Pharmac.*, **6**, 129.
Casteels, R. (1966). *J. Physiol., Lond.*, **184**, 131.
Casteels, R. (1969). *J. Physiol., Lond.*, **205**, 193.
Casteels, R. (1971). *J. Physiol., Lond.*, **214**, 225.
Casteels, R., Droogmans, G. & Hendrickx, H. (1971). *J. Physiol.*, **217**, 281.
Casteels, R. & Kuriyama, H. (1965). *J. Physiol., Lond.*, **177**, 263.
Casteels, R. & Kuriyama, H. (1966). *J. Physiol., Lond.*, **184**, 120.
Coombs, J. S., Eccles, J. C. & Fatt, P. (1955). *J. Physiol., Lond.*, **130**, 326.
del Castillo, J. & Katz, B. (1955). *J. Physiol., Lond.*, **128**, 157.
Dewey, M. M. & Barr, L. (1962). *Science, N.Y.*, **137**, 670.
Durbin, R. P. & Jenkinson, D. H. (1961a). *J. Physiol., Lond.*, **157**, 74.
Durbin, R. P. & Jenkinson, D. H. (1961b). *J. Physiol., Lond.*, **157**, 90.
Fatt, P. & Katz, B. (1951). *J. Physiol., Lond.*, **115**, 320.
Feltz, A. & Mallart, A. (1970). *Brain Res.*, **22**, 264.
Feltz, A. & Mallart, A. (1971). *J. Physiol., Lond.*, **218**, 85.
Fewtrell, C. M. S. & Rang, H. P. (1971). *Br. J. Pharmac.*, **43**, 417P.
Fewtrell, C. M. S. & Rang, H. P. (1973). This symposium.

FURCHGOTT, R. F. (1966). In: *Advances in Drug Research*, Vol. 3, ed. Harper, N. J. & Simmons, A. B., p. 21. London: Academic Press.
FURCHGOTT, R. F. & BURSZTYN, P. (1967). *Ann. N.Y. Acad. Sci.*, **144**, 882.
GINSBORG, B. L. (1967). *Pharmac. Rev.*, **19**, 289.
HOLMAN, M. E. (1970). In: *Smooth Muscle*, ed. Bülbring, E., Brading, A. F., Tomita, T. & Jones, A. W., p. 244. London: Arnold.
HERRLINGER, J. D., LÜLLMANN, H. & SCHUH, F. (1967). *Arch. exp. Path. Pharmak.*, **256**, 348.
HIDAKA, T. & KURIYAMA, H. (1969). *J. gen. Physiol.*, **53**, 471.
HURWITZ, L. (1960). *Am. J. Physiol.*, **198**, 94.
HURWITZ, L. (1965). In: *Muscle*, ed. Paul *et al.*, p. 239. Oxford: Pergamon Press.
HURWITZ, L., TINSLEY, B. & BATTLE, F. (1960). *Am. J. Physiol.*, **199**, 107.
JENKINSON, D. H. (1960). *J. Physiol., Lond.*, **152**, 309.
JENKINSON, D. H. & NICHOLLS, J. G. (1961). *J. Physiol., Lond.*, **159**, 111.
KASAI, M. & CHANGEUX, J.-P. (1971). *J. Membrane Biol.*, **6**, 24.
KOBAYASHI, M., PROSSER, C. L. & NAGAI, T. (1967). *Am. J. Physiol.*, **213**, 275.
KOESTER, J. & NASTUK, W. L. (1970). *Fedn Proc.*, **29**, 716.
KURIYAMA, H. (1970). In: *Smooth Muscle*, ed. Bülbring, E., Brading, A. F., Tomita, T. & Jones, A. W., p. 366. London: Arnold.
LEMBECK, F. & STROBACH, R. (1956). *Arch. exp. Path. Pharmak.*, **228**, 130.
ROBERTSON, P. A. (1960). *Nature, Lond.*, **186**, 316.
SCHATZMANN, H. J. (1961). *Pflügers Arch. ges. Physiol.*, **274**, 295.
SCHATZMANN, H. J. (1964a). *Ergebn. Physiol.*, **55**, 28.
SCHATZMANN, H. J. (1964b). In: *Pharmacology of Smooth Muscle*, ed. Bülbring, E., p. 57. Oxford: Pergamon Press.
SETEKLEIV, J. (1970). In: *Smooth Muscle*, ed. Bülbring, E., Brading, A. F., Tomita, T. & Jones, A. W., p. 343. London: Arnold.
SPERELAKIS, N. & TARR, M. (1965). *Am. J. Physiol.*, **208**, 737.
TAKEUCHI, A. & TAKEUCHI, N. (1960). *J. Physiol., Lond.*, **154**, 52.
TAKEUCHI, N. (1963a). *J. Physiol., Lond.*, **167**, 128.
TAKEUCHI, N. (1963b). *J. Physiol., Lond.*, **167**, 141.
TOMITA, T. (1970). In: *Smooth Muscle*, ed. Bülbring, E., Brading, A. F., Tomita, T. & Jones, A. W., p. 197. London: Arnold.
WEISS, G. B., COALSON, R. E. & HURWITZ, L. (1961). *Am. J. Physiol.*, **200**, 789.
WEISS, G. B. & HURWITZ, L. (1963). *J. gen. Physiol.*, **47**, 173.

## DISCUSSION

*Jenkinson (London)*

Have you any information on the extent and rate of chloride entry during the action of carbachol? Also, how quickly does chloride leave the cells when the bathing fluid is changed to chloride-free solution, and how do $E_K$ and $E_{Na}$ alter as the internal chloride concentration falls?

*Bolton (Oxford)*

You raise the very interesting possibility that if the chloride permeability was sufficiently large during the action of carbachol, then chloride might be so quickly redistributed that $E_{Cl}$ and the membrane potential would be very similar at all times, with the result that removing chloride from the external solution might have no detectable effect.

However, the response to submaximal concentrations of carbachol is unaffected in chloride-deficient solution and the increase in conductance produced by such concentrations must be two to four times the resting membrane conductance or less. Now Casteels (1971), Brading (1971a), and yourself (Durbin & Jenkinson, 1961a) have shown that the slow phase of chloride exchange between taenia and its bathing solution has a half-time of about 10 min ($K \approx 0{\cdot}05\ \text{min}^{-1}$) which suggests that the movement of chloride across the cell membrane is two orders of magnitude slower than would be required by this hypothesis, even allowing for a 2–4-fold increase in chloride conductance when carbachol is applied.

The efflux by chloride from taenia to chloride-free solutions, where chloride is replaced by propionate or benzenesulphonate, has a half-time of about 10 min, that is to say, the efflux of $^{36}Cl$ is unaffected by replacing chloride with an impermeant anion. According to Casteels (1971), who worked on taenia, after 1 h in chloride-free solution the internal chloride is about 1 mM but $E_{Na}$ and $E_K$ are unchanged.

*Noble* (*Oxford*)

If acetylcholine produces roughly equal increases in sodium and potassium conductances, as your reversal potential measurement suggests, then the slope of the relation between reversal potential and log $[Na^+]_o$ should be about 30 mV per 10-fold change in concentration. Is this the case? I ask the question because this might be another way of determining whether other ions contribute to the conductance change.

*Bolton* (*Oxford*)

I think the method you suggest depends on the assumption that the relative conductances to various ions do not change when the external concentration of any ion is varied. This may not be so. The apparent change in the equilibrium potential when sodium was replaced by Tris was about 22 mV for a 10-fold change. The few experiments I have done in which sodium and chloride were replaced by sucrose suggested that in this case a value of about 30 mV may be appropriate. You will notice that when chloride is also replaced the shift is increased whereas, if chloride enters the cell through the receptor-operated channels, a decreased shift would be expected. Apart from changes in the relative conductances of the channels to sodium and potassium ions, the results using Tris replacement could also be explained if $\Delta G_K/\Delta G_{Na}$ was larger than unity.

*Barnard* (*New York*)

Your curve relating conductance change to carbachol concentration covered most of the range of receptor occupancy (calculated from an apparent affinity constant for carbachol). Does this imply that there are few spare receptors in this smooth muscle?

*Bolton* (*Oxford*)

If you are defining 'spare receptors' as those not occupied or activated by carbachol when a maximal conductance change is produced, then my evidence does not enable me to give any answer to your question. In Fig. 2 the vertical scale chosen for the increase in conductance is arbitrary and the line overlies the lower part of the receptor-occupancy curve only by chance. It is not possible to measure the maximal conductance change of which the tissue is capable with the technique used (see Bolton, 1972, for details and limitations). Nor can it be assumed that fractional receptor-occupancy and increase in conductance are directly proportional, as cooperative mechanisms may be operating.

# DESENSITIZATION AT THE MOTOR ENDPLATE

L. G. MAGAZANIK AND F. VYSKOČIL

*Sechenov Institute of Evolutionary Physiology and Biochemistry, Academy of Sciences of the USSR, Leningrad, Soviet Union and Institute of Physiology, Czechoslovak Academy of Sciences, Prague, Czechoslovakia*

## *I. General characteristics and methods*

The transience of the effect of acetylcholine (ACh) was described more than thirty-five years ago, almost simultaneously with the experimental evidence about the key role of ACh in neuromuscular transmission (Brown, Dale & Feldberg, 1936; Cowan, 1936). The depolarization induced by ACh at the postjunctional membrane of the muscle fibre reaches a maximum and then begins to fall gradually, despite the fact that the ACh concentration remains constant. This phenomenon, named 'desensitization' (Thesleff, 1955, 1960), has been observed not only in skeletal muscle but also at other kinds of chemosensitive tissue such as electroplax and nerve cells.

At present the desensitization of postjunctional membrane might be phenomenologically defined as a progressive decline of the induced increase in conductance during prolonged contact with ACh or other cholinomimetics.

The nature of desensitization is still unknown. This is partly due to the lack of knowledge of the precise mechanism of activation by which combination of ACh with the receptor induces an abrupt increase in membrane conductance. This mechanism appears to involve a number of successive events, and theoretically each of them might be considered as a bottle-neck limiting the whole process during the prolonged action of ACh (Magazanik, 1970a,b; 1971a,b; Magazanik & Vyskočil, 1970). The molecular events in activation and desensitization are reflected only indirectly in changes in membrane conductance and membrane potential, or in contraction of the whole muscle, and the absence of direct experimental tools presents the main difficulty for studies on desensitization.

At present there are three principal methods for evoking desensitization at the motor endplate, which differ in the manner in which the ACh or other activators are applied to postjunctional membrane.

(1) Addition of drug to the muscle bath. This method makes it possible to regulate accurately the concentration of agonist in the bath and then to

measure muscle contraction (Rang & Ritter, 1969; 1970a,b), changes of potential difference between the endplate zone and nerve-free part of muscle (Fatt, 1950; Jenkinson, Stamenovic & Whitaker, 1968; Magazanik, 1969; Rang & Ritter, 1970a), changes of the membrane potential of muscle fibre (Thesleff, 1955), or changes of input resistance (Karlin, 1967). With this method all of the receptors are acted upon by the drug, but appreciable time is required for equilibrium of agonist concentration near the postjunctional membrane. Moreover, the prolonged action of drug can cause not only desensitization but also some ionic changes inside the cell (Karlin, 1967; Jenkinson & Terrar, 1973). The question also remains to be answered why the recovery of sensitivity after washing away the agonist often takes more than 10 times as long as the onset of the desensitization (unpublished observation).

(2) Irrigation of a part of the endplate zone by a small pipette ($\sim 50\ \mu m$ in diameter) filled with agonist (Manthey, 1966; Nastuk, 1967; Parsons, 1969). In this method the effect of agonist is usually monitored by changes of input resistance of the fibre. The method appears to give reproducible results, but suffers from the disadvantage that it is not possible to elicit brief test responses to compare the postjunctional sensitivity before and during desensitization.

(3) Ionophoretic application from a double micropipette (Katz & Thesleff, 1957). One of the channels is used for brief (5–20 ms) test pulses of ACh, while the second channel is used to deliver a prolonged (10–20 s) desensitizing pulse of ACh (Fig. 1). Such a prolonged conditioning application of ACh results in desensitization which can be estimated by changes in the amplitude of both the test response and conditioning response. The amplitude of test response is gradually restored after switching off the conditioning current. This method has some advantages as compared with the above technique: (a) the rate of desensitization onset and recovery are rather high (a few seconds); (b) the area affected by ACh is comparatively small, which means that no appreciable ionic changes occur; (c) using multibarrel micropipettes one can compare the effect of various cholinomimetics at the same place; (d) good reproducibility of the phenomenon during one experiment makes it possible to study the influence of various factors on desensitization (changes of temperature, ionic composition, pH, chemical agents etc.). However, this method has also some limitations since the concentration of agonist at the site of action is unknown and non-uniform. Furthermore, the area of agonist action during ejection from different channels of the multibarrel micropipette does not always coincide completely, especially if one of these agonists is delivered by short pulses and the other continuously.

## *II. Theoretical models of desensitization*

The ACh effect is mediated by a complex system consisting probably of several functional elements. One of these elements, the 'receptor', may be regarded as a detector which recognizes the transmitter molecule and reacts with it. The receptor site is localized only at the outer surface of the cell membrane (del Castillo & Katz, 1955). Changes of the receptor molecule are transmitted to subsequent parts of this system, and as a result, the state of the ionophore changes. It appears that with prolonged activation one or more steps of this functional chain prove insufficient and cause desensitization. The majority of previous hypotheses about the mechanism of desensitization involve a modification of the receptor (Waud, 1968).

At present the hypothesis of desensitization proposed by Katz & Thesleff (1957) seems to be the most plausible. It is based on the following experimentally observed features of the kinetics of desensitization (Katz & Thesleff, 1957): (1) the rate of desensitization depends on the amount (concentration) of ACh acting on the postjunctional membrane; (2) the rate of recovery of sensitivity after withdrawal of the agonist is constant and does not depend either on the agonist concentration or on the degree of desensitization it induces; (3) the rate of recovery is independent of the rate of onset of desensitization. According to this hypothesis the receptor may exist in two forms; active R and inactive R′. Two fundamental assumptions underly this hypothesis: (1) agonist A can react both with R and R′: conversion of the agonist–receptor complex from the active AR into inactive AR′ form proceeds slowly at a rate similar to the conversion of agonist-free inactive receptor R′ into the active form R. The processes which take place in this instance are described by the following cycle of reactions:

$$\begin{array}{ccc} \mathrm{A}+\mathrm{R} & \underset{k_2}{\overset{k_1}{\rightleftharpoons}} & \mathrm{AR} \\ k_r \uparrow & & \downarrow k_d \\ \mathrm{A}+\mathrm{R}' & \underset{k'_2}{\overset{k'_1}{\rightleftharpoons}} & \mathrm{AR}' \end{array}$$

When comparing experimental results with the cyclic model Katz & Thesleff (1957) made the following assumptions. (1) Agonists usually exhibit a higher affinity for R′ (desensitized receptor) than for R (normal receptor), that is:

$$\frac{k'_1}{k'_2} > \frac{k_1}{k_2}$$

(2) The rate constants for association and dissociation and for transition between R and R′ are related by:

$$\frac{k'_1 \times k_2}{k'_2 \times k_1} \gg \frac{k_d}{k_r}$$

The comparison of the cyclic model with other receptor models (parallel reactions, sequential reactions, two-site model and rate theory model) demonstrated its advantages (Rang & Ritter, 1970a). If it is assumed that changes in the receptor molecule are the sole mechanism of desensitization, then the cyclic model accounts very well for various features, such as the constancy of the rate of recovery from desensitization, irrespective of the rate of onset, and of the chemical structure of the agonist used to induce desensitization.

### *III. Effect of antagonists on desensitization*

The cyclic receptor model describes satisfactorily the evidence obtained by Katz & Thesleff (1957) for a relatively simple system of only one agonist but without any antagonist. We studied the effect of ACh antagonists ((+)-tubocurarine and atropine) on the desensitization rate. It was found that in the presence of (+)-tubocurarine ($5 \times 10^{-7}$ M) the amplitude of ACh responses declines to 50% and simultaneously with this the desensitization rate decreases. This slowing down of desensitization corresponds perfectly to the rate that can be attained without tubocurarine merely by diminishing the ACh-conditioning dose twofold. Alternatively, when the conditioning dose of ACh is raised to overcome the blocking effect of (+)-tubocurarine present, the desensitization rate is the same as that produced by the lower dose in the absence of any antagonist (Magazanik, 1968). The same results were obtained in the experiments with atropine (Fig. 1).

In accordance with the cyclic receptor model, however, some increase of desensitization is predicted, irrespective whether (+)-tubocurarine and/or atropine have affinity for the desensitized receptor, R′, as well as for the normal receptor, R (Rang & Ritter, 1970a). On the other hand, our results are explicable on the assumption that the only effect of (+)-tubocurarine or atropine is to reduce activation, so that by overcoming the decrease of activation induced by antagonists we restore the former rate of desensitization.

Rang & Ritter (1970a,b) found that some antagonists are potentiated when applied in combination with agonists. The so-called metaphilic effect of these drugs was explained by a greater affinity of the antagonist for the desensitized receptor than for the normal one. It appeared to us that such an interpretation could be applied to a group of cholinolytics which affect the rate of desensitization at concentrations much lower than those needed to inhibit endplate potentials (e.p.ps) (Magazanik, 1970a,b; 1971a,b). For example, mesphenal (I.1) increases desensitization and inhibits ACh potentials

I. 1. Mesphenal

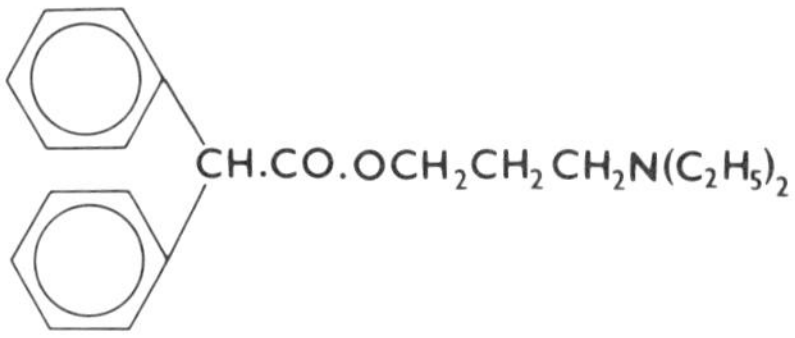

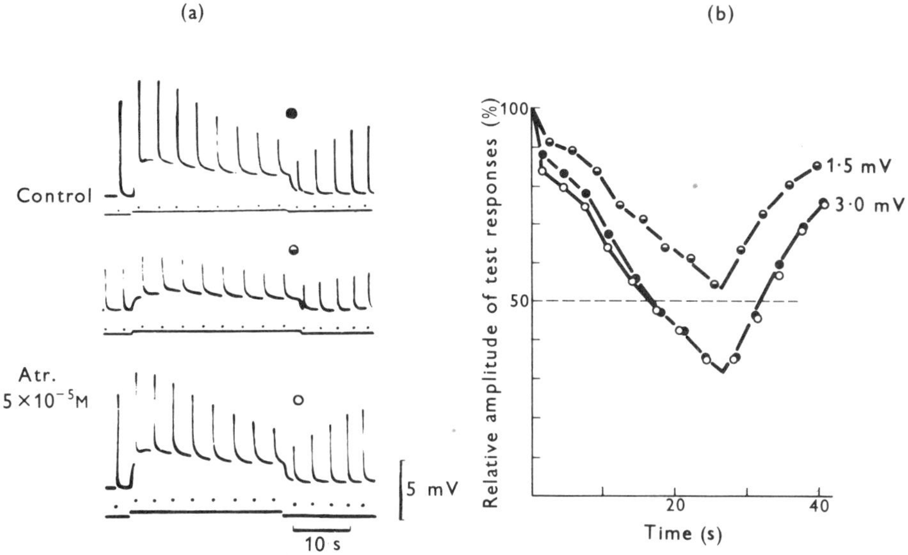


FIG. 1. The effect of atropine sulphate (Atr.) on the rate of desensitization. The double-barrel micropipette technique was used. (a), Records of desensitization caused by prolonged conditioning pulse of ACh from one barrel of micropipette. Desensitization of the small part of postjunctional membrane where the pipette was placed, resulted in the gradual diminution of the short test responses, which recover after the conditioning pulse is switched off. Middle record: 20 min after application of atropine ($5 \times 10^{-5}$ M). Note the decrease in amplitude of both test and conditioning responses due to the blocking action of atropine and the slowing down of desensitization. Bottom records: the restoration of the original rate of desensitization in the presence of atropine when the conditioning and test pulses were increased (see lower trace) so as to overcome the blocking action of atropine. When the test responses were increased to the control level by increasing the amplitude of the ionophoretic pulse a similar picture to that of the control was obtained. (b), Results shown in graphical form. Desensitization is expressed as % decrease of the test responses (100%=amplitude before desensitization). Numbers in mV indicate the peak amplitude of the conditioning response. (●), Control; (◒), atropine, small test pulses; (○), atropine, large test pulses. All experiments described in this and other figures were performed on isolated sartorius muscle of the frog *Rana temporaria*, at 20–22° C unless otherwise stated.

at a concentration of $5 \times 10^{-7}$–$1 \times 10^{-6}$ M (Fig. 2), whereas $10^{-5}$ M or more is required to inhibit e.p.ps. In the presence of mesphenal, desensitization was observed even in the experiments with single micropipette (Fig. 2, upper part). When ACh is applied by a single ionophoretic micropipette in the presence of mesphenal the degree of inhibition of ACh potentials increases as the frequency of application of the ACh pulses is increased. If the repetitive application of ACh is interrupted, the first response after the period of rest has a larger amplitude, but then the amplitude decreases progressively down to the former equilibrium level. It is of interest that agents that increase desensitization do not influence e.p.ps even when the frequency of stimulation is increased to 50–100 cycles/s. It therefore appears that desensitization does not occur during the generation of e.p.ps, possibly because the

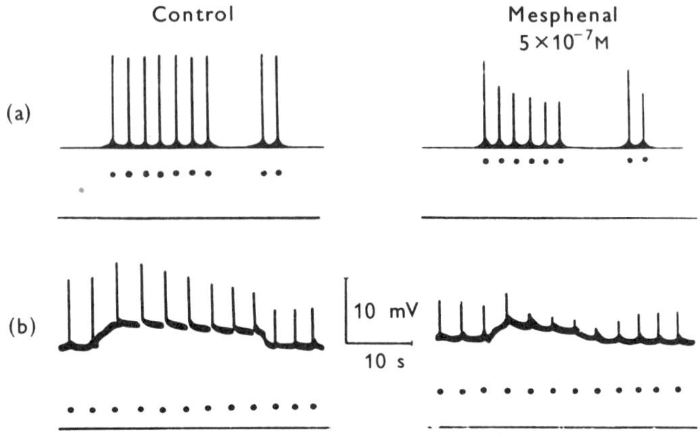


FIG. 2. Effect of mesphenal on desensitization. Right-hand records were obtained 15 min after adding $5\times10^{-7}$ M mesphenal. (a), ACh potentials elicited by ionophoretic pulses every 2·5 s. In the presence of mesphenal, but in the control experiment, interruption of the ionophoretic pulses transiently increases the response. (b), Double-barrel micropipette technique (for details see Fig. 1). In the presence of mesphenal the conditioning pulse of ACh causes a greater and more rapid decline of the response to the brief test pulses. (Magazanik, 1971b.)

action of the released ACh is very much briefer than it is with an ACh potential.

When more diverse substances such as diphenhydramine and SKF-525A (I.2) were studied we obtained results that cannot readily be interpreted in

I. 2. SKF–525A

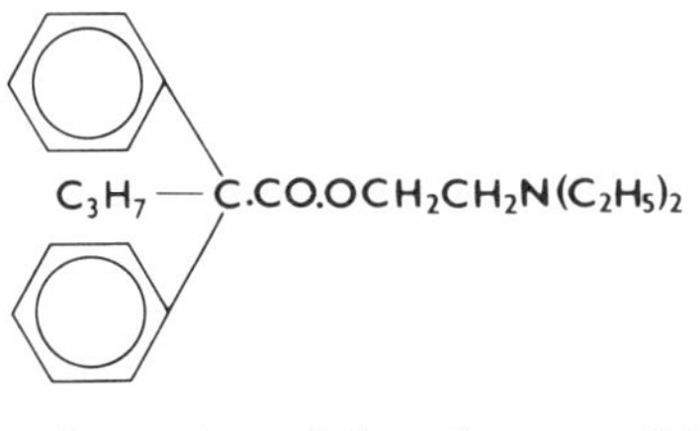


terms of the receptor hypothesis. It was found that the rate of desensitization can be increased by substances showing practically no cholinolytic activity. This might mean that these compounds can interact only with the desensitized receptor and have no affinity for normal receptors. It is, however, very difficult to distinguish this mechanism from a mechanism in which the antagonist acts not directly on the receptor but elsewhere on the chain of events leading to desensitization.

To explore the possibility that these substances influence some other step in the cholinolytic system (Magazanik, 1970a, 1971a), we performed experiments with intracellular application of SKF-525A and its quarternary methiodide. A few minutes after passing current through the micropipette ($1\times10^{-8}$ A, inside positive) desensitization was greatly enhanced (Fig. 3): the amplitudes

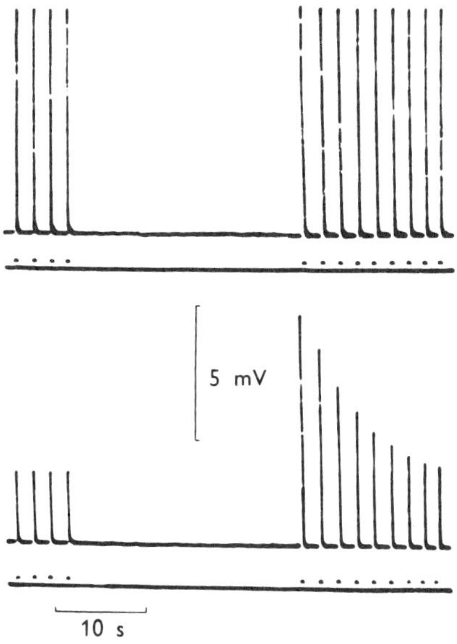


FIG. 3. The effect of SKF-525A applied intracellularly on desensitization. Upper pair of oscillographic records—control. ACh potentials recorded every 2 s. The pulses were switched off for 26 s (see monitor on lower beam). The amplitude of ACh potentials was unaffected by the resting period. Lower pair—after 10 min of the intracellular injection of SKF-525A at a distance of about 50 $\mu$m from the ACh pipette. The injection pipette was filled with $10^{-2}$ M SKF-525A + 1 M KCl, and positive current of about $10^{-8}$ A (which decreased the membrane potential by no more than 4–5 mV) was applied through it. The amplitude of the train of potentials on the left is reduced by desensitization. When the train is interrupted for 26 s, the amplitude recovers and decreases again as desensitization occurs. (With permission of *Brain Research*.)

of consecutive ACh potentials decreased, but they recovered after a short period of rest (Vyskočil & Magazanik, 1972).

The fact that these compounds can affect desensitization from inside the fibre, though the receptors are known to be accessible only from the outside makes it unlikely that they are acting by combining with the receptor sites.

## *IV. Other factors influencing desensitization*

The receptor hypothesis of desensitization does not readily account for the influence of the ionic medium on desensitization. It is known that desensitization depends on calcium concentration (Manthey, 1966; Magazanik, 1968; Magazanik & Shekhirev, 1970), the rate of desensitization increasing with an increase in calcium concentration. Other multivalent cations also affect desensitization (Magazanik & Vyskočil, 1970) and their relative activity can be arranged as follows:

$$Mg^{2+} \ll Ca^{2+} \leqslant Ba^{2+} < Sr^{2+} \ll Al^{3+} < La^{3+}$$

Nastuk & Liu (1966) suggested a direct competition between ACh and calcium for the receptor. This suggestion contradicts, however, the well-known fact that miniature e.p.ps can be recorded from a muscle immersed in isotonic $CaCl_2$ (Katz & Miledi, 1967). In terms of the cyclic model it could be postulated that calcium and other multivalent cations act by virtue of their extremely high affinity to the desensitized receptor. But taking into account the well-known diversity of effects of these ions on excitable membranes one would expect interaction of calcium during desensitization with a site different from the receptor (Magazanik & Vyskočil, 1970).

The rate of desensitization can be affected by current passed through a second intracellular microelectrode (Fig. 4) (Magazanik & Vyskočil, 1970).

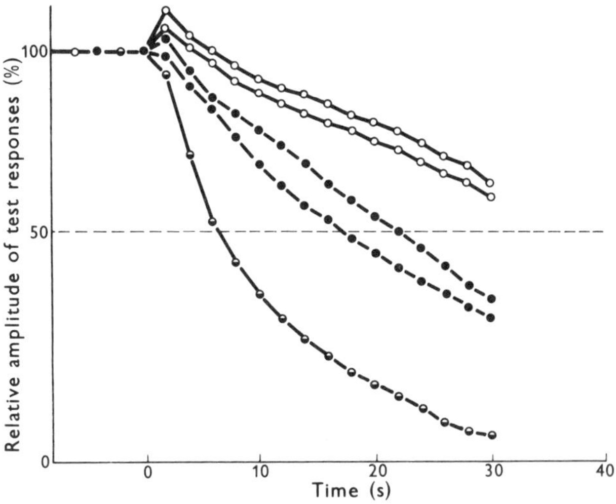


FIG. 4. The relationship between the rate of desensitization and the membrane potential. Desensitization was first recorded at a normal membrane potential, −79 mV (●, control), then after artificial depolarization to −58 mV (○) and hyperpolarization to −100 mV (◒) and finally again at −79 mV. A second intracellular electrode was used for polarizing the muscle fibre. (With permission of *J. Physiol., Lond.*)

The desensitization rate increases when the muscle fibre is hyperpolarized and decreases when it is depolarized. Such alteration of the desensitization rate was also observed (Fig. 5) when the muscle fibre was depolarized to about 50 mV by increasing the potassium concentration to 15 mM (Magazanik & Vyskočil, 1970). Both the amplitude of the test response and the rate of desensitization decreased when the membrane potential was reduced. The restoration of the former level of responses either by increasing the amount of applied ACh or by artificially restoring the membrane potential to the original level led to restoration of the desensitization rate.

It has been found that the rate of desensitization decreases markedly when the preparation is cooled from 20° C to 10° C. The decrease was even more

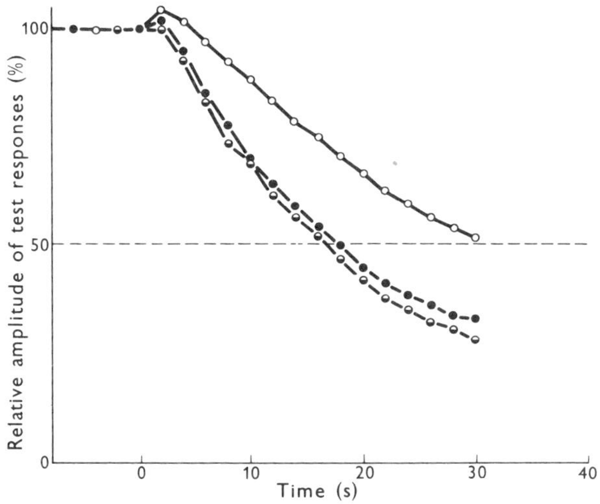


FIG. 5. Effect of depolarization by potassium on the rate of desensitization. (◒), Control (membrane potential −88 mV). (○), After 14 min in a solution with 15 mM potassium (membrane potential −52 mV). The rate of desensitization was decreased. (●), Membrane potential was restored to the control (−90 mV) by passing current through a second intracellular microelectrode. The rate of desensitization returned approximately to the initial value. (With permission of *J. Physiol., Lond.*)

strongly pronounced at 2° C (Fig. 6). It is interesting that the amplitude of miniature e.p.ps (taking into account changes in cable properties) is less dependent on temperature (Li & Gouras, 1958; Jensen, 1972) than is desensitization. This permits the suggestion that the molecular processes participating in the desensitization mechanism differ from those in the activation mechanism of the postsynaptic membrane.

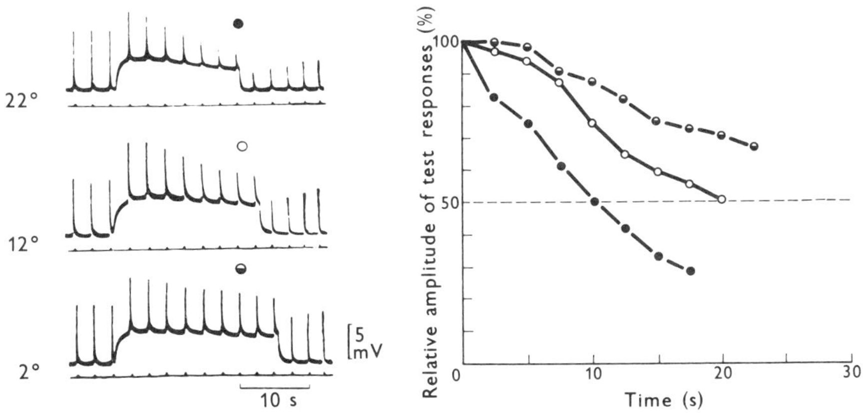


FIG. 6. Effect of temperature on the rate of desensitization. Records as in Fig. 1. The rate of desensitization was measured on the same area of postjunctional membrane at 22°, (●); 12°, (○); and 2° C, (◒).

## *V. Neurotoxins and desensitization*

Recently the interest in desensitization mechanism has increased as a result of studies with irreversible cholinergic receptor blocking agents—bungarotoxin (BuTX) and cobra toxin (Changeux, Kasai & Lee, 1970; Changeux, Meunier & Huchet, 1971; Lester, 1970, 1972; Miledi, Molinoff & Potter, 1971; Barnard, Wieckowski & Chiu, 1971; Miledi & Potter, 1971). Miledi & Potter (1971) found that prolonged immersion of muscles in solutions containing ACh and neostigmine could protect against irreversible receptor block by BuTX, and they concluded that BuTX cannot interact with the desensitized receptor The relationship between BuTX and desensitization is thus used as evidence of the specific action of BuTX on the receptor as well as the receptor origin of desensitization (Miledi & Potter, 1971).

Since desensitization may occur during generation of ACh potentials (Magazanik, 1970a,b; 1971a,b), one could suggest that BuTX ought to inhibit e.p.ps more rapidly than ACh potentials where desensitization should protect the receptors somewhat. This was not found to be the case, however; as shown in Fig. 7 ACh potentials decrease even more rapidly than e.p.ps in the presence of BuTX.

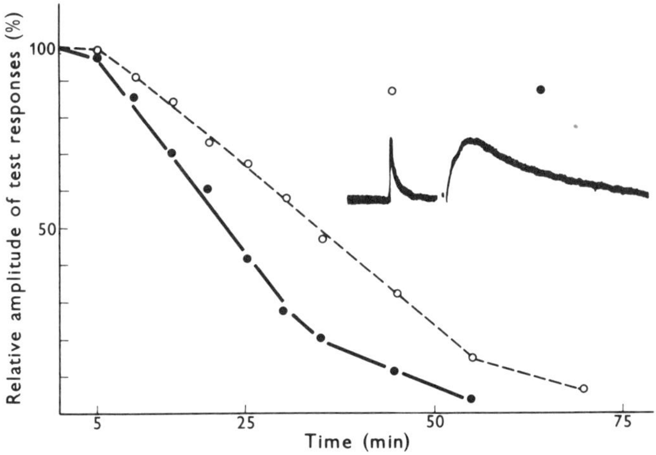


FIG. 7. Effect of $5 \times 10^{-7}$ g/ml α-bungarotoxin (BuTX) on endplate potential (○) and ACh potential (●) in a single muscle fibre. Each potential was evoked every 2 s. The % decrease of the two responses is plotted against the time of exposure to BuTX. (With permission of *Brain Research*.)

This result led us to perform direct experiments to check the effect of BuTX on desensitization using the double-barrel micropipette technique. The amplitude of both short-lasting test responses and the depolarization caused by long-lasting pulses of ACh decline progressively. In spite of the diminished depolarization produced by the conditioning pulse, the rate of desensitization

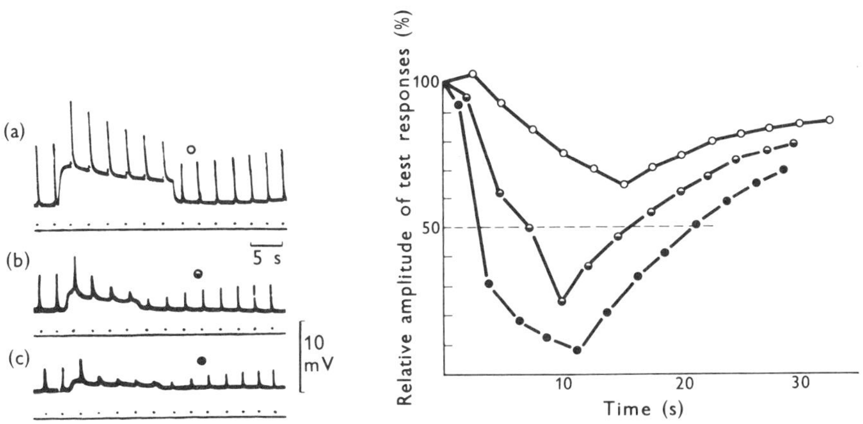


FIG. 8. Effect of bath-applied $\alpha$-bungarotoxin (BuTX) on the rate of desensitization. Records as in Fig. 1. (a), (○), Control; (b), (◒), BuTX $5 \times 10^{-7}$ g/ml for 5 min; (c), (●), BuTX $5 \times 10^{-7}$ g/ml for 15 min.

markedly increased, the half-time of decline of the test responses being several times shorter in the presence of BuTX (Fig. 8). Both the blocking action of BuTX and its effect on desensitization are irreversible, and persist long after the toxin is washed out.

It is interesting that the rate of recovery from desensitization does not change either in experiments with BuTX (see Fig. 8) or during the action of other substances (chlorpromazine, SKF-525A, etc.) which increase the rate of onset of desensitization.

From the viewpoint of the cyclic model for desensitization, the increase in the rate of desensitization during the action of BuTX could be interpreted in terms of a higher affinity of BuTX for the desensitized receptor. But in this case one could expect that the rate of recovery would be decreased (Rang & Ritter, 1970a), which did not happen. Hence, either the cyclic model of desensitization is not applicable in this particular case or the receptor is not the only site of action of BuTX.

In order to examine other possible sites of action we injected BuTX ionophoretically into the muscle fibre from a micropipette (tip diameter about 1 $\mu$m) filled with $1 \times 10^{-3}$ g/ml BuTX and 1 M KCl introduced near the nerve ending. A current of about $10^{-8}$ A was passed depolarizing the fibre by not more than 2–4 mV. As shown in Fig. 9 ACh potentials and e.p.ps recorded from the endplate of the fibre decrease progressively some time after switching on the current carrying BuTX. The intracellularly applied BuTX also enhances desensitization just as it does when applied in the bathing medium (Fig. 10). These effects of intracellularly applied BuTX varied considerably from cell to cell: the half-time of the decrease of the e.p.p. varied from 1 to 20 min, possibly because of variation in the distance between

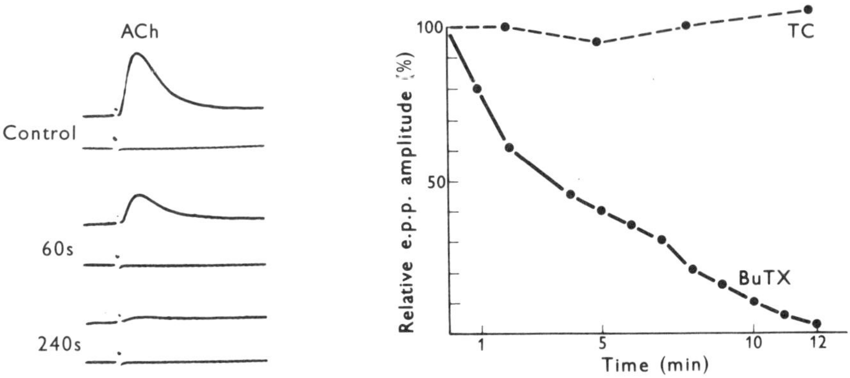


FIG. 9. Intracellular microapplication of α-bungarotoxin (BuTX) and (+)-tubocurarine (TC) at the endplate zone. Left: decrease of the ACh potential after 60 and 240 s of intracellular injection of BuTX (BuTX pipette positive). Right: % decrease of e.p.p. amplitude during BuTX and TC application into the muscle fibre. No change in the ACh potential was observed when BuTX was injected into the neighbouring fibre. (With permission of *Brain Research*.)

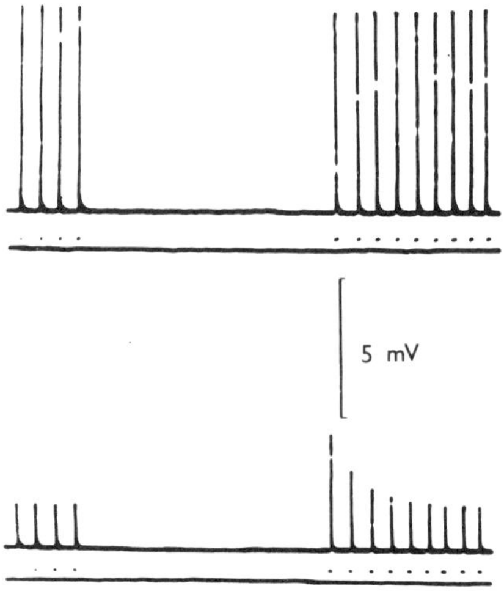


FIG. 10. Effect of α-bungarotoxin (BuTX) applied intracellularly on desensitization. Experimental arrangement is the same as in Fig. 3. Intracellular ionophoretic micropipette was filled with $10^{-3}$ g/ml BuTX+1 M KCl. Note that after period of rest the amplitude of the first ACh potential (lower record) does not reach the amplitude of the control potentials (upper record), which means that not only desensitization but also block of the response is occurring. Both the blocking effect and the enhancement of desensitization are irreversible, and persist after washing away the toxin or after reversing the direction of the ionophoretic current. (With permission of *Brain Research*.)

the BuTX pipette and the source of ACh. Various possibilities might account for the action of intracellularly applied BuTX in such experiments.

(1) BuTX might leak in sufficient amounts from the pipette as it approaches

the membrane just before the impalement. This is unlikely, however, because the effect of BuTX was seen only when positive current was passed through the intracellular pipette.

(2) BuTX might leak from the cell around the inserted pipette tip. However, we observed in similar experiments that the intracellular application of (+)-tubocurarine produced no effect (Fig. 8, see also del Castillo & Katz, 1957), so appreciable leakage seems unlikely.

(3) BuTX might diffuse through the membrane. In control experiments however BuTX was introduced into the cell adjacent to that from which recordings were made, and no effect of BuTX was observed. This enables us to reject the suggestion that BuTX leaving the cell can create a sufficient concentration to act extracellularly.

(4) Disregarding special mechanisms whereby intracellular BuTX might be transported to extracellular receptor sites, it therefore seems most likely that BuTX can act on the inner surface of the membrane (Magazanik & Vyskočil, 1972a,b).

## *VI. Conclusions*

The experimental results show that: (1) desensitization can be influenced by factors which do not produce a direct effect on the receptor; (2) some of the agents affecting desensitization exert their effects also when applied inside the muscle fibre, and their site of action can be localized to the inner side of the cell membrane.

These findings suggest that the desensitization mechanism cannot be restricted only to the R–R′ transition. Thus, desensitization may reflect not only the state of the receptor but also that of the subsequent steps in the activation mechanism. Nevertheless the cyclic scheme of Katz & Thesleff (1957) can be used successfully for a formal description of the desensitization mechanism, if the following possibilities are taken into account.

(1) Not the receptor (R) itself but the subsequent step of the system (S) becomes inactive, that is, $R\text{–}S^A \rightarrow R\text{–}S^I$.

(2) The various factors that influence desensitization do so by altering the rate constant ($k_d$) for transition of the system from the active ($R\text{–}S^A$) into inactive ($R\text{–}S^I$) state without affecting the rate constant ($k_r$) for recovery of the system to the original state.

$$\begin{array}{ccc} A + R\text{–}S & \underset{k_2}{\overset{k_1}{\rightleftharpoons}} & AR\text{–}S^A \\ k_r \uparrow & & \downarrow k_d \\ A + R\text{–}S^I & \underset{k'_2}{\overset{k'_1}{\rightleftharpoons}} & AR\text{–}S^I \end{array}$$

The virtue of this description is that it explains satisfactorily the properties of desensitization presented by Katz & Thesleff, as well as recently obtained facts. The physical nature of the $R\text{–}S^{A} \rightarrow R\text{–}S^{I}$ transition is not quite clear. Taking into consideration close relationships between the rate of desensitization and the concentration of calcium in the surrounding medium, the following hypothesis can be proposed to explain this process. The interaction of ACh with the receptor activates the system, namely, the ionophore is converted to a conducting state. This process is accompanied by dissociation of calcium ions (Watkins, 1965) the concentration of which in the membrane determines the state of ionophore gates. If ACh acts for a sufficiently long time or is applied very frequently, free calcium accumulates near the ionophore and inhibits activation. This binding of calcium at certain parts of the ionophore might be the cause of desensitization. Factors that are able either to increase the calcium concentration in the membrane or to compete with calcium for binding to appropriate sites in the system lead to changes of the desensitization rate. After brief exposure to ACh (as in the case of e.p.ps) these processes do not take place (Magazanik & Vyskočil, 1970). It is not quite clear what duration and intensity of ACh response are required to initiate desensitization.

The proposed nonreceptor mechanism of desensitization does not exclude alterations of the receptor macromolecule in the process of desensitization. At present, however, direct methods of measuring changes of the receptor are not available. Therefore, it is difficult to assess the significance of interactions between ACh or its antagonists with desensitized receptors. The solution of this question may be found when attempts to isolate components of the receptor system and to analyse their function prove successful.

Finally, it remains to say that the nature of desensitization is interesting not only as a significant membrane phenomenon, but also as a possible tool for investigation of a more important problem—the arrangement and sequence of events in the activation of the postsynaptic membrane.

## REFERENCES

BARNARD, E. A., WIECKOWSKI, J. & CHIU, T. H. (1971). *Nature, Lond.*, **234**, 207.
BROWN, G. L., DALE, H. H. & FELDBERG, W. (1936). *J. Physiol., Lond.*, **87**, 394.
CHANGEUX, J.-P., KASAI, M. & LEE, C.-Y. (1970). *Proc. natn. Acad. Sci., U.S.A.*, **67**, 1241.
CHANGEUX, J.-P., MEUNIER, J.-C. & HUCHET, M. (1971). *Mol. Pharmac.*, **7**, 538.
COWAN, S. L. (1936). *J. Physiol., Lond.*, **88**, 3P.
DEL CASTILLO, J. & KATZ, B. (1955). *J. Physiol., Lond.*, **128**, 157.
DEL CASTILLO, J. & KATZ, B. (1957). *Proc. Roy. Soc.*, B, **339**, 146.
FATT, P. (1950). *J. Physiol., Lond.*, **111**, 408.
JENKINSON, D. H., STAMENOVIC, B. A. & WHITAKER, B. D. L. (1968). *J. Physiol., Lond.*, **195**, 743.
JENKINSON, D. H. & TERRAR, D. (1973). *Br. J. Pharmac.*, in press.
JENSEN, D. W. (1972). *Comp. Biochem. Physiol.*, **41**A, 685.
KATZ, B. & MILEDI, R. (1967). *Nature, Lond.*, **215**, 651.
KATZ, B. & THESLEFF, S. (1957). *J. Physiol., Lond.*, **138**, 63.
KARLIN, A. (1967). *Proc. natn. Acad. Sci., U.S.A.*, **58**, 1162.

LESTER, H. A. (1970). *Nature, Lond.*, **227**, 727.
LESTER, H. A. (1972). *Mol. Pharmac.*, **8**, 632.
LI, C.-L. & GOURAS, P. (1958). *Am. J. Physiol.*, **192**, 464.
MAGAZANIK, L. G. (1968). *Biofisica*, **13**, 199 (in Russian).
MAGAZANIK, L. G. (1969). *Sechenov J. Physiol.*, **56**, 582 (in Russian).
MAGAZANIK, L. G. (1970a). *Bull. exp. Biol. & Med.*, n. **3**, 10 (in Russian).
MAGAZANIK, L. G. (1970b). *Proc. XI USSR Physiol. Soc. Meet.*, **1**, 13 (in Russian).
MAGAZANIK, L. G. (1971a). *Sechenov J. Physiol.*, **57**, 1313 (in Russian).
MAGAZANIK, L. G. (1971b). *Pharmacol. a. Toxicol.*, n. **3**, 292 (in Russian).
MAGAZANIK, L. G. & SHEKHIREV, N. N. (1970). *Sechenov J. Physiol.*, **56**, 582 (in Russian).
MAGAZANIK, L. G. & VYSKOČIL, F. (1970). *J. Physiol., Lond.*, **210**, 507.
MAGAZANIK, L. G. & VYSKOČIL, F. (1972a). *J. evolut. Biochem. a. Physiol.*, **8**, 555 (in Russian).
MAGAZANIK, L. G. & VYSKOČIL, F. (1972b). *Brain Res.*, **48**, 420.
MANTHEY, A. A. (1966). *J. gen. Physiol.*, **49**, 963.
MILEDI, R., MOLINOFF, P. & POTTER, L. T. (1971). *Nature, Lond.*, **229**, 554.
MILEDI, R. & POTTER, L. T. (1971). *Nature, Lond.*, **233**, 599.
NASTUK, W. L. (1967). *Fedn Proc.*, **26**, 1639.
NASTUK, W. L. & LIU, J. H. (1966). *Science, N.Y.*, **154**, 266.
PARSONS, R. L. (1969). *Am. J. Physiol.*, **217**, 805.
RANG, H. P. & RITTER, J. M. (1969). *Mol. Pharmac.*, **5**, 394.
RANG, H. P. & RITTER, J. M. (1970a). *Mol. Pharmac.*, **6**, 357.
RANG, H. P. & RITTER, J. M. (1970b). *Mol. Pharmac.*, **6**, 383.
THESLEFF, S. (1955). *Acta physiol. scand.*, **34**, 218.
THESLEFF, S. (1960). *Physiol. Rev.*, **40**, 734.
VYSKOČIL, F. & MAGAZANIK, L. G. (1972). *Brain Res.*, **48**, 417.
WATKINS, J. C. (1965). *J. Theor. Biol.*, **9**, 37.
WAUD, D. R. (1968). *Pharmac. Rev.*, **20**, 49.

# FUNCTIONAL PROPERTIES OF RECEPTORS IN STRIATED MUSCLE

S. THESLEFF

*Institute of Pharmacology, University of Lund, Lund, Sweden*

A mammalian striated muscle has cholinergic receptors for chemical stimulation and an action potential mechanism for electrical excitation. With chemical stimuli the receptors are activated and this causes a graded membrane depolarization through the simultaneous opening of channels for sodium and potassium ions across the membrane. With electrical stimulation on the other hand, the membrane depolarization produced by the electric current, triggers a selective, voltage-dependent and short-lasting increase in the permeability of the muscle membrane to sodium ions followed in time by an opposite potassium current. Chemical and electrical stimuli thus produce in some respects similar effects, that is, both cause the opening of membrane channels for sodium and potassium ions, but in other aspects they are markedly different.

Despite fundamental differences between the chemical activation of cholinergic receptors and the electrically induced action potential the experimental results which I will present indicate that a connection exists between the mechanisms underlying the two types of membrane permeability increase.

In innervated mammalian skeletal muscle cholinergic receptors are present only in the limited area of the synaptic region, and therefore occupy a very minor part of the muscle membrane. Following denervation, however, cholinergic receptors develop in the entire muscle membrane and the muscle cell becomes highly sensitive to applied acetylcholine (Axelsson & Thesleff, 1959). We have examined how the electrical excitability of the muscle fibre, that is, the action potential, is modified when cholinergic receptors develop in denervated mammalian muscle (Redfern & Thesleff, 1971a). As a measure of action current we used the rate of rise of the action potential in fibres locally polarized to −90 mV, a voltage level at which maximal rates of rise are recorded (Redfern & Thesleff, 1971a). Fig. 1 shows that the average maximal rate of rise of the action potential is reduced on the 2nd day following denervation from 630 V/s to 370 V/s. During the subsequent week the rate of rise of the spike remains at about this low level. Denervation not only reduces the rate of rise of the action potential but also reduces its rate of

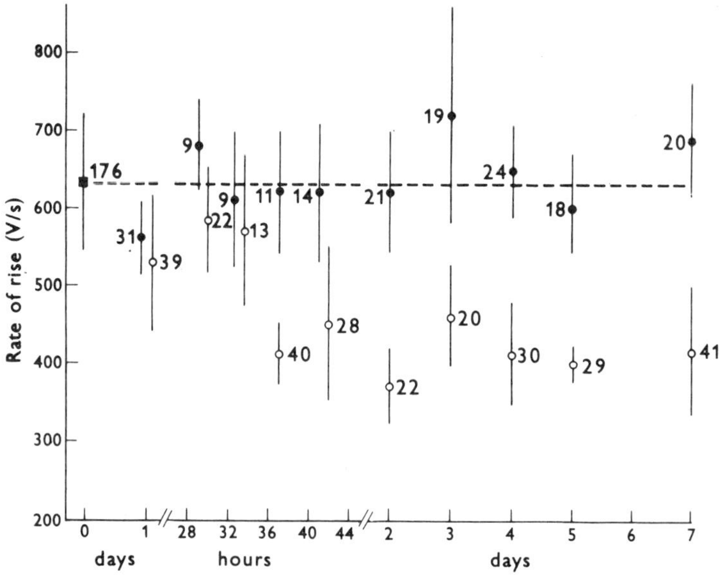


FIG. 1. The maximal rate of rise of action potential (ordinate) in extensor digitorum longus muscles of the rat. (○), Values from muscles denervated for the time shown by the abscissa; (●), values from the contralateral innervated muscle. Each value is the mean ± S.D. and the adjacent figure indicates the number of fibres examined. The mean value for all the innervated muscles is shown by the value at zero time and by the broken line. (Redfern & Thesleff, 1971a.)

repolarization and prolongs its duration (Fig. 2). Apparently denervation reduces either the number or the efficiency of the membrane channels responsible for the action current.

In addition to reducing the action current, denervation also alters the physicochemical properties of the membrane sites responsible for spike generation. Tetrodotoxin (TTX) is an agent that selectively blocks the inward sodium current of the action potential, thus completely blocking spike generation in skeletal muscle and in nerve. Following denervation, however, skeletal muscle fibres develop action potentials resistant to even very high concentrations of TTX ($10^{-6}$ M) as shown in Fig. 2. It should be mentioned that in spite of being TTX-resistant the action current of these potentials is still carried by sodium ions (Redfern & Thesleff, 1971b). In rat muscle TTX-resistant action potentials appear on the 2nd day following denervation, that is, at about the same time that the reduction in the rate of rise of the action current is observed. As shown by the graph in Fig. 3 the TTX-resistant action potentials reach a maximum rate of rise close to 300 V/s by the 4th–5th day after denervation.

The reduction in action current and the appearance of TTX-resistant action potentials occurred 2–3 days after denervation, which is the time when extrajunctional cholinergic receptors are known to start to form in the

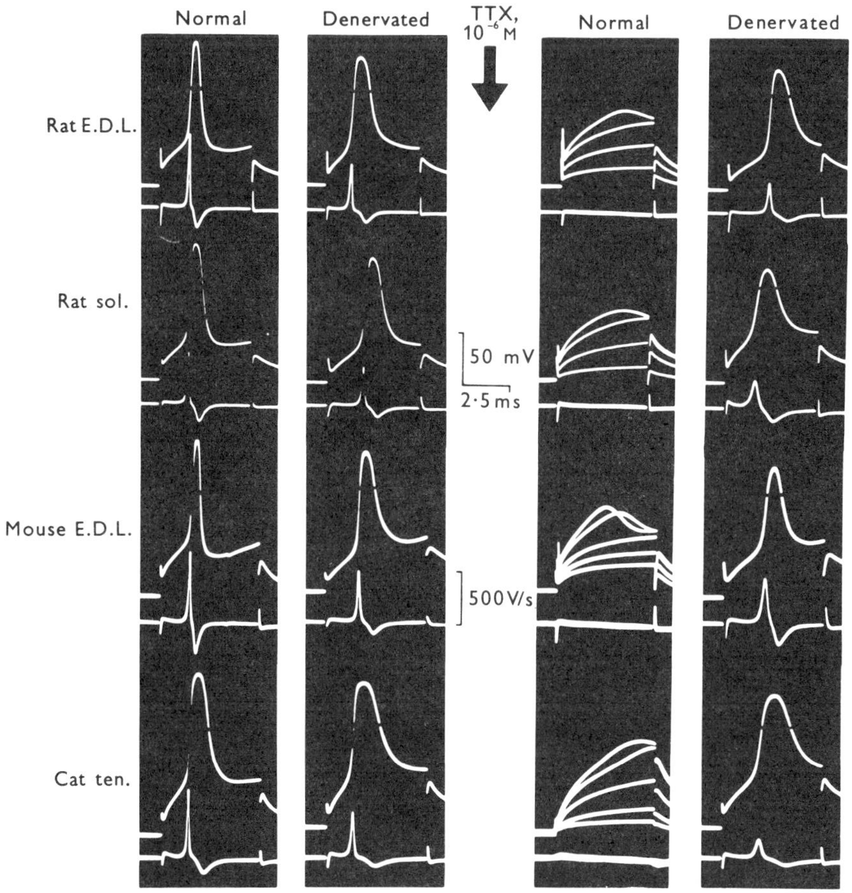


FIG. 2. Intracellular recordings of a typical action potential (upper trace) and its first derivative (lower trace) in innervated and in 6–7 days denervated rat extensor digitorum longus (E.D.L.), soleus (sol.), mouse E.D.L. and cat tenuissimus (ten.) muscles. The records in the left-hand panel were obtained in the absence of TTX and those in the right-hand panel in the presence of $10^{-6}$ M TTX. The break in the action potential tracing indicates the zero potential level of the cell.

membrane. It was therefore of interest to examine whether a temporal and spatial relationship existed between the formation of cholinergic receptors and the changes in the action potential. In Fig. 4 is plotted the time course of the development of TTX-resistant action potentials and of extrajunctional cholinergic sensitivity as determined by microionophoretic application of the drug to membrane 'spots'. From these experiments it appears that TTX resistance precedes the development of cholinergic receptors by about 24 h. A more quantitative measure of the development of extrajunctional cholinergic receptors is the determination of the number of binding sites for a purified

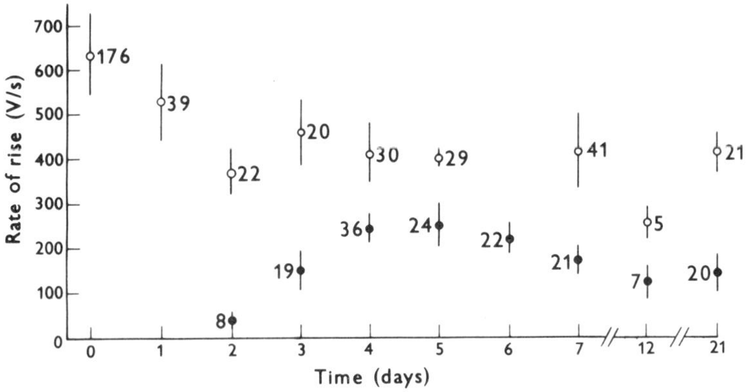


FIG. 3. The time course of the development of TTX-resistant action potentials in the denervated extensor digitorum longus muscle of the rat. (●), Values from muscles in the presence of $10^{-6}$ M TTX; (○), values from muscles in the absence of this drug. The values are the means ± S.D. and the adjacent figures indicate the number of fibres examined.

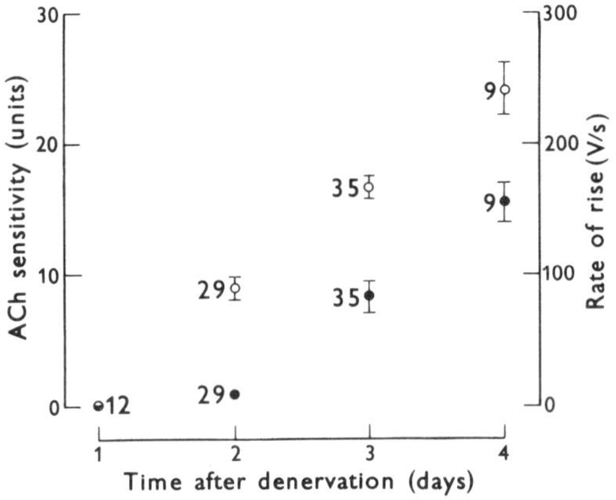


FIG. 4. The time course of the development of TTX-resistant action potentials (○) and extrajunctional cholinergic 'spot' sensitivity (●) during the first 4 days after denervation in the extensor digitorum longus muscle of the rat. The values are the means ± S.E. and the figure next to the mean shows the number of fibres examined. One unit of acetylcholine sensitivity equals 1 mV depolarization produced by $10^{-9}$ coulombs passed through the pipette. (Harris & Thesleff, 1971.)

cobra (*Naja naja siamensis*) toxin. This neurotoxin binds, in an apparently irreversible manner, and with high specificity, to cholinergic receptors in muscle (Lester, 1970; Eaker, Harris & Thesleff, 1971; Grampp & Thesleff, unpublished observation). As shown by Fig. 5 a close correlation is observed between the increase in the number of binding sites for the neurotoxin in the denervated mouse extensor muscle and the rate of rise of the action potential in the presence of TTX $10^{-6}$ M. Table 1 gives the particulars of the action

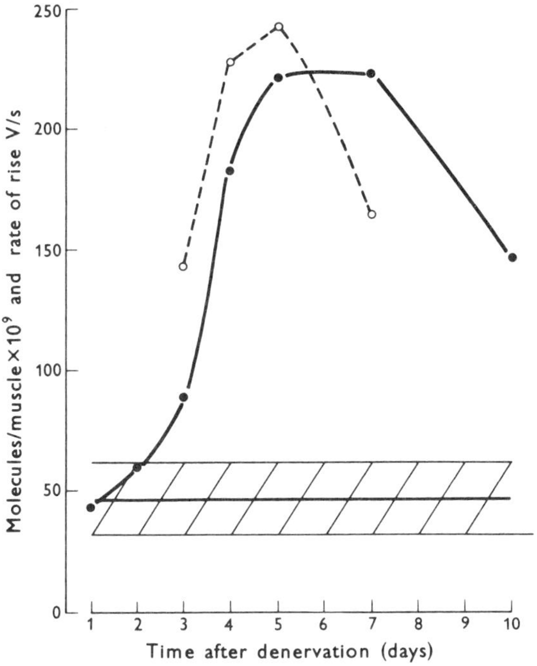


FIG. 5. The mean number of molecules of the acetylated *Naja naja* toxin (●) bound to the extensor digitorum longus muscle of the mouse, denervated for 1–10 days (abscissa). The mean ±S.E. number of molecules bound to the contralateral innervated muscle is indicated by the solid line and the hatched area. Each value is the mean of 6 muscles. (○), The mean maximal rate of rise of the action potential in the presence of TTX $10^{-6}$ M. Each value is the mean of 20 fibres in 3 muscles, see Table 1. Two days after denervation a TTX-resistant action potential was recorded in only one fibre out of 45 examined.

TABLE 1. *Effective denervation on membrane properties of muscle fibres*

| Days after denervation | Resting membrane potential mV | Rate of rise V/s | Threshold potential mV | Overshoot mV |
|---|---|---|---|---|
| 3 | 59·5±0·91 | 143·5±17·1 | 42·9±0·65 | 19·4±1·75 |
| 4 | 59·3±0·85 | 227·2±13·3 | 48·8±0·56 | 28·0±1·24 |
| 5 | 63·4±0·96 | 242·1± 5·4 | 50·6±0·50 | 31·7±0·67 |
| 7 | 64·4±1·00 | 164·1±10·9 | 52·4±0·80 | 21·2±1·16 |

The mean values ±S.E. ($n$=20) of resting membrane potential, maximal rate of rise of the action potential, the threshold potential for spike generation and the 'overshoot' of the action potential in denervated mouse extensor digitorum longus muscle in the presence of TTX $10^{-6}$ M.

potential in the mouse extensor digitorum longus muscle in the presence of TTX, 3–7 days after denervation.

In the rat diaphragm muscle the acetylcholine sensitive area of the endplate region starts to increase in size on the 2nd day following denervation. The acetylcholine sensitivity spreads gradually away from the endplate towards the ends of the muscle fibre and by one week after denervation the entire cell has a high sensitivity to applied acetylcholine (Elmqvist & Thesleff, 1960). To study a possible spatial correlation between the appearance of cholinergic receptors and the presence of TTX-resistant action potentials experiments were made in which action potentials were recorded in the endplate region and 3–4 mm away from the endplate in hemidiaphragm muscles denervated 2, 3 and 7 days previously (Redfern & Thesleff, 1971b). Fig. 6 shows that 2 days after denervation in the presence of TTX, a regenerative response is recorded in the endplate region but not in other parts of the fibre. By 3 days the generation of TTX-resistant action potentials improved in the endplate region and the first indication of a regenerative response was observed outside this region. One week following denervation TTX-resistant spikes were recorded along the entire length of the muscle fibre, although the rate of rise was still somewhat higher in spikes recorded from the endplate region. It thus appears that in the denervated muscle fibre TTX-resistant action potentials have the same spatial and temporal distribution as cholinergic receptors.

Denervation is not a prerequisite for the formation of extrajunctional

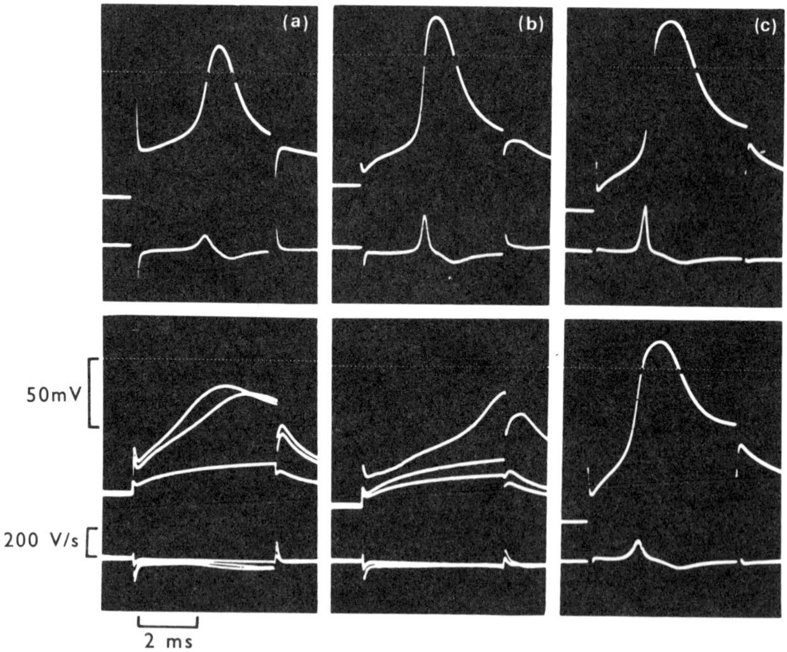


FIG. 6. The upper records are typical action potentials from the endplate region of rat diaphragm muscles denervated for 2 days (a), 3 days (b) and 7 days (c). The lower records show the responses obtained in fibres 3–4 mm away from the endplate. The dotted line shows the zero potential level of the cell. (Redfern & Thesleff, 1971b.)

receptors. Katz & Miledi (1964) have shown that local injury to innervated muscles induces acetylcholine sensitivity in the membrane areas close to the site of injury. When fibres of such muscles were examined for the presence of acetylcholine sensitivity and for their ability to produce TTX-resistant action potentials it was observed that whenever a part of the membrane was sensitive to acetylcholine it also produced a TTX-resistant spike. In other parts of the fibre TTX blocked the action potential (Redfern & Thesleff, 1971b).

Cholinergic receptors are associated with membrane proteins and their appearance in denervated muscle is prevented by inhibitors of protein synthesis (Fambrough, 1970). Experiments were therefore made to determine if protein synthesis inhibitors like actinomycin D, chloramphenicol and cycloheximide, in addition to blocking receptor formation in denervated muscle, would also prevent the reduction in action current and the development of TTX-resistant action potentials (Grampp, Harris & Thesleff, 1972). Administration of a single intraperitoneal injection of actinomycin D (0·5 mg/kg) to adult mice blocked the development of TTX-resistant action potentials as shown in Fig. 7. The blocking effect of this dose of actinomycin D lasted about 4 days as shown in Fig. 8. The development of extrajunctional cholinergic receptors was inhibited for a similar length of time. The post-denervation fall in the maximum rate of rise of the muscle fibre action potential was, however, relatively little affected. Chloramphenicol and cycloheximide in appropriate dosages had effects similar to those of actinomycin D.

From these results it seems reasonable to conclude that, following denervation, the formation of cholinergic receptors as well as of TTX-resistant action potentials depends upon the synthesis of new proteins.

It was of interest that actinomycin D was capable of inhibiting the denervation changes only when given within the first 2 days after denervation (Fig. 9). When actinomycin D was given on the 3rd day after denervation TTX-resistant action potentials and cholinergic receptors developed exactly as in denervated muscles from untreated animals. Similarly, actinomycin D treatment failed to affect cholinergic receptors and TTX-resistant spikes once they were present in the muscle. These findings show that it is the early stage of denervation that provides the induction for the synthesis of the proteins that lead to the formation of extrajunctional cholinergic receptors and of TTX-resistant action potentials.

The results reported can be summarized by saying that denervation of mammalian striated muscle causes a reduction of the maximal rate of rise of the action potential and that at the same time the action potential becomes resistant to the blocking effect of TTX. These changes in the action potential coincide temporally as well as spatially with the development of extrajunctional cholinergic receptors in the muscle membrane. Furthermore, the development of TTX-resistant action potentials and of cholinergic receptors is dependent upon the synthesis of proteins.

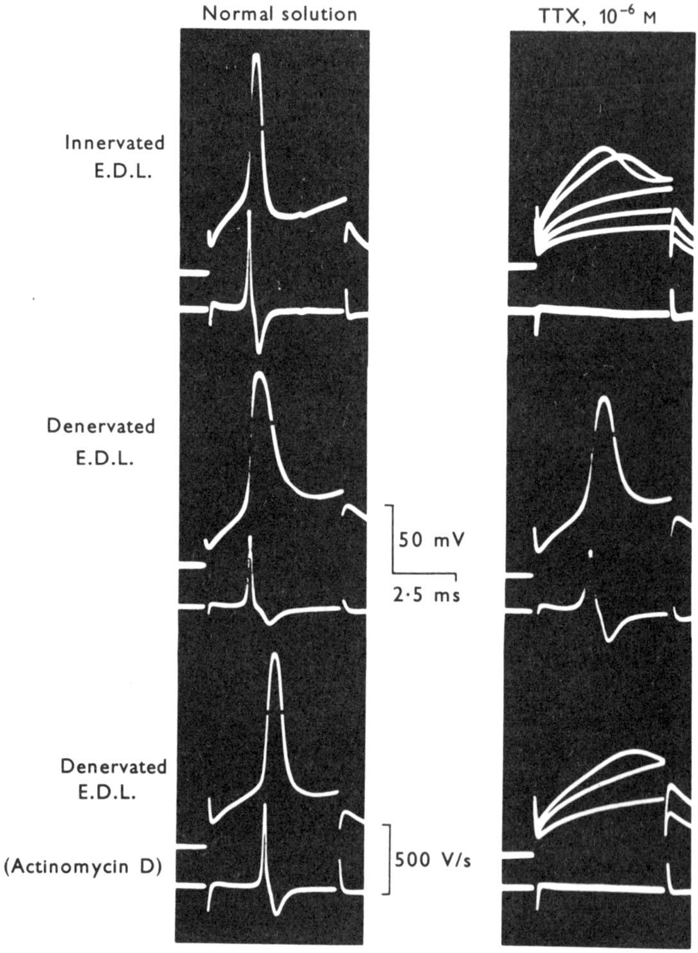


FIG. 7. Action potentials and their first derivative recorded in innervated and 4 days denervated extensor digitorum longus (E.D.L.) muscles of the mouse. Note that TTX blocks action potentials in the innervated muscle and in the denervated muscle from actinomycin D treated animals. The break in the action potential tracing indicates the zero potential level of the cell. Actinomycin D was given 1 day after denervation. (Grampp, Harris & Thesleff, 1972.)

Assuming that the observed relationship between action potential changes and the appearance of cholinergic receptors is not coincidental several possible explanations can be advanced.

A relatively simple explanation would be that cholinergic receptors, when developing in extrajunctional regions, might cover or otherwise interfere with the ionophores responsible for the action potential and thereby reduce their efficiency as well as protect them from the access of the TTX molecule.

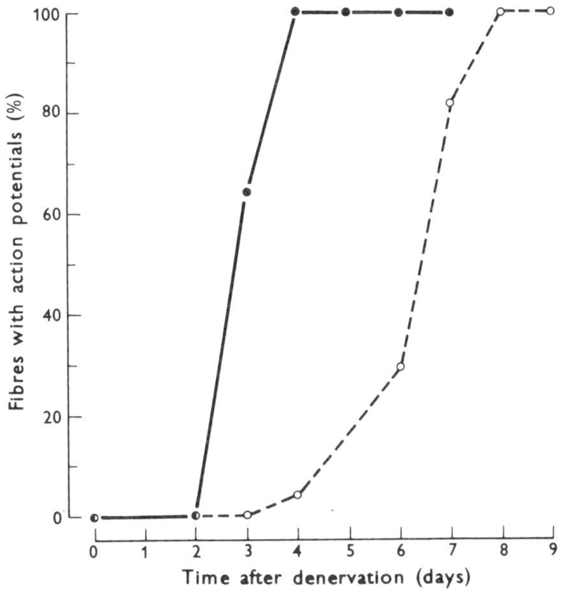


FIG. 8. The effect of actinomycin D on the development of TTX-resistant action potentials in denervated extensor digitorum longus (E.D.L.) muscles of the mouse. The number of fibres responding with TTX-resistant action potentials is expressed as % of the fibres investigated. (○), Actinomycin D treated animals; (●), untreated animals. (Grampp, Harris & Thesleff, 1972.)

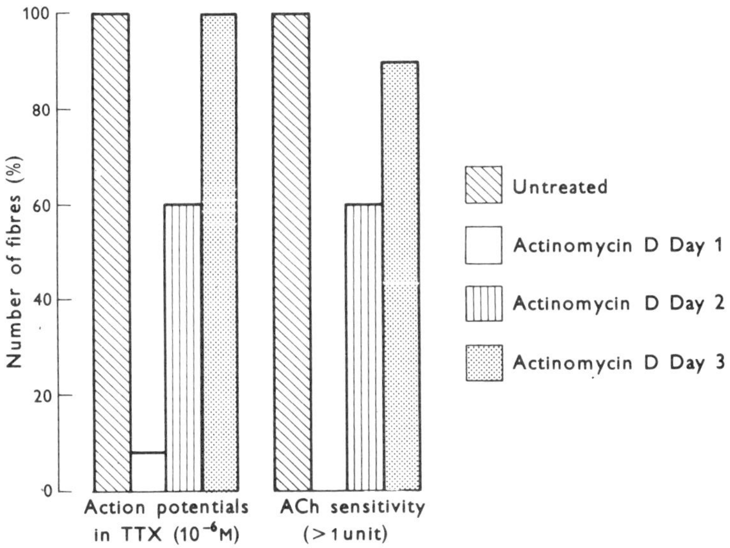


FIG. 9. Effect of actinomycin D administered 1, 2 and 3 days after denervation on the development of TTX-resistant action potentials (left-hand panel) and extrajunctional acetylcholine sensitivity (right-hand panel) in the extensor digitorum longus muscle of the mouse.

However, the findings of Miledi & Potter (1971) with α-bungarotoxin, as well as our own studies with the cobra neurotoxin (Grampp & Thesleff, unpublished observations), indicate that the number of cholinergic receptors in extrajunctional regions is unexpectedly small. Our estimates from measurements on the extensor digitorum longus muscle of the mouse (see Fig. 5) gave an average of $4{\cdot}3 \times 10^7$ binding sites per innervated fibre (presumably confined to the endplate region) and is thus similar to the values obtained by Miledi & Potter (1971) and Barnard, Wieckowski & Chiu (1971). Three days after denervation each fibre contained $8{\cdot}1 \times 10^7$ binding sites and by 5 days about $2 \times 10^8$ sites, which represents only a 5-fold increase as compared with an innervated fibre. These numbers give an estimated receptor density of roughly 10 000/$\mu$m$^2$ in the endplate membrane and of 100/$\mu$m$^2$ at extrajunctional membrane sites in the muscle 5 days after denervation. With such a low receptor density in extrajunctional regions possibly only $10^{-4}$ of the total membrane area is covered by receptors and it is therefore difficult to see how the presence of receptors could structurally interfere with action potential ionophores. To maintain the hypothesis one would have to postulate that receptors preferentially form in close proximity to existing ionophores for the action current.

Another, but more speculative, possibility is that, following denervation, action potential generating structures change so that they also function as extrajunctional cholinergic receptors. Such a dual function could only characterize extrajunctional cholinergic receptor molecules, since TTX blocks spike generation in the innervated endplate despite its high receptor density. It should be mentioned that extrajunctional receptors have physicochemical properties that apparently differ from those of junctional ones (Beránek & Vyskočil, 1967; Feltz & Mallart, 1971a,b). Of particular interest is that Lømo & Rosenthal (1972) have observed that electrical stimulation of denervated rat muscle prevents the formation of extrajunctional cholinergic receptors, or reduces their number towards normal once they have appeared. Former junctional receptors were unaffected by electrical stimulation. Against the hypothesis of a dual function speaks, however, the observation that drugs which reversibly or irreversibly block cholinergic receptors fail to affect the TTX-resistant action potential (Harris & Thesleff, 1971).

Obviously, our knowledge of receptor mechanisms and of the physicochemical nature of the action potential is too rudimentary to allow anything but speculations as to the cause of the apparent connection between the two types of excitation processes.

Irrespective of the basis for the postdenervation changes in the action potential, the TTX-resistant spike is an important and apparently specific sign of denervation. It has the advantage over the increase in extrajunctional cholinergic sensitivity that it is an all-or-none phenomenon which is readily observed in the muscle. We have used the presence of TTX-resistant action potentials as a tool for studying the importance of neurotrophic influences

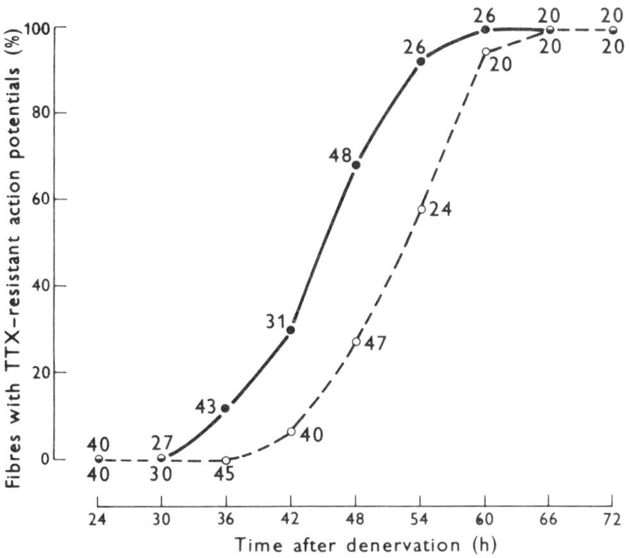


FIG. 10. Number of TTX-resistant action potentials (as %) in the rat extensor digitorum longus muscle at various times after denervation. The muscles were denervated 'close' (●——●) or 'distant' (○----○). (Harris & Thesleff, 1972.)

(Harris & Thesleff, 1972). Experiments were made in which the nerve to the extensor digitorum longus muscle of adult rats was cut either 'close' to the muscle at the knee or 'distant' by cutting the sciatic nerve in the sciatic foramen. The difference in nerve stump length achieved by cutting at the two levels was approximately 3 cm. In 'close' denervated muscles TTX-resistant action potentials appeared about 6 h earlier than in 'distant' denervated ones (Fig. 10). Since electrical and mechanical inactivity resulted in the muscle at the moment when the nerve was cut the results imply that a neurotrophic influence was exerted by the longer nerve stump.

## REFERENCES

Axelsson, J. & Thesleff, S. (1959). *J. Physiol., Lond.*, **149**, 178.
Barnard, E. A., Wieckowski, J. & Chiu, T. H. (1971). *Nature, Lond.*, **234**, 207.
Beránek, R. & Vyskočil, F. (1967). *J. Physiol., Lond.*, **188**, 53.
Eaker, D., Harris, J. B. & Thesleff, S. (1971). *Eur. J. Pharmac.*, **15**, 254.
Elmqvist, D. & Thesleff, S. (1960). *Acta pharmac. toxic.*, **17**, 84.
Fambrough, D. M. (1970). *Science, N.Y.*, **168**, 372.
Feltz, A. & Mallart, A. (1971a). *J. Physiol., Lond.*, **218**, 85.
Feltz, A. & Mallart, A. (1971b). *J. Physiol., Lond.*, **218**, 101.
Grampp, W., Harris, J. B. & Thesleff, S. (1972). *J. Physiol., Lond.*, **221**, 743.
Harris, J. B. & Thesleff, S. (1971). *Acta physiol. scand.*, **83**, 382.
Harris, J. B. & Thesleff, S. (1972). *Nature, New Biol., Lond.*, **236**, 60.
Katz, B. & Miledi, R. (1964). *J. Physiol., Lond.*, **170**, 389.
Lester, H. A. (1970). *Nature, Lond.*, **227**, 727.

Lømo, T. & Rosenthal, J. (1972). *J. Physiol., Lond.*, **221**, 493.
Miledi, R. & Potter, L. T. (1971). *Nature, Lond.*, **233**, 599.
Redfern, P. & Thesleff, S. (1971a). *Acta physiol. scand.*, **81**, 557.
Redfern, P. & Thesleff, S. (1971b). *Acta physiol. scand.*, **82**, 70.

## DISCUSSION

*Vrbová (Birmingham)*

Why do you suggest that new receptors are synthesized after denervation? Is it not possible that pre-existing receptors are 'uncovered' after denervation?

*Thesleff (Lund)*

Our results indicate that the formation of extrajunctional cholinergic receptors depends upon protein synthesis. The results, however, give no clue as to whether new receptor molecules were synthesized, 'uncovered' or otherwise made available for the interaction with acetylcholine.

*Changeux (Paris)*

Is the action potential of embryonic muscle sensitive to block by TTX?

*Thesleff (Lund)*

Embryonic muscle contracts spontaneously and these contractions are not abolished by TTX, so it appears that the action potential is resistant to the blocking effect. We have not made a quantitative study.

*Barnard (New York)*

Does your estimate of 100 sites/$\mu m^2$ on the surface of denervated muscle represent a uniform distribution, or are the receptors more abundant at the original endplates?

*Thesleff (Lund)*

Our estimates of receptor densities in denervated muscle are based upon averages for the whole muscle and give no information as to the density at the original endplate.

*Karlin (New York)*

Is the TTX-resistant spike in denervated muscle affected by agents which specifically block the ACh-receptor?

*Thesleff (Lund)*

A number of drugs capable of blocking or modifying the response to acetylcholine have been studied for their effect on the TTX-resistant action potential (Harris & Thesleff, 1971). None of these agents affected the TTX-resistant action potential. As long as we do not know how the receptor is coupled to the ionophore these negative results can be considered only as circumstantial evidence against the possibility that the TTX-resistant action potential generating site is identical or closely related to the extrajunctional cholinergic receptor.

# COOPERATIVITY OF THE ELECTROPLAX MEMBRANE

T. R. PODLESKI

*Section of Neurobiology and Behavior, Cornell University, Ithaca, N.Y. 14850, USA*

Considerable attention has been given to the molecular basis of 'cooperativity' in macromolecules (Hill, 1910; Adair, 1925; Monod, Wyman & Changeux, 1965; Koshland & Neet, 1968; Perutz, 1969; Edelstein, 1971) and in biological membranes (Changeux, 1969). Cooperativity is defined generally as a reaction of order greater than one, and, in biology, possibly the best known example of a cooperative reaction is the binding of oxygen to haemoglobin. The binding curve for this reaction is sigmoid, and sigmoid binding curves have proved often to be the first indication of a cooperative reaction.

In the area of membrane physiology there are many examples of high-order reactions. One example is the Hodgkin–Huxley ionic model for the action potential of excitable cells (Hodgkin & Huxley, 1952). These authors showed that, with the giant axon of *Sepia*, the rise in sodium and potassium conductances occurred only after a delay following a step depolarization of the membrane. Furthermore, the rise in both conductances as a function of time was sigmoid. These general features have now been observed with many electrically excitable membranes (Grundfest, 1966), and it is likely that such cooperative phenomena are due to some general molecular property of these membranes.

While several molecular interpretations have been suggested for the cooperativity observed in both macromolecules and membranes, no one model has been proven experimentally. A model of general interest for the discussion on membranes is illustrated in Fig. 1. The first model (Model 1) resembles the one proposed by Hodgkin & Huxley, that is, the high-conductance form of a carrier system requires the activation of more than one carrier molecule. In the second model (Model 2) depicted in Fig. 1 two subunits of a carrier or receptor molecule are shown. In the case under consideration, the inactive form is the low-conducting conformation and the active form is the high-conducting conformation. Cooperativity will occur if the conformational transition of the two subunits is linked. In the limiting case where the two subunits must be occupied in order to cause the transition,

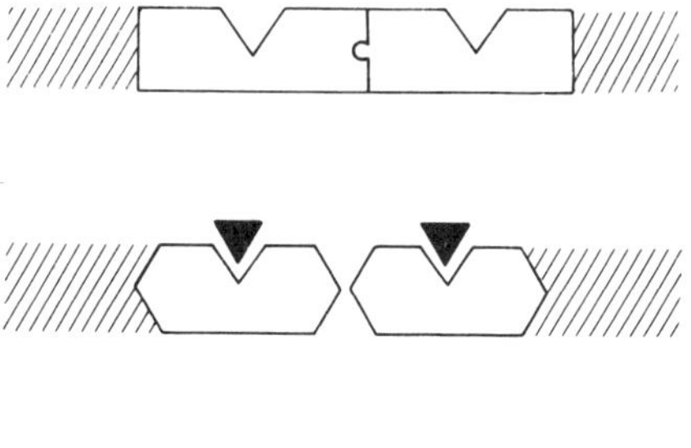


FIG. 1. Schematic drawing of a carrier or receptor that has two binding sites. The two sites are coupled together through molecular interactions of the type discussed in the text.

the reaction in terms of the ligand will be second-order (Model 1). On the other hand, cooperativity will also occur if the two conformations are in equilibrium in the absence of ligand and the ligand has a higher affinity for one state as opposed to the other (Model 2). Model 2 is the one developed by Monod, Wyman & Changeux (1965) in the well-known model for allosteric transitions. Both of these models are of the two-state variety since no intermediate states appear, that is, the carrier is either active or inactive.

To study the cooperative behaviour of a membrane it is convenient to study the changes in membrane properties resulting from the action of well-defined substances. The cases to be discussed in this paper will be examples of changes in membrane permeability elicited by chemical ligands. In these instances it will be shown that the membrane response plotted against concentration of ligand, is sigmoid. In order to quantify the magnitude of the cooperativity it will be convenient to use a method of plotting the data that is referred to as the Hill plot (Hill, 1910). An example of this type of plot is shown in Fig. 2. $\bar{Y}$ is the fraction of the total number of sites bound occupied by ligand molecules. In the region near 50% ligand bound the curve is nearly linear and the slope of this region is greater than 1·0 (Wyman, 1964). In the case shown in Fig. 2 the slope of the broken line is 1·8 and the slope is referred to as the Hill coefficient, $n_H$. For a hyperbolic binding curve $n_H$ is 1·0, whereas for sigmoid curves $n_H$ is greater than 1·0.

The Hill coefficient gives us a method for distinguishing between the two models. Model 1 predicts that the data plotted in the Hill plot will be linear throughout the entire binding region, that is, between 0 and 100% binding. In addition, the Hill coefficient cannot be a non-integer. For the case giving a second-order reaction the Hill coefficient must be equal to 2·0. The second model makes quite different predictions. The data plotted in the Hill plot will not be linear but will follow the solid curve shown in Fig. 2. In addition, the restraint of non-integral numbers for the Hill coefficient does not exist. The maximum Hill coefficient for this model will be 2, but lower values can be anticipated (Wyman, 1964).

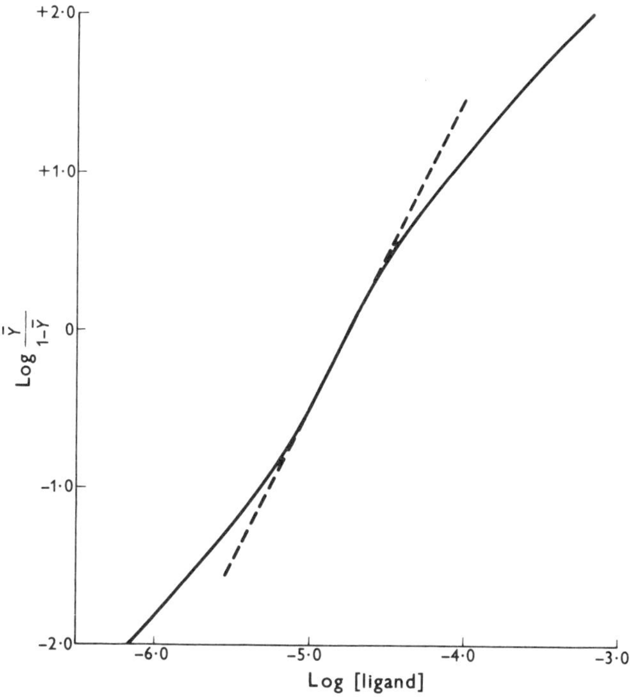


FIG. 2. Hill plot of the binding of a ligand to an oligomeric molecule with two binding sites. $\bar{Y}$ is the fraction of sites occupied by ligand molecules. The solid line represents the binding data; the broken line represents the region where the Hill coefficient is determined. The slope of the solid line at either extreme of binding approaches 1·0.

Fig. 3 shows the membrane response of a single cell (electroplax) isolated from the organ of Sachs of the electric fish *Electrophorus electricus* (Schoffeniels & Nachmansohn, 1957; Higman, Podleski & Bartels, 1963; Karlin, 1967; Changeux & Podleski, 1968). The changes in membrane potential in response to various concentrations of phenyltrimethylammonium (PTA) are shown in the upper portion of this figure. The relationship between potential change and concentration is definitely sigmoid, as is confirmed in the lower portion of this figure where the data are plotted in a Hill plot. The Hill coefficient is about 1·8. This observation has been confirmed with many cells and different ligands, for example, carbachol and decamethonium. The concentration–effect curves are always sigmoid and have Hill coefficients between 1·6 and 1·9 (Changeux & Podleski, 1968). We have rarely observed a Hill coefficient of 2·0 or greater.

The concentration–effect curves for different ligands on other chemosensitive membranes have also been studied, and Fig. 4 shows the results of Takeuchi & Takeuchi (1969). The biological preparation in this case is

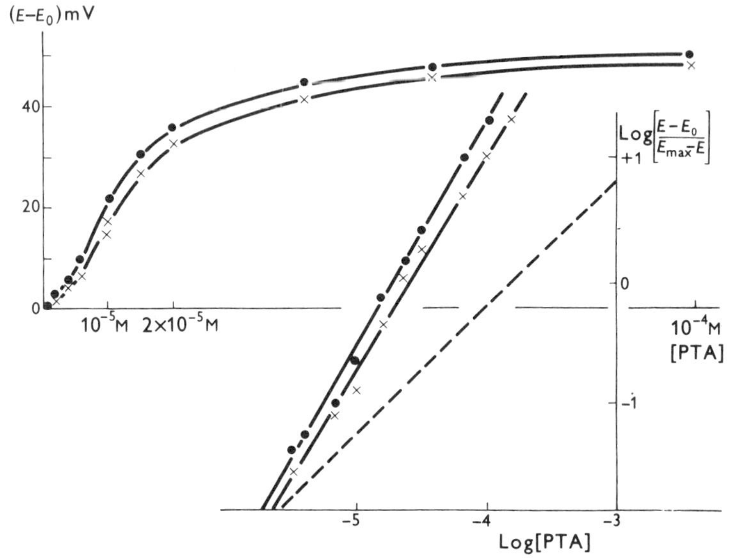


FIG. 3. Upper: the concentration–effect curves of two electroplax cells to phenyltrimethylammonium (PTA). $E_0$ is the membrane potential when no drug is present; $E$ is the potential in the presence of the depolarizing drug; $E_{max}$ is the potential in the presence of a large excess of the depolarizing drug. Lower: the Hill plot of the data shown in the upper figure. The Hill coefficients for the two lines are 1·7. The broken line is a theoretical curve giving a Hill coefficient of 1·0.

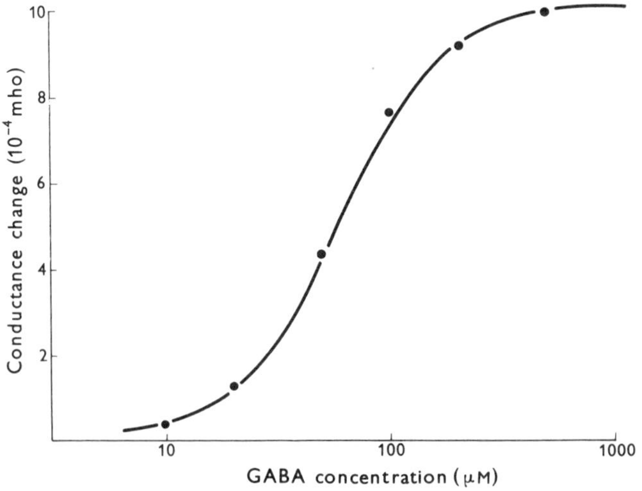


FIG. 4. γ-Aminobutyric acid (GABA) increases the conductance of the postsynaptic membrane of the crayfish neuromuscular junction. The relationship between concentration of GABA and the change in membrane conductance is illustrated. (Reprinted with permission of *J. Physiol., Lond.*)

crayfish muscle and the compound used is $\gamma$-aminobutyric acid. This concentration–effect curve is sigmoid, as is demonstrated in Fig. 5. As with the electroplax data, the Hill plot gives a coefficient larger than 1·0, and according to the observations of Takeuchi & Takeuchi the Hill coefficient is $1{\cdot}9 \pm 0{\cdot}03$. Recently Feltz (1971) has found values for the Hill coefficient between 2·0 and 3·5 for this preparation. Similarly, Rang (1971) reported that the relationship between conductance and concentration of one cholinergic ligand at the neuromuscular junction is definitely sigmoid. This experiment was performed by the use of voltage-clamp procedures and is very strong support for the conductance change being cooperative. There is, therefore, considerable evidence from the study of pharmacological agents that the shape of many concentration–effect curves is not hyperbolic, as had previously been assumed (Clark, 1937), but that the curves are sigmoid.

The two interpretations of these observations that have been suggested correspond to the two models discussed in Fig. 1. The one favoured by

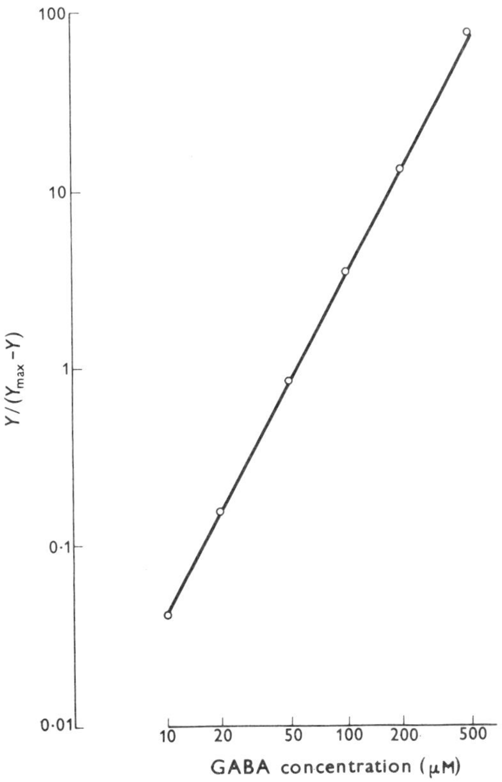


FIG. 5. Hill plot of conductance change produced by GABA at the crayfish neuromuscular junction. $Y$ is the increase in conductance produced by GABA, $Y_{max}$ the maximal increase obtained at high concentrations of GABA. The Hill coefficient is close to 2·0. (Redrawn from Takeuchi & Takeuchi, 1969.)

Takeuchi & Takeuchi (1969) and Feltz (1971) is the one that requires two or more molecules of ligand to be bound to the receptor in order to cause the conformational change giving rise to the increase in conductance. The other interpretation is the allosteric one and two different molecular mechanisms may be proposed to account for the cooperativity. The basic difference between the two allosteric mechanisms is in the structure that takes part in the conformational coupling. In one instance the structure is the receptor molecules themselves and in the other the membrane structure couples the two subunits together (Changeux, Thiery, Tung & Kittel, 1967; Karlin, 1967). In the first case the receptor is proposed to exist as a dimer in the membrane, whereas in the latter case the number of subunits coupled to one another may be larger. In both cases it is assumed that the receptor exists, in the absence of the ligand, in two conformational states. One state is the high-conductance state and the other is the low-conductance state. Ligands that depolarize, such as phenyltrimethylammonium shown in Fig. 2, have a higher affinity for the high-conductance state, and by virtue of this affinity, displace the equilibrium between these two states in favour of the high-conductance state. Different maximum depolarization (Fig. 6) produced

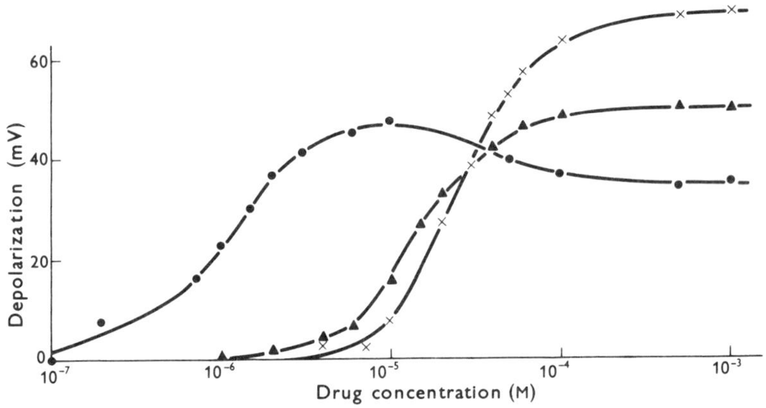


FIG. 6. The concentration–effect curves of the electroplax to three different ligands, carbachol (×), phenyltrimethylammonium (▲), and decamethonium (●).

by different ligands would then be due to the relative affinities that the ligands have for the two states. This difference cannot, incidentally, be attributed, to differences in the permselective change elicited by the three different ligands, since the evidence indicates that the reversal potentials for these ligands are identical (Changeux, Podleski, Kasai & Blumenthal, 1970; Feltz & Mallart, 1971).

There are difficulties in the direct application of these models to the membrane responses described in Figs. 3, 4 and 5. It is difficult, for example, to apply the test suggested by Fig. 2. The Hill coefficients of the data obtained from both the electroplax and crayfish muscle are rarely whole integers, which supports the allosteric model. On the other hand, the Hill plots seem to be perfectly linear; that is, there is no noticeable change in the slope at either end of the concentration–effect curves. The deviations expected on the basis of the allosteric model are, however, small and could possibly fall within the error of the measurements. Additional difficulties arise from our present inability to determine the exact relationship between binding and conductance. In the allosteric model, for example, a clear distinction exists between the 'binding' and 'state' functions (Monod, Wyman & Changeux, 1965). The binding function is the percentage saturation of the receptor sites, whereas the state function refers to the fraction of the protein molecules in one conformation, generally the biologically active conformation. Several authors have suggested that the proper reference between conductance and concentration of ligand is the state function, and several attempts have been made to utilize the behaviour of the state function for predictive purposes (Karlin, 1967; Kasai & Changeux, 1971c; Edelstein, personal communication). At the moment, however, this problem has not been resolved, and undoubtedly new types of experimentation will be needed to resolve it.

Both models proposed in Fig. 1 do, however, require some type of interaction to occur between the two subunits. In the case of the allosteric model the types of interactions expected are well known because of the number of studies done on allosteric proteins (Koshland & Neet, 1968; Perutz, 1969; Edelstein, 1971). One such type of experiment is to determine whether there are conditions in which one can alter the interaction between the subunits. Fig. 7 shows that treatment of the electroplax membrane with dithiothreitol, an agent that reduces disulphide bonds, reduces the cooperative behaviour of the membrane (Karlin, 1967). This experiment can be readily interpreted on the basis of disulphide bonds playing a role in the interaction between subunits. To determine whether this is indeed the proper interpretation will necessitate further experimentation.

A second type of experiment in which it was possible to reduce the Hill coefficient from 1·8 to 1·0 is shown in Fig. 8. In this instance it was shown that very low concentrations of decamethonium were able to reduce the Hill coefficient to 1·0 (Changeux & Podleski, 1968). This experiment has been interpreted as being not only an indication of interaction between sites but also as an indication that decamethonium and carbachol are bound to allosteric sites.

Other experiments have been performed with the idea that decamethonium and carbachol bind to topographically different sites. Figs. 9, 10 and 11 lend support to the idea that the sites for decamethonium and the mono-quaternary ligands, such as carbachol, might be very different from one another.

Firstly, Fig. 9 demonstrates that, while (+)-tubocurarine appears to be a

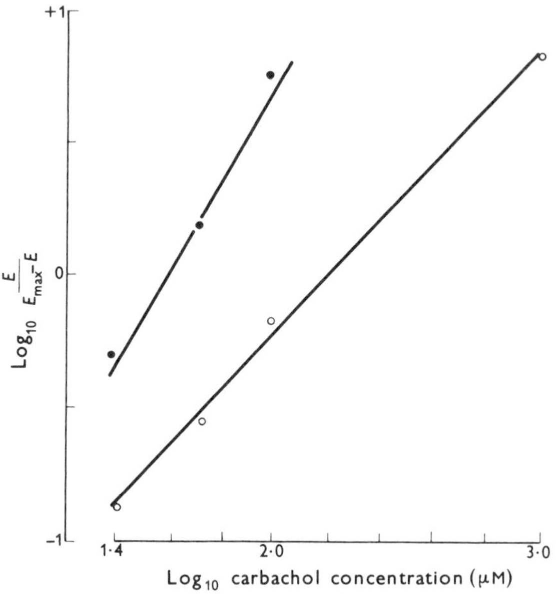


FIG. 7. Hill plot of depolarization of eel electroplax by carbachol. $E$ is the depolarization measured 75 s after addition of carbachol to the solution bathing the innervated surface of the cell; $E_{max}$ is the maximum effect obtainable with a large concentration of carbachol. (●), Control. Hill coefficient = 1·8. (○), After treatment with 1 mM dithiothreitol for 10 min. Hill coefficient = 1·3. (Redrawn from Karlin, 1967.)

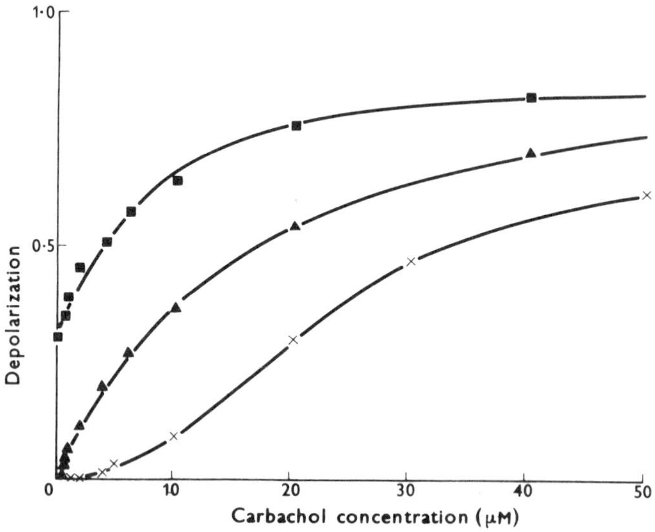


FIG. 8. The effect of two concentrations of decamethonium on the shape of the concentration–effect curve of carbachol. The maximum depolarization obtainable with carbachol is taken as 1·0, and decamethonium does not change the maximum response to carbachol. (×), Control; (▲), in presence of $1{\cdot}5\times10^{-7}$ M decamethonium; (■), in presence of $7{\cdot}5\times10^{-7}$ M decamethonium. (Reprinted with permission of *Proc. natn. Acad. Sci.*)

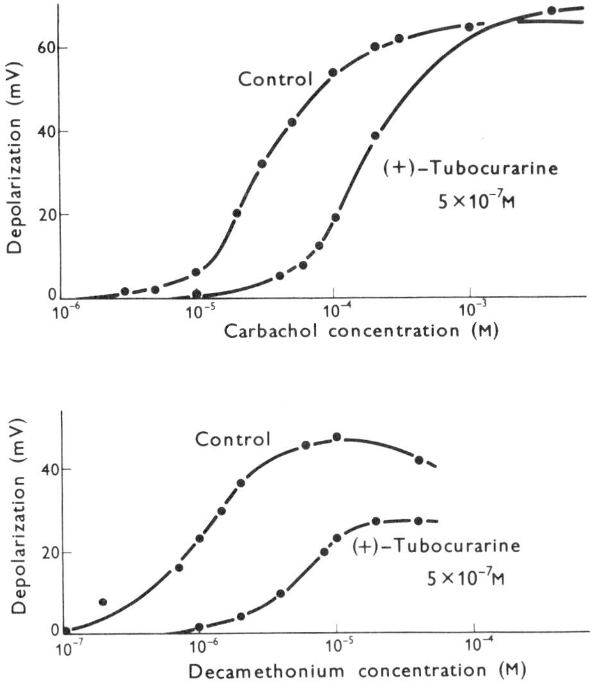


FIG. 9. The response of the electroplax to decamethonium or carbachol in the presence of $5 \times 10^{-7}$ M (+)-tubocurarine.

competitive inhibitor of carbachol, the competition between (+)-tubocurarine and decamethonium is distinctly noncompetitive. This fact is indicated by the reduction in the maximum response of decamethonium in the presence of (+)-tubocurarine. These observations are not, however, incompatible with the sites for decamethonium and carbachol being the same. Recently Edelstein (personal communication) has shown that a similar set of data could be fitted very accurately with the allosteric model (see also Karlin, 1967). Following the formulation of Edelstein, I have found that the data shown in Fig. 9 can also be fitted on the basis of a simple modification of the conformational isomerization constant *L*, which represents the equilibrium constant for the transition from one state to the other in the absence of ligand (Monod, Wyman & Changeux, 1965). This model also predicts that at higher concentration of (+)-tubocurarine the maximum response for carbachol should be reduced. This prediction seems to be supported by the observations of Higman, Podleski & Bartels (1963), although the same may not be true for all cells. The allosteric model is, therefore, successful in predicting the behaviour of some ligands, and similar comparisons may prove useful in determining which of the proposed models is correct.

As yet, however, the allosteric model has not been successful in accounting for several important observations. For example, as shown in Fig. 7, dithiothreitol reduces the activity of carbachol and reduces the Hill coefficient from 1·8 to 1·0. This reducing agent has a markedly different behaviour on the activity of decamethonium (Karlin, 1967; Podleski, Meunier & Changeux, 1969). In Fig. 10, the effects of dithiothreitol on both carbachol and decamethonium are shown. While carbachol is inhibited, decamethonium initially

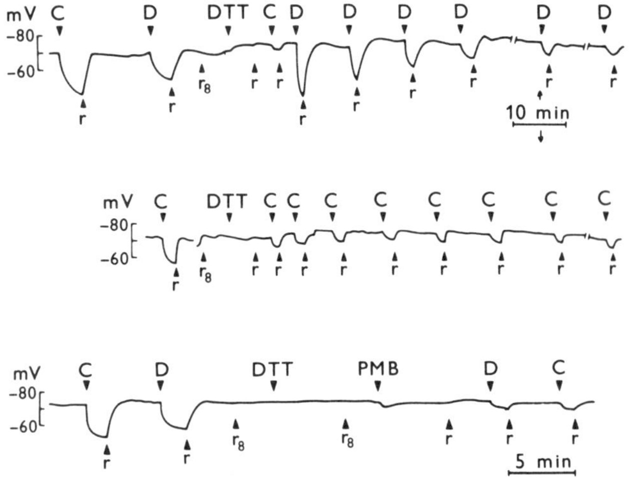


FIG. 10. The tracings show the membrane potential of the electroplax when its innervated surface was exposed to the compounds shown. (C), Carbachol $2 \times 10^{-5}$ M; (D), decamethonium $10^{-6}$ M; (DTT), dithiothreitol $10^{-3}$ M; (PMB), *p*-hydroxymercuribenzoate $10^{-4}$ M. (▲), Wash in control solution. The pH was raised to 8·0 in the washes preceding the application of DTT and PMB. Upper tracing: the response to decamethonium is initially potentiated but then slowly declines after application of DTT. Middle tracing: the response to carbachol is inhibited after DTT and does not change with time. Lower tracing: PMB following DTT inhibits the response to both decamethonium and carbachol. This concentration of PMB does not affect cells that have not been treated with DTT.

is potentiated about twofold. Following the potentiation, however, the response to decamethonium slowly decreases until the response becomes stabilized in an inhibited state. If one treats the membrane with *p*-chloromercuribenzoate after dithiothreitol, the response to decamethonium is inhibited and no potentiation occurs. Since this concentration of *p*-chloromercuribenzoate had no effect on the response to either decamethonium or carbachol in the absence of prior treatment with dithiothreitol, the most likely interpretation of this result is that *p*-chloromercuribenzoate reacts with the liberated sulphydryl groups. It should be noted that the treatment with *p*-chloromercuribenzoate under these conditions did not result in further inhibition of the carbachol response. These results indicate that the sulphydryl groups resulting from the reduction of the disulphide bonds with dithiothreitol are not homogeneous, and that those groups responsible for the potentiation of decamethonium are not the ones responsible for the inhibition of carbachol.

Fig. 11 shows a complete concentration–effect curve to decamethonium before, immediately after and 30 min after dithiothreitol treatment. The Hill coefficients for these three curves are 1·8, 1·8 and 1·0. The initial increase in the response to decamethonium is not accompanied by a change in the Hill coefficient nor in the maximum response. The inhibited response to decamethonium shows both a decrease in the maximum response and the Hill coefficient. Karlin & Bartels (1966) showed that there was no reduction in the maximum response to carbachol after dithiothreitol treatment.

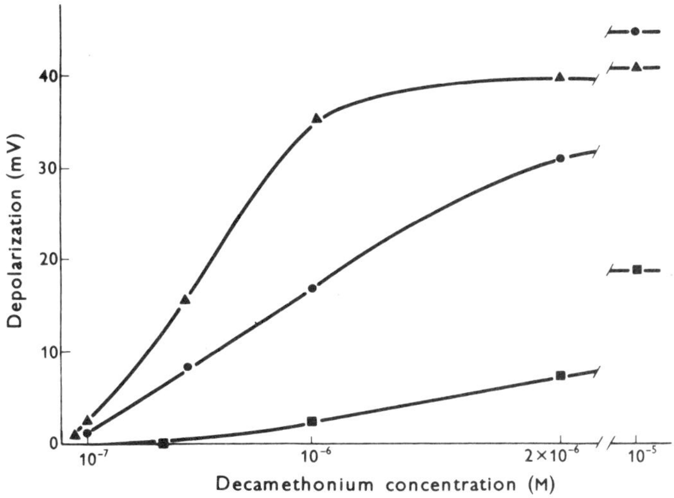


FIG. 11. The response of the electroplax to decamethonium following a 5 min exposure to $10^{-3}$ M dithiothreitol (DTT) at pH 8·0. (●), Control; (▲), immediately after DTT; (■), 30 min after DTT.

The behaviour of the decamethonium and carbachol response with time is shown in Fig. 12. This figure emphasizes the differential effects of dithiothreitol on responses to carbachol and decamethonium. These observations support the suggestion made before concerning the possible separate sites for decamethonium and carbachol. Definite results on this possibility, however, are in all likelihood dependent upon the isolation and characterization of the molecules associated with the membrane. Karlin (1969) has, for example, suggested that decamethonium binds to one of the sulphydryl groups liberated by dithiothreitol.

It might also be mentioned that, while an attractive hypothesis for the effect of time on decamethonium would be the spontaneous oxidation of the sulphydryl groups to incorrect disulphide bonds, possibly even accelerated

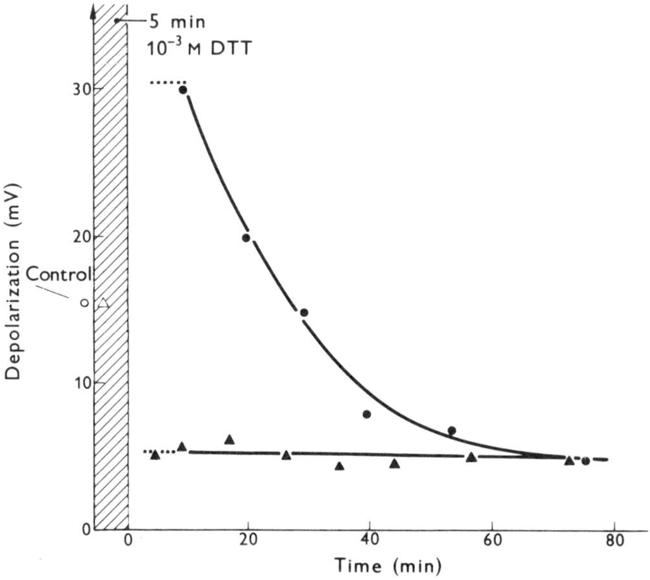


FIG. 12. The response of the electroplax to decamethonium (●), (○) and carbachol (▲), (△) at various times following the treatment with $10^{-3}$ M dithiothreitol. The control responses are indicated at the left margin.

by decamethonium, we were unable to demonstrate any effect of decamethonium on the rate of inactivation. The potentiation, however, does not occur in the presence of dithiothreitol, and the inactivated response seems to be completely restored by oxidizing agents, such as 5,5′-dithio-*bis*(2-nitrobenzoic acid) (DTNB), which makes it unlikely that any oxidation of the sulphydryl bonds has occurred during the application of decamethonium.

In addition to the strictly pharmacological type of experiments, it has become possible to study similar membrane phenomena by using a biochemical preparation of membranes. Changeux, Gautron, Israel & Podleski (1969) and Karlin (1965) have reported techniques for isolating plasma membranes from the electric organ of *Electrophorus electricus*. Two general categories of membranes are isolated and these membranes have different enzymatic activities associated with them (Bauman, Changeux & Benda, 1970) as well as marked differences in the protein patterns observed when using sodium dodecyl sulphate-solubilized membranes on acrylamide gels (Podleski, unpublished observation). Kasai & Changeux (1971a,b,c) have shown that one category of membrane vesicles can be loaded with radioactive sodium and that the flux of sodium is accelerated by the ligands used in Fig. 6. These authors have been able to duplicate most of the observations discussed in Figs. 3, 6, 8 and 9 that were made on single isolated cells, and the correlation between the two types of experiments is very good. For example, the curve relating flux to concentration of ligand is sigmoid and the midpoints of the curves for the various ligands are the same as those observed on the cells.

There does seem to be a paradox, however, in that recently it has become possible to measure the binding of ligands to putative receptor molecules (Kasai & Changeux, 1971c; Eldefrawi, Eldefrawi, Seifert & O'Brien, 1972). In most instances there is no indication of cooperative binding.

It appears, therefore, that the binding of ligands to the sites on the membrane may not in itself account for the cooperativity observed when membrane permeability is the parameter being measured. There are several interpretations of these results (Kasai & Changeux, 1971c). One is that the binding studies result in measuring only the binding to one state of the receptor. This interpretation suggests that some modification in the receptor occurs in the course of its purification. Other interpretations imply that conformational coupling between the receptor sites and some other event might account for the cooperativity. Nachmansohn (1971) has suggested, for example, that the binding of the ligand to the site is just the first step in a multistepped reaction involving the displacement of calcium ions. Changeux (Podleski & Changeux, 1970; Kasai & Changeux, 1971c) has suggested that the receptor is made up of two molecular structures, one being associated with the binding site of the ligand and the second termed the 'ionophore' that is responsible for the actual translocation of the ions. At the present time there is no evidence that would allow us to provide a definitive explanation of the observed cooperativity in molecular terms. Anticipation that a correct molecular interpretation is not too far off seems warranted by the progress being made on the isolation and characterization of receptor molecules.

The author wishes to acknowledge the stimulating collaboration of J.-P. Changeux, with whom the experiments described in this paper were performed. At Cornell University the author's work is supported in part by grants from the National Science Foundation, No. GB-24475, and the Muscular Dystrophy Associations of America.

## REFERENCES

ADAIR, G. S. (1925). *J. biol. Chem.*, **63**, 529.

BAUMAN, A., CHANGEUX, J.-P. & BENDA, P. (1970). *F.E.B.S. Letters*, **8**, 145.

CHANGEUX, J.-P. (1969). In: Nobel Symposium II. *Symmetry and Function in Biological Systems at the Molecular Level*, ed. Engström, A. & Strandberg, B., p. 235. New York: John Wiley.

CHANGEUX, J.-P., GAUTRON, M., ISRAEL, M. & PODLESKI, T. R. (1969). *C. R. Acad. Sci. (Paris)*, **269**, 1788D.

CHANGEUX, J.-P. & PODLESKI, T. R. (1968). *Proc. natn. Acad. Sci., U.S.A.*, **59**, 944.

CHANGEUX, J.-P., PODLESKI, T. R., KASAI, M. & BLUMENTHAL, R. (1970). In: *Excitatory Synaptic Mechanisms*, ed. Andersen, P. & Jansen, J. K. S., p. 123. Oslo: Universitetsforlaget.

CHANGEUX, J.-P., THIERY, J., TUNG, Y. & KITTEL, C. (1967). *Proc. natn. Acad. Sci., U.S.A.*, **57**, 335.

CLARK, A. J. (1937). In: *Handbuch Exp. Pharmak.*, Ergänzungswerk, ed. Heffer, A., Vol. 4, p. 62. Berlin: Springer Verlag.

EDELSTEIN, S. J. (1971). *Nature, Lond.*, **230**, 224.

ELDEFRAWI, M. E., ELDEFRAWI, A. T., SEIFERT, S. & O'BRIEN, R. D. (1972). *Archs Biochem. Biophys.*, **150**, 210.
FELTZ, A. (1971). *J. Physiol., Lond.*, **216**, 391.
FELTZ, A. & MALLART, A. (1971). *J. Physiol., Lond.*, **218**, 85.
GRUNDFEST, H. (1966). *Ann. N.Y. Acad. Sci.*, **137**, 901.
HIGMAN, H. B., PODLESKI, T. R. & BARTELS, E. (1963). *Biochim. biophys. Acta*, **75**, 187.
HILL, A. V. (1910). *J. Physiol., Lond.*, **40**, 190.
HODGKIN, A. L. & HUXLEY, A. F. (1952). *J. Physiol., Lond.*, **117**, 500.
KARLIN, A. (1965). *J. cell Biol.*, **25**, 159.
KARLIN, A. (1967). *J. Theor. Biol.*, **16**, 306.
KARLIN, A. (1969). *J. gen. Physiol.*, **54**, 245s.
KARLIN, A. & BARTELS, E. (1966). *Biochim. biophys. Acta*, **126**, 525.
KASAI, M. & CHANGEUX, J.-P. (1971a). *J. Memb. Biol.*, **6**, 1.
KASAI, M. & CHANGEUX, J.-P. (1971b). *J. Memb. Biol.*, **6**, 24.
KASAI, M. & CHANGEUX, J.-P. (1971c). *J. Memb. Biol.*, **6**, 58.
KOSHLAND, D. E. & NEET, K. E. (1968). *A. Rev. Biochem.*, **37**, 359.
MONOD, J., WYMAN, J. & CHANGEUX, J.-P. (1965). *J. Mol. Biol.*, **12**, 88.
NACHMANSOHN, D. (1971). *Proc. natn. Acad. Sci., U.S.A.*, **68**, 3170.
PERUTZ, M. F. (1969). *Proc. Roy. Soc.*, B, **173**, 113.
PODLESKI, T. R. & CHANGEUX, J.-P. (1970). In: *Fundamental Concepts in Drug Receptor Interactions*, ed. Danielli, J. F., Moran, J. F. & Triggle, D. J. New York: Academic Press.
PODLESKI, T. R., MEUNIER, J.-C. & CHANGEUX, J.-P. (1969). *Proc. natn. Acad. Sci., U.S.A.*, **63**, 1239.
RANG, H. P. (1971). *Nature, Lond.*, **231**, 91.
SCHOFFENIELS, E. & NACHMANSOHN, D. (1957). *Biochim. biophys. Acta*, **26**, 1.
TAKEUCHI, A. & TAKEUCHI, N. (1969). *J. Physiol., Lond.*, **205**, 377.
WYMAN, J. (1964). *Adv. Protein Chem.*, **19**, 224.

## DISCUSSION

*Rang* (*Southampton*)

What interpretation do you put on the conversion by decamethonium of the concentration–effect curve for carbachol from a sigmoid to a hyperbolic form? Does it imply that the two compounds bind to separate sites? As a matter of information, I have looked for but failed to demonstrate this type of interaction between decamethonium and carbachol at the frog motor endplate.

*Podleski* (*New York*)

The interpretation originally given to this observation by J.-P. Changeux and myself implied that these two ligands combine with different sites. I think we are in need of accurate binding data to either the membrane or the receptor to resolve the question of separate sites. It is possible that completely separate sites may not be necessary. The fact, however, that Kasai and Changeux were able to observe a similar phenomenon on the isolated membrane fragments does emphasize the validity of the experiment. The fact that you did not observe this type of interaction on the frog endplate under voltage-clamp conditions may imply either a species difference or the possibility that a voltage-dependent event is responsible for the interaction we observed on the electroplax.

# THE RELATION BETWEEN CLASSICAL AND COOPERATIVE MODELS FOR DRUG ACTION

D. COLQUHOUN*

*Department of Pharmacology, Yale University School of Medicine, New Haven, Connecticut 06510, USA*

It is not my purpose to advocate any particular model for drug action as being the truth. And, *a fortiori*, the particular values of parameters used here in numerical examples are chosen for illustration only, though they are chosen to be not grossly incompatible with experimental results (see p. 163). My intention is merely to discuss the extent to which some new observations are compatible with the substantial body of quantitative evidence that is consistent with the classical ideas about drug action. These new observations suggest that some form of cooperative step is involved in the response to certain agonists, whereas no cooperativity was postulated in the classical ideas about drug action.

## *I. Classical ideas about drug action*

The classical theory of drug antagonism was developed by Gaddum (1937), Schild (1949) and Arunlakshana & Schild (1959), on the basis of the work of Langley (1905), Hill (1909) and Clark (1933, 1937). The classical theory of the action of agonist drugs was developed mainly by Stephenson (1956), alternative models being proposed by Ariens *et al.* (1964) whose group subsequently adopted, in essence, Stephenson's view (van Rossum, 1966).

In all of this work the drug was assumed to react with identical, independent binding sites, the receptors, and occupation of the receptor by an agonist was supposed to activate it, the activation ceasing when the drug dissociated. The reaction may be written

$$A + R \rightleftharpoons AR \qquad (1)$$

where A represents the drug, R the receptor, and AR the complex. The

* Present address: Department of Physiology and Biochemistry, University of Southampton, Southampton SO9 3TU, England.

model implies that binding at equilibrium will follow the simple hyperbolic Langmuir (1918) curve (Fig. 1), which was first described by Hill (1909). The Langmuir equation is

$$p_A = \frac{x_A}{x_A + K_A} = \frac{c_A}{c_A + 1} \tag{2}$$

where the subscript indicates the drug referred to, and

$p$ = fraction of receptors occupied (the *occupancy*)
$x$ = drug concentration
$K$ = equilibrium dissociation constant (with the dimensions of concentration) (3)
$c = x/K$ the normalized (dimensionless) concentration; concentration expressed as a multiple of the equilibrium constant.

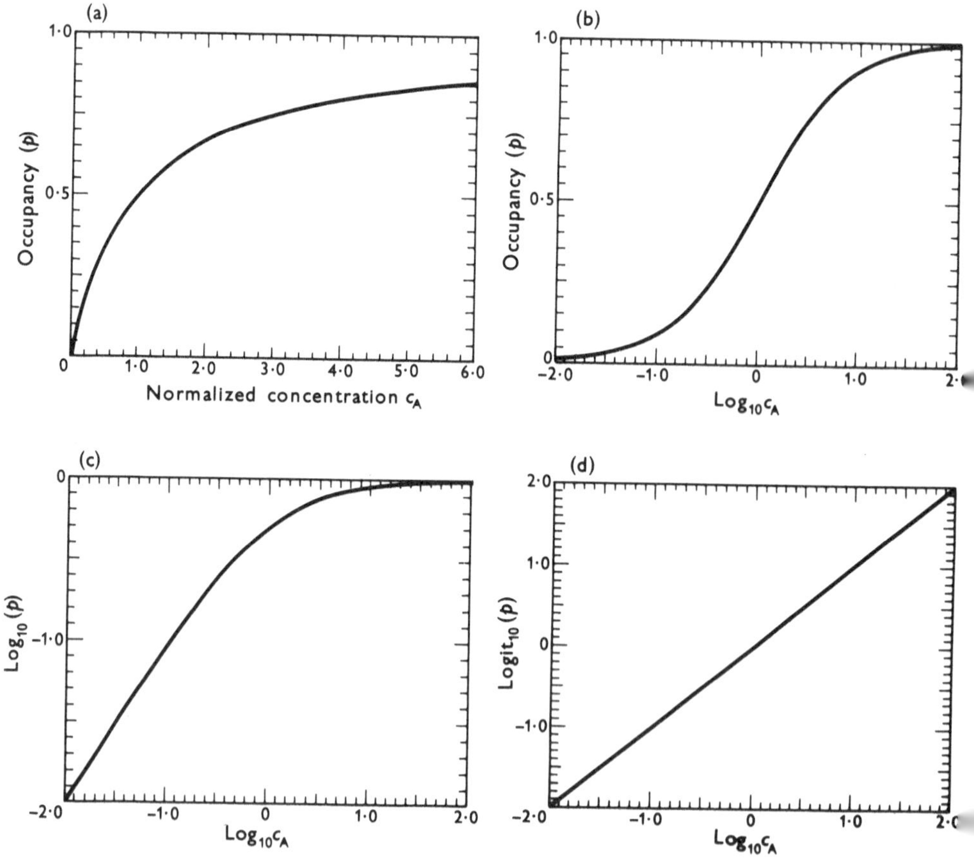


FIG. 1. The Langmuir curve (equation 1) plotted in various ways. (a), Occupancy, $p$, against normalized concentration, $c_A$. (b), $p$ against log $c_A$. (c), $\log_{10} p$ against $\log_{10} c_A$. (d), Hill plot, that is, logit $(p) \equiv \log [(p(c)-p(0))/(p(\infty)-p(0))]$ against log $c_A$.

If several drugs are allowed to equilibrate simultaneously with the binding sites we get

$$p_{\mathrm{A}} = \frac{c_{\mathrm{A}}}{1+\sum c} \qquad \text{where} \quad \sum c = c_{\mathrm{A}} + c_{\mathrm{B}} + c_{\mathrm{C}} \ldots \text{etc.} \tag{4}$$

*Efficacy*

The effectiveness of a competitive antagonist (at equilibrium) is described by its equilibrium constant alone. In the case of agonists, Stephenson (1956) postulated that, in addition to the equilibrium constant, one more drug-dependent variable, the efficacy, $e$, was needed to account for their action. Efficacy is an empirical constant, ranging from 0 (for an antagonist) upwards, and may be regarded as a measure of the effectiveness with which the drug, once combined, activates the receptor. Stephenson defined a *stimulus*, $S = e \times p$, and postulated that any drug producing a given value of the stimulus would produce the same tissue response, that is, the relationship between stimulus and response is characteristic of the tissue and does not depend on the drug used. Drugs with high efficacy can produce the maximum response of which the tissue is capable while occupying only a small fraction of receptors. In this case there is said to be a substantial number of spare receptors. The stimulus–response relationship is, in general, unknown, and calculations of drug affinities and efficacies depend on comparisons of drug concentrations producing equal responses, that is, by the use of a *null method.* This means that one needs to assume only that if an agonist produces a certain stimulus (or opens a certain fraction of ion channels in the models discussed below), the same response will always result, regardless of whether, for example, some other receptors are occupied by an antagonist.

Various null methods have been devised, within the framework of the classical theory, for the estimation of efficacies and equilibrium constants for antagonists, partial agonists and full agonists. The four main approaches used are the following:

1. Analysis of competitive reversible antagonism (Gaddum, 1937; Schild, 1949; Arunlakshana & Schild, 1959). The usual procedure is to measure the agonist dose ratio as a function of antagonist concentration. In most cases, the predicted linear relationship is obeyed with great accuracy (see Rang, 1971 and Fig. 8b) enabling the equilibrium constant to be calculated for the antagonist.
2. Comparison of concentration–effect curves for agonists of differing efficacies (Stephenson, 1956). If equiactive concentrations of drugs of different efficacy are plotted against each other as reciprocals, a linear relationship is predicted, from which (provided the difference in their efficacies is large) the equilibrium constant for the drug of lower efficacy can be calculated (for examples see Barlow, Scott & Stephenson, 1967; Mackay, 1966; Waud, 1969).

3. Interaction between drugs of different efficacy (Stephenson, 1956). In this type of test, the concentration of an agonist tested on its own is compared with the concentration that gives the same effect when applied together with a known concentration of a second agonist of lower efficacy. In a variant of this approach Furchgott & Bursztyn (1967) used an irreversible blocking agent to obtund completely the stimulation by the weaker agonist, and then measured its equilibrium constant as a competitive antagonist of the more efficacious drug.
4. The use of irreversible antagonists (Stephenson, 1966; Furchgott, 1966; van Rossum, 1966). In this method the concentrations of an agonist giving equal responses before and after irreversible block of a proportion of the receptors are compared and plotted on a reciprocal scale. The predicted linear reciprocal plot is usually obtained, and the resulting estimates of equilibrium constants agree quite well with those obtained by other methods (Furchgott & Bursztyn, 1967; Parker, 1972).

In addition to these measurements at equilibrium, kinetic experiments on the rate of approach to equilibrium (for example, Hill, 1909; Paton, 1961; Paton & Rang, 1965; Rang, 1966; Stephenson & Ginsborg, 1969; Colquhoun, 1968; Colquhoun & Ritchie, 1972b; Colquhoun, Henderson & Ritchie, 1972) also gave results that were in striking agreement with the predictions of the classical theories. However, the increasing realization that diffusion in the presence of binding may closely mimic the classical kinetic behaviour of the drug–receptor interaction has complicated the interpretation of kinetic experiments (see, for example, Rang, 1966; Thron & Waud, 1968; Waud, 1968; Colquhoun, Henderson & Ritchie, 1972).

*More direct approaches*

None of the experiments referred to so far give *direct* information about whether the relationship between drug concentration and occupancy (or number of receptors activated) in fact follows the postulated Langmuir curve in Fig. 1, though they are consistent with this model. Unfortunately, as is well known (for example, Stephenson, 1956; Waud, 1968; Rang, 1971), the complexity of the events between drug binding and response prevents any detailed analysis of the shape of the concentration–effect curve, when complex responses such as muscle tension are measured. The most fundamental response that can be measured at the moment is the ionic conductance change produced in postsynaptic membranes by transmitter analogues, where presumably this change is *directly* proportional to the number of ionic channels opened by the drug. It is from such measurements that the main difficulties for the classical model have arisen; these difficulties have led to the proposal of alternative cooperative models.

## *II. Reasons for modifying the classical ideas*

### *Evidence for cooperativity in the relation between concentration and conductance increase*

It was noticed by Katz & Thesleff (1957) and Jenkinson (1960) that the depolarization produced by carbachol at the frog neuromuscular junction was not related to concentration by the simple hyperbolic Langmuir curve, which the classical ideas would predict if occupation of a receptor opened a channel, but by a distinctly sigmoid curve. This sigmoidicity is accompanied by values for the slope of the Hill plot in the region of 2, rather than 1·0 expected for the Langmuir curve (Figs. 1 and 2). Similar sigmoid depolarization curves have been observed in the electroplax of the electric eel, in response to drugs such as carbachol, decamethonium and phenyltrimethylammonium (Karlin, 1967; Changeux & Podleski, 1968).

The sigmoid curve is still observed when the primary phenomenon, conductance increase, is measured in voltage-clamped preparations. This has been shown for the action of $\gamma$-aminobutyric acid (GABA) on insect muscle (Werman & Brookes, 1969) and crayfish muscle (Takeuchi & Takeuchi, 1969; Feltz, 1971), as illustrated in Fig. 2. (In this case the voltage change is small because GABA increases the chloride conductance and the chloride equilibrium potential is close to the resting potential.) Similar results were found at the voltage-clamped frog neuromuscular junction by Rang (1973), who observed sigmoid concentration–effect curves for cholinergic agonists. It does not seem that the sigmoidicity can be attributed to an artifact of the electrical measurement method, for Kasai & Changeux (1971a) obtained very similar results in measurements of the efflux of radiosodium from isolated sacs of membrane prepared from eel electroplax cells.

### *Can the receptor exist in only two conformations?*

Many explanations for the observed cooperativity are, of course, possible. The choice could be narrowed a little if it were known whether or not the response to all agonists were qualitatively similar. For example, cholinergic agonists are known to increase the conductance of the postsynaptic membrane to both sodium and potassium. If the relative conductance increased to the two ions were not the same for all drugs, then it is obvious that more than one variable, in addition to an equilibrium constant, would be necessary to describe the differences between various agonists. So the qualitative similarity of responses was implicit in the classical theory which postulated a single variable, the efficacy. It has been shown by Rang (1972), at the frog neuromuscular junction, that the current flow induced by the drug is related to the voltage at which the membrane is clamped, in just the same way for a number of cholinergic agonists. The current–voltage curves could be superimposed by merely altering the drug concentration. There is evidence that

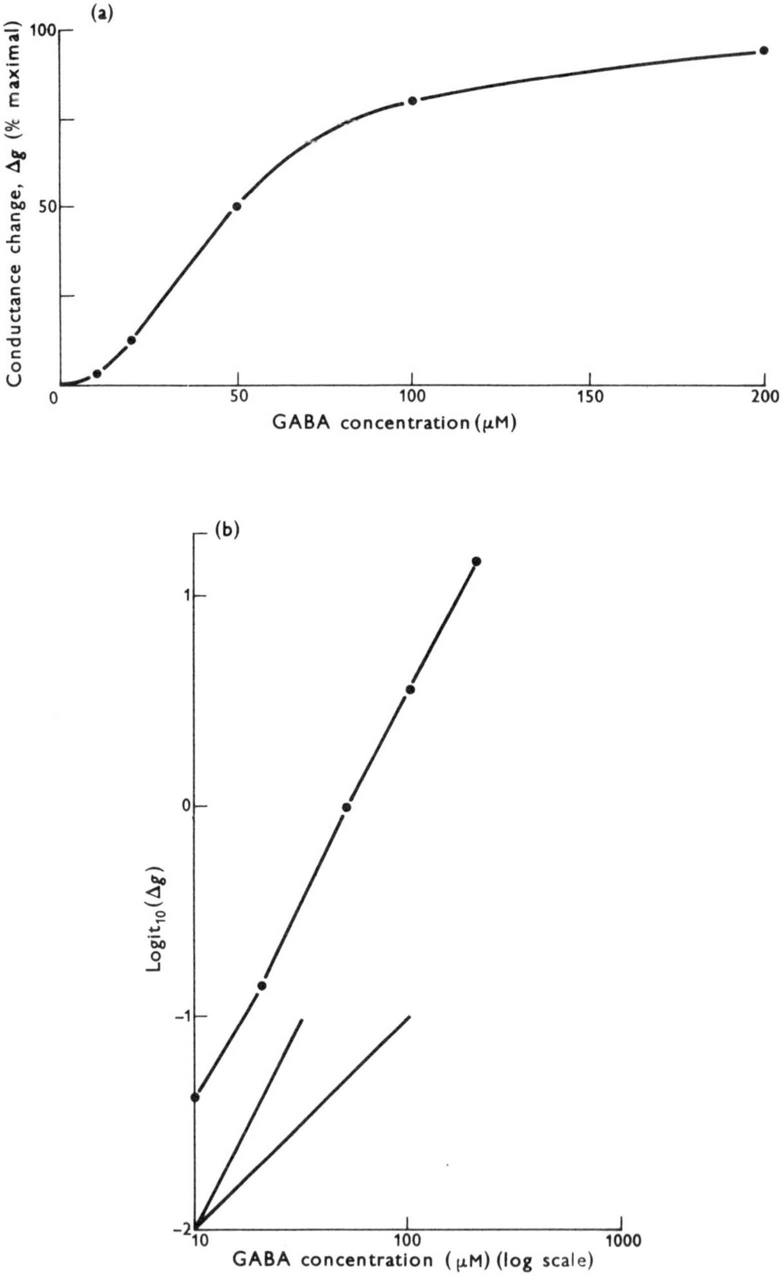


FIG. 2. Experimental sigmoid concentration–effect curves. (a), Conductance change at the crustacean neuromuscular junction produced by $\gamma$-aminobutyric acid (GABA). (b), Hill plot (defined in Fig. 1) of the same results. Replotted from Takeuchi & Takeuchi (1967). The lines at the foot have slopes equal to 1·0 and 2·0.

this relation extends up to the voltage at which no current flows; that is, that the reversal potentials, and hence the relative conductance increases to sodium and potassium, are the same for different cholinergic agonists (Manalis & Werman, 1969; Koester & Nastuk, 1970; Feltz & Mallart, 1971). In eel electroplax cells, Changeux & Podleski (1968) found that altering the external potassium concentration produced an equal modification of the depolarization caused by carbachol and decamethonium, which also suggests that both drugs act by the same ionic mechanism. These observations suggest that all the drugs tested produce channels with the same ionic conductance properties, namely, that the 'activated' receptor is the same, even though the efficacies of the drugs tested vary considerably. In other words, it now seems reasonable to postulate that the channel may exist in only two states,* open or shut, which are the same whatever drug is used. Only the length of time for which it is open and shut are dependent on the drug. This is in contrast with the classical view in which efficacy was usually thought of as representing a more-or-less continuously variable extent of opening of the channel, according to the nature of the ligand used. It is implicit in the rate theory of drug action proposed by Paton (1961) that the elementary quantum of stimulus to the tissue was independent of the drug used (see Furchgott, 1964; Paton & Rang, 1965; Waud, 1968). However, this model does not account for cooperativity: some two-state models that do will now be mentioned.

### *III. Explanations for the observed cooperativity*

The sigmoid curves shown in Fig. 2 bear an obvious resemblance to the sigmoid oxygen binding curves seen with haemoglobin, or the sigmoid velocity/substrate concentration curve seen with enzymes such as aspartate transcarbamylase. A similar sigmoid relationship would result if several *independent* subunits had to be simultaneously in the correct conformation in order to open a channel; this sort of mechanism was used by Hodgkin & Huxley (1952) to describe the potassium channel in squid axon (in this case the equilibrium between different subunit conformations is controlled by membrane potential rather than drug concentration). These resemblances suggest certain simple models for drug action which are generally called allosteric though the term is rather ambiguous. The interaction between the binding site and the ionophore can, in a rather trivial sense, be described as allosteric, but homotropic and heterotropic interactions between separate binding sites have also been suggested, and these mechanisms closely resemble those postulated for allosteric enzymes. The present discussion will be restricted to drugs that act at the same site, or at least sufficiently nearly the

* The phenomenon of desensitization may require a third conformational state, in addition to the resting and activated states of the receptor (see Katz & Thesleff, 1957; Rang & Ritter, 1970a,b) but this added complication is not discussed further in this article.

same site for their binding to be mutually exclusive. A large part of the experimental evidence is most economically accounted for by this sort of mechanism, without having to postulate actions at more than one sort of site.

### *Two-state models in general*

It will be found in Sections IV–VI that a large class of two-state models is compatible with the experimental results, that is, this class predicts results of the same form as the classical model. This phenomenon is a direct consequence of the fact that the experiments have, necessarily, been done using null methods (see above and p. 167). The models to be discussed all suppose that the receptor consists of one or more protomers. Each protomer bears a drug binding site, and can exist in only two conformations, for which the affinity of drug molecules may be different. The conformations corresponding to the open and closed states of the ion channel will be denoted R and T, respectively. The class of models compatible with the type of experimental observation referred to earlier (p. 153) includes all of those for which the fraction of open channels at equilibrium, in the presence of any number of drugs which all compete for the same binding site, is given by an expression of the form

$$p_{open} = f\left(\frac{1+\sum c}{1+\sum Mc}\right) \qquad (5)$$

where $\sum$ indicates summation of the values for each sort of ligand present, and

$p_{open}$ = fraction of channels in the open state.
$f$ = is any monotonic increasing function.
$c = x/K_R$. The normalized concentration; the concentration, $x$, expressed as a multiple of the microscopic equilibrium constant for the interaction of the drug with binding site on a protomer in the R (open) conformation. (6)
$M = K_R/K_T$. The affinity of the drug for the binding site on the T conformation of a protomer, relative to that for the R conformation. This will be small for drugs which favour the R conformation, and thus tend to open the channels. Likewise, $Mc = x/K_T$, is concentration normalized with respect to the equilibrium constant for the T conformation.

The argument in parentheses in equation (5) is very closely related to Stephenson's 'stimulus'*. Some examples of mechanisms of this class will

* If the right-hand side of equation (5) is written for a single drug as

$$f\left(\frac{1+c}{1+Mc}-1\right)$$

now be considered in detail, and then the relation between this class of model and the classical model, and the relation of both to experimental results, will be discussed. Equation (5) implies that relations similar to the classical ones will be predicted if all of the variables that change during the experiment are included in the argument in parentheses. This is not so for the method in which concentration–effect curves are compared before and after an irreversible antagonist is applied. Therefore predictions for this type of experiment are less simple, and will be discussed separately (section VII).

*The independent subunit model*

The explanation of the observed cooperativity need not involve any interaction between binding sites. Following the analogy of the Hodgkin–Huxley (1952) model for the axonal potassium channel (see also Hill & Chen, 1971), we could postulate that in order for a channel to open a certain number ($n$ say), of associated subunits must all be in the R conformation, and that the conformation (and hence affinity for drug) of each subunit is independent of that of all the others. Following Monod, Wyman & Changeux (1965), the reaction postulated, with a ligand A, for a single subunit is

$$\begin{array}{ccc} \mathrm{T} & \underset{}{\overset{L}{\rightleftharpoons}} & \mathrm{R} \\ K_{\mathrm{AT}}\ \updownarrow & & \updownarrow\ K_{\mathrm{AR}} \\ \mathrm{TA} & & \mathrm{RA} \end{array} \qquad (7)$$

---

the argument can be written as

$$\left(\frac{1}{M}-1\right)\left(\frac{Mc}{Mc+1}\right)$$

or

$$\left(\frac{1}{M}-1\right)\left(\frac{x}{x+K_{\mathrm{T}}}\right).$$

This is analogous with Stephenson's model

$$\text{Response}=f(S)=f(e\times p),$$

with the factor

$$\left(\frac{1}{M}-1\right)$$

corresponding with $e$, and the occupancy, $p$, corresponding with

$$\frac{x}{x+K_{\mathrm{T}}}$$

which is a Langmuir occupancy function, though it is at best only an approximation to the actual occupancy in cooperative models. For the two-state model, $K_{\mathrm{T}}$ represents the equilibrium constant for the T conformation, and it will be shown (p. 180) that experimental measurements of equilibrium constants do in fact give, approximately, estimates of $K_{\mathrm{T}}$.

where $L=[T]/[R]$=equilibrium constant for the $T \rightleftharpoons R$ transition. The other symbols are defined in (6) above. Notice that $L$ will be large when most channels are closed in the resting state. It makes no difference to predictions at equilibrium whether the $TA \rightleftharpoons RA$ transition takes place at a finite rate or not, because the equilibrium constant for this transition is defined by the other equilibrium constants, being $LM$. The fraction of protomers in the R conformation in the presence of a number of ligands that compete for the same binding site will be, at equilibrium,

$$p_R = \frac{1}{1+L\left(\dfrac{1+\Sigma Mc}{1+\Sigma c}\right)} \tag{8}$$

If we assume that a channel opens only when all of its $n$ protomers are in the R conformation, then the fraction of channels that are open, $p_{open}$ is equal to the fraction of sets of $n$ protomers that are all in the R conformation. This fraction follows from the multiplication rule of probability (see, for example, Colquhoun, 1971, pp. 20, 380–85). Because of the independence of subunits it is

$$p_{open} = p_R^n = \left(\frac{1}{1+L\left(\dfrac{1+\Sigma Mc}{1+\Sigma c}\right)}\right)^n \tag{9}$$

This is seen to be an example of equation (5).

As illustrated in Fig. 3, this model shows sigmoidicity and Hill slopes greater than 1·0, as found experimentally (Fig. 2).

The fraction of open channels in the absence of ligand ($c=0$) is, of course, in general, not zero, but from (9),

$$p_{open}(0) = \left(\frac{1}{1+L}\right)^n \tag{10}$$

and the maximum fraction of channels that can be opened by a large concentration of drug A ($c_A \to \infty$) is, in general, less than one, and is

$$p_{open}(\infty) = \left(\frac{1}{1+LM_A}\right)^n \tag{11}$$

The fraction of sites occupied by drug molecules as a function of drug concentration deviates from equation (9); it follows a hyperbolic curve with an apparent equilibrium constant of $K_R(L+1)/(LM+1)$, which approximates to $LK_R$ for a strong agonist ($M \ll 1$) and to $K_T$ for an antagonist ($M \geqslant 1$). It is clear from (10) and (11) that if $L$ is very large $p_{open}(0) \simeq 0$, that is, hardly any channels are open in the resting state, and if $M$ is very small (that is, the ligand combines only with the R conformation, and $LM \ll 1$), $p_{open}(\infty) \simeq 1$, that is, all the channels can be opened by a sufficient drug concentration. In

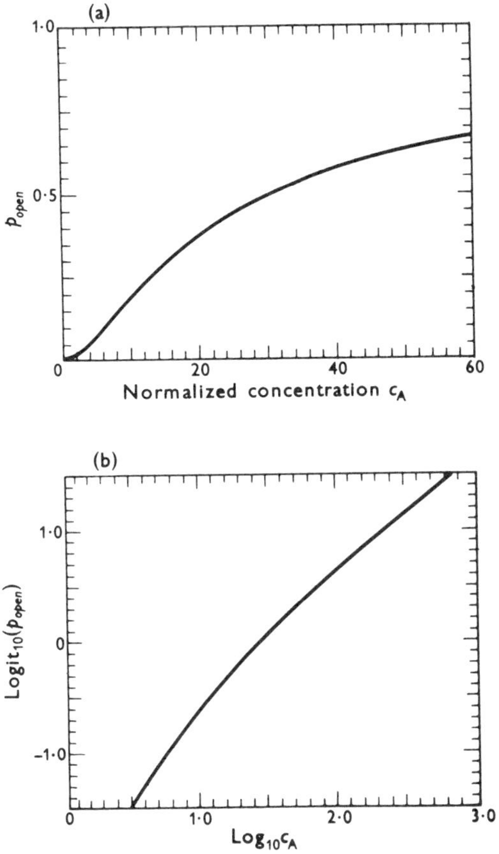


FIG. 3. Theoretical sigmoid concentration–effect curves. Independent model, $n=4$. Fraction of channels open in resting state $p_{open}(0)=0\cdot5\times10^{-3}$; fraction opened by very high drug concentration, $p_{open}(\infty)=0\cdot96$ ($L=5\cdot6$, $M=0\cdot0018$). (a), $p_{open}$ against $c$ (see equation 6); (b), Hill plot (maximum slope in range plotted is 1·8).

this special case only, virtually all the protomers in the R conformation will be occupied by a drug molecule, and virtually all those in the T conformation will be vacant. It, therefore, *looks as though* the act of occupancy has induced the conformation change. This special case is, therefore, referred to as the *induced fit case*. In this case, considering a single ligand for simplicity, equation (9) reduces to

$$p_{open}=\left(\frac{x}{x+LK_R}\right)^n \tag{12}$$

and the binding to individual subunits follows the simple Langmuir equation with an apparent equilibrium constant $LK_R$, which, because $L$ is large, is much higher than the real equilibrium constant, $K_R$; that is, the affinity is underestimated.

Furthermore, models that postulate that it is necessary to have $m$ or more of the $n$ independent subunits in the R conformation in order to open a channel are also special cases of equation (5) and, therefore, predict the same sort of behaviour, described below, in experiments based on null methods. This model, having an additional arbitrary parameter, can describe an even wider range of behaviour than equation (9).

### *The Monod–Wyman–Changeux (MWC) model*

Monod, Wyman & Changeux (1965) proposed a model to account for the cooperative behaviour of haemoglobin and certain enzymes. Its application to drug receptors has been discussed by Karlin (1967) and Podleski & Changeux (1970). This model also postulates the existence of $n$ subunits (protomers) of the sort symbolized in (7), but instead of the subunits being independent, they are linked in such a way that all $n$ are constrained to adopt the same conformation, so there are still only two states, $R_n$ (open) or $T_n$ (shut). The transition between these states is referred to as a concerted transition. The reactions with a ligand, A, will be

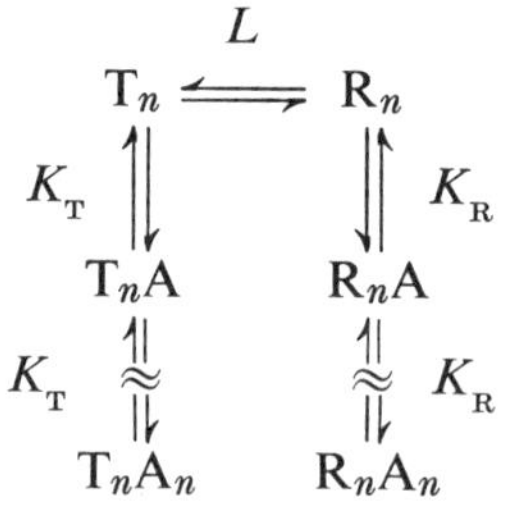


where $L=[T_n]/[R_n]$ is the equilibrium constant for $T_n \rightleftharpoons R_n$ transition in the absence of ligand (which will, as before, be large if most channels are closed at rest). $K_R$ and $K_T$ are the *microscopic* equilibrium constants for the interaction with binding sites on protomers in the R and T conformations.

As in the independent case, it makes no difference to predictions at equilibrium whether the transitions $T_nA_i \rightleftharpoons R_nA_i$ $(i>0)$ take place at a finite rate, because the equilibrium constants for these reactions are defined by the other equilibrium constants, being $LM^i$.

The application of this model to drug receptors has been discussed by Karlin (1967). The fraction of channels in the open state (that is, $R_n$, $R_nA, \ldots R_nA_n$) is

$$p_{open}=p_R=\frac{1}{1+L\left(\dfrac{1+\sum Mc}{1+\sum c}\right)^n} \tag{13}$$

which is once again an example of the general case, equation (5). This model, also, predicts sigmoid binding curves and Hill plots* of slope greater than 1 as illustrated in Fig. 4. As in the independent case, a ligand that binds preferentially to the R state ($M < 1$) will tend to shift the equilibrium towards

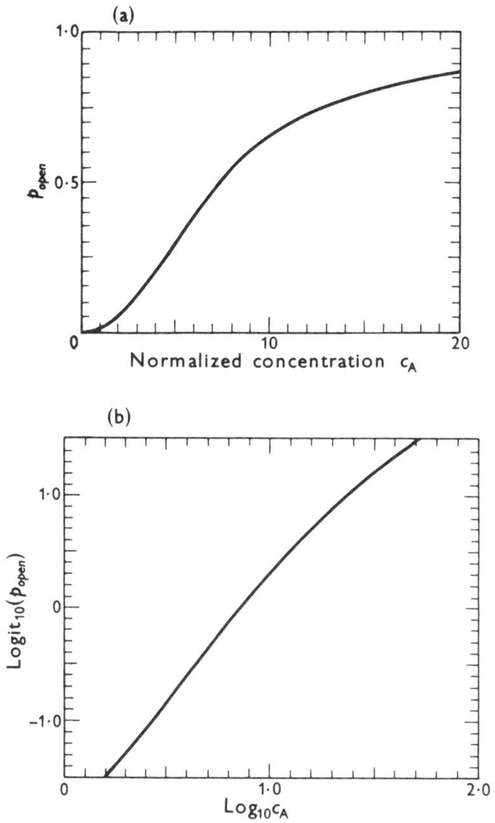


FIG. 4. Theoretical sigmoid concentration–effect curves. MWC model, $n=4$. $p_{open}(0)=10^{-3}$, $p_{open}(\infty)=0{\cdot}98$ ($L=1000$, $M=0{\cdot}067$). (a), $p_{open}$ against $c$ (see equation 6); (b), Hill plot (maximum slope in range plotted is 2·1).

* As with other models the Hill plot is not, in general, straight. The maximum slope is not more than $n$, being

$$n\sum_{i=0}^{n-1} M^i \Big/ \left(\sum_{i=0}^{n-1} M^{i/2}\right)^2$$

This maximum occurs at

$$c_R = 1/\sqrt{M}$$

and

$$p_R = 1/(1+LM^{n/2})$$

a point which may be outside the observable range of $p_R$.

this state. In this case, the concerted change of all $n$ protomers means that this transition generates new high affinity (R) sites, which accounts for the cooperativity. In the absence of ligand

$$p_{open}(0)=p_{R}(0)=\frac{1}{1+L} \tag{14}$$

and at very high concentrations

$$p_{open}(\infty)=p_{R}(\infty)=\frac{1}{1+LM^{n}} \tag{15}$$

As in the independent case, the fraction of sites occupied will, in general, be different from $p_{open}$. But, again as in the independent case, when $M$ is near zero (the ligand combines only with the open state) and $L$ is very large, we approach a situation in which the receptors are either in the closed, vacant state ($T_n$) or in the open, occupied state ($R_nA_n$). Under these 'induced-fit' conditions

$$p_{open}=p_{R}=\frac{x^{n}}{x^{n}+LK_{R}^{n}} \tag{16}$$

which is the form of the Hill equation, proposed by Brown & Hill (1923) to account for the sigmoid binding of oxygen to haemoglobin. It has a linear Hill plot with a slope of $n$. The apparent equilibrium constant is seen to be increased (that is, affinity decreased) by a factor of $L^{1/n}$. Because of the slightly different definitions (cf. equations 10 and 14), this factor will have about the same numerical value as the factor $L$ encountered in the independent case.

## *The lattice model*

Changeux, Thiéry, Tung & Kittel (1967) proposed a model for cooperativity based on the proposition that the excitable membrane resembles a two-dimensional crystalline lattice made up of protomers (subunits), each with one or more binding sites. Suppose each protomer incorporates a channel, and can exist in R (open) and T (shut) conformations, with equilibrium constants $K_R$ and $K_T$ for the ligand. The equilibrium constant for the $R \rightleftharpoons T$ transition must as before be quite large in order that most channels are shut in the absence of ligand. For a protomer whose neighbours are all in the T conformation this equilibrium constant is defined as $L_0=[T]/[R]$. The origin of cooperativity in this model lies in the postulate that the energy needed for promotion of any protomer from the T to the R conformation decreases according to the number of neighbouring protomers in the R conformation. A simple assumption about the nature of the interaction between protomers then gives the equilibrium constant between unoccupied R and T protomers as

$$L = L_0 \Lambda^{p_R} \tag{17}$$

where $\Lambda$ is a measure of the interaction between protomers (Changeux *et al.*, 1967). The reaction scheme is thus exactly like (7), except that $L$ is no longer a constant, but now depends on the fraction of protomers in the R conformation. This fraction is accordingly

$$p_R = \frac{1}{1 + L_0 \Lambda^{p_R} \left( \frac{1 + \sum Mc}{1 + \sum c} \right)} \tag{18}$$

This reduces to (8) when there is no interaction between protomers ($\Lambda = 1$). When $\Lambda < 1$ it predicts sigmoid curves and steep Hill plots like the other models (Changeux *et al.*, 1967). Although (18) is a transcendental equation, which has to be solved numerically for $p_R$, it is nevertheless of the general form of equation (5),* and so is consistent with the experimental observations.

## *Distinction between models, and estimation of parameters*

No attempt has been made to distinguish between the models mentioned. This seems wise in view of the considerable controversy that still surrounds the basis of the cooperativity in such a well-studied molecule as haemoglobin (see, for example, Perutz, 1970; Edelstein, 1971; Minton, 1971; Hewitt, Kilmartin, Ten Eyck & Perutz, 1972; Ogata & McConnell, 1972). As shown below, a large part of the evidence is compatible with all of them. Of techniques in use at present, two are clearly potentially useful in distinguishing between models.

The first is the measurement of the conductance changes in response to various combinations of drugs. This has given useful results, but is limited by the technical difficulty of measuring large conductance changes. This often means that Hill plots can be obtained only for weak agonists, where the maximum response is in the observable range of conductance. It also means that it is not known whether even the most potent agonists can open *all* channels, so $M$ cannot be estimated accurately. For numerical examples, values of $M$ producing $p_{open}(\infty) = 0{\cdot}8 - 1{\cdot}0$ have been used for full agonists, and $p_{open}(\infty) \simeq 0{\cdot}05$ for partial agonists, these values being plausible guesses for the values at the frog neuromuscular junction. At the frog neuromuscular junction, it appears (Rang, personal communication) that no more than about 0·1 % of channels can be open at rest, so $L$ must be at least 1000 in

* As long as $\Lambda$ is not so small that the membrane undergoes an all-or-nothing phase transition (Changeux *et al.*, 1967). Such transitions are not seen in the experiments under discussion.

the MWC model, or $1000^{1/n}$ in the independent model. This may be compared with haemoglobin A for which $L$ (MWC model) is thought to be at least 3000 and possibly much greater (see references above). Appropriate values of $n$ are also uncertain. Numerical calculations have been done with $n=2$ and $n=4$, the latter being used here, arbitrarily, for numerical illustrations.

The second experimental approach is to measure the binding of labelled drug. The binding curve should show no sigmoidicity for the independent model, whereas for the MWC model and the lattice model, it could show sigmoidicity, as haemoglobin does (Monod *et al.*, 1965; Changeux *et al.*, 1967). Moderately precise results are available for binding of some antag-

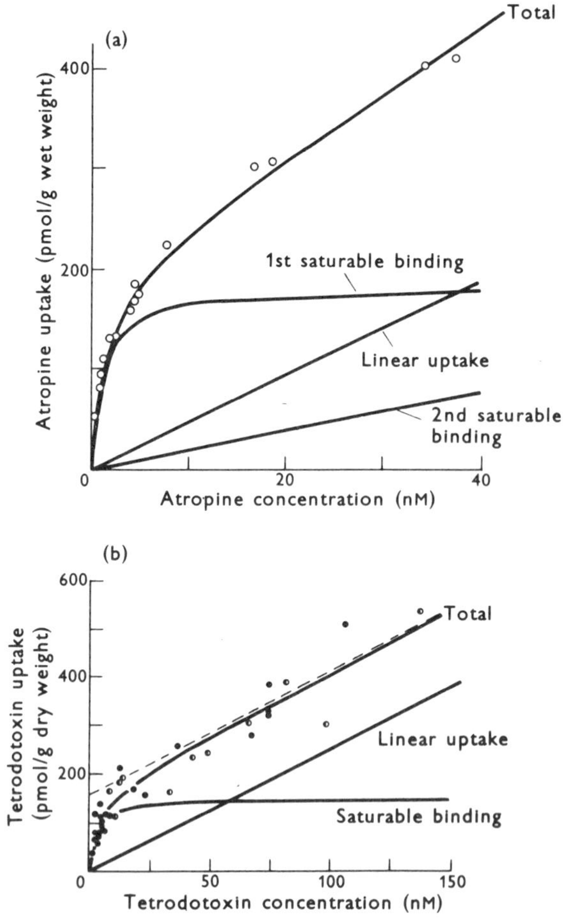


FIG. 5. Binding to intact tissues. (a), Binding of labelled atropine to smooth muscle of guinea-pig ileum, with postulated components of binding (Paton & Rang, 1965). (b), Binding of tetrodotoxin to rabbit vagus nerve, with postulated components of binding (Colquhoun, Henderson & Ritchie, 1972).

onist drugs. As shown in Fig. 5, no sigmoidicity is visible, but even according to the cooperative models, little would be expected for antagonists; with large $L$ values, roughly hyperbolic binding, with equilibrium constant $K_T$ would be expected. Unfortunately, there are still no precise enough experiments on the binding of agonists for a clear distinction to be made (see, for example, Paton & Rang, 1965; Kasai & Changeux, 1971b).

## *IV. Efficacy as selectivity*

Fig. 6a shows the experimental results of Stephenson (1956), which show the transition from partial to full agonist in the alkyltrimethylammonium series of compounds acting on the guinea-pig ileum. Stephenson postulated that variation of a single drug-dependent parameter, efficacy, could account for the type of effect—antagonist, partial agonist, full agonist—produced by any particular drug, and showed that his results were quantitatively consistent with this hypothesis. Figure 6b shows theoretical curves calculated by Stephenson (1956) to illustrate the effect of changing efficacy, $e$, when the equilibrium constant (affinity) for the drug–receptor interaction was kept constant.

In the cooperative models discussed above, the selectivity, or relative affinity, $M$, of a ligand for the T and R conformations plays the role of efficacy (Changeux & Podleski, 1968), and unlike the original arbitrary parameter, this has a simple physical interpretation. Fig. 6 shows curves calculated for various values of $M$. Because it is shown below that the affinity (in classical terms) is much the same as $K_T$ (in cooperative models), reducing $M$ at constant affinity, means reducing $K_R$ (that is, increasing the affinity for the open state), with $K_T$ constant. The curves resemble those from the classical model. Clearly, the same general pattern will result from all two-state models of the class defined in (5). The maximum response, $f(1/M)$, will decrease as $M$ increases, as in Fig. 6. Moreover, for a potent agonist ($M$ very small), (5) reduces to $p_R \simeq f(1+x/K_R)$ so reducing $K_R$ reduces the concentration for a given response by the same factor, thus producing the parallel shift to the left of the response–log concentration curve seen in Fig. 6.

The arguments in Section V, and in the footnote on pp. 156–7, suggest that the nearest that can be got to an analogue of the efficacy, $e$, is the quantity $(1/M)-1$. This becomes infinite for the most potent agonists, that is, when $M$ becomes zero, as expected. And, again as expected, it is zero when $M=1$, so that the ligand occupies sites but has no effect on the open–shut equilibrium, that is, it is an ideal competitive antagonist. In the cooperative model a ligand could have $M$ greater than 1 (so $1/M-1$ could be as little as $-1$). In this case the ligand would actively *close* channels, a sort of antagonist not included in the classical model (see Section V).

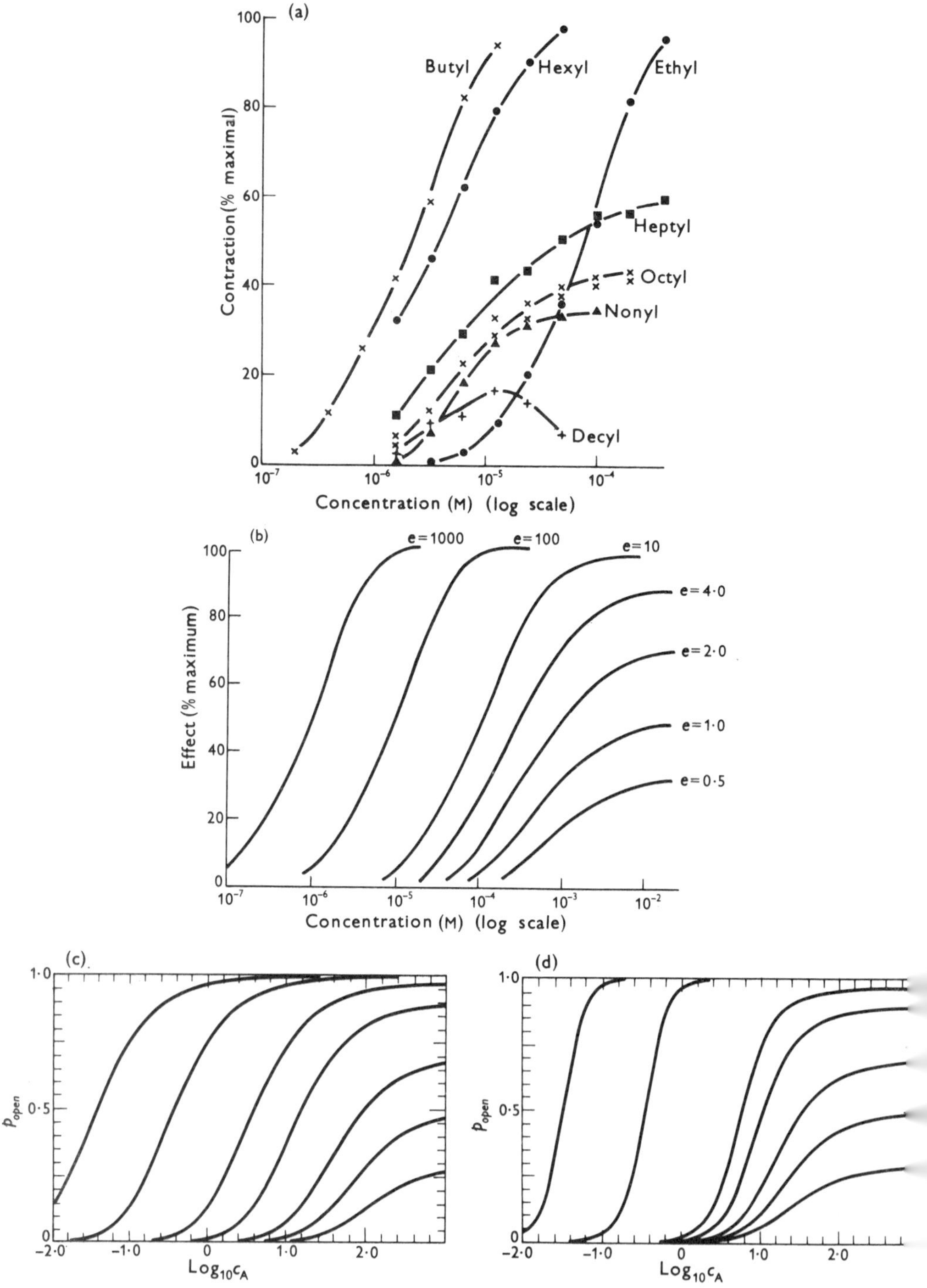
(a)
Butyl
Hexyl
Ethyl
Heptyl
Octyl
Nonyl
Decyl
Contraction(% maximal)
Concentration (M) (log scale)
(b)
e=1000
e=100
e=10
e=4·0
e=2·0
e=1·0
e=0·5
Effect (% maximum)
Concentration (M) (log scale)
(c)
(d)
$p_{open}$
$Log_{10}c_A$

### *V. Interaction of full agonists with partial agonists and antagonists acting at the same site*

Methods have been devised for measuring, in the framework of classical theory, the equilibrium constants for antagonists (Gaddum, Hameed, Hathway & Stephens, 1955; Schild, 1949; Arunlakshana & Schild, 1959), and for measuring the equilibrium constants and relative efficacies of partial agonists (Stephenson, 1956). All of these methods are necessarily null methods (see Section I). They involve measuring the concentrations of agonist, A, needed to produce *equal responses* in the absence and presence of the antagonist or partial agonist.

*Partial agonists*

If equal responses are produced by concentration $x_A$ of a full agonist on its own, and by concentration $x'_A$ in the presence of the partial agonist at concentration $x_B$, then the classical theory indicates that, the following relationship should hold (Stephenson, 1956)

$$x_A = x'_A \left( \frac{1}{\frac{x_B}{K_B}\left(1 - \frac{e_B}{e_A}\right) + 1} \right) + e_B K_A x_B \tag{19}$$

where $e_A$ and $e_B$ are the efficacies for the full and partial agonists. This predicts that a plot of $x_A$ against $x'_A$ should be linear, and the experimental results in Fig. 7 show that this is the case.

Provided that the efficacy of the full agonist is much greater than that of the partial agonist ($e_A \gg e_B$), $K_B$ can be estimated from the slope of the plot as

$$K_B \approx K_{est} = \frac{x_B}{\frac{1}{slope} - 1} \tag{20}$$

$K_{est}$ actually estimates $K_B/(1-e_B/e_A)$, which is close to $K_B$ if $e_A \gg e_B$. This analysis is equivalent to the method described by Stephenson (1956).

It is shown in Fig. 7 (c and d) that behaviour similar to that observed is predicted by the MWC model. According to any cooperative model of the class defined by equation (5) (examples of these were discussed in Section III), assuming as usual that equal responses to A in the presence and absence of B

FIG. 6. The interpretation of efficacy. (a), Concentration–effect curves for alkyltrimethylammonium compounds on guinea-pig ileum from Stephenson (1956). (b) Theoretical curves for the classical model found by changing efficacy with constant equilibrium constant ($10^{-3}$ M for all curves). From Stephenson (1956). (c), Independent model, $n=4$, $L=5{\cdot}6$. $K_T=100$ for all curves, $K_R$ reduced such that (from right to left) $M=0{\cdot}063$, $0{\cdot}034$, $0{\cdot}017$, $0{\cdot}0048$, $0{\cdot}0013$, $0{\cdot}00013$, $0{\cdot}000013$. (d), MWC model, $n=4$, $L=1000$. $K_T=10$ for all curves, $K_R$ reduced such that (from right to left) $M=0{\cdot}22$, $0{\cdot}18$, $0{\cdot}14$, $0{\cdot}10$, $0{\cdot}075$, $0{\cdot}0075$, $0{\cdot}00075$.

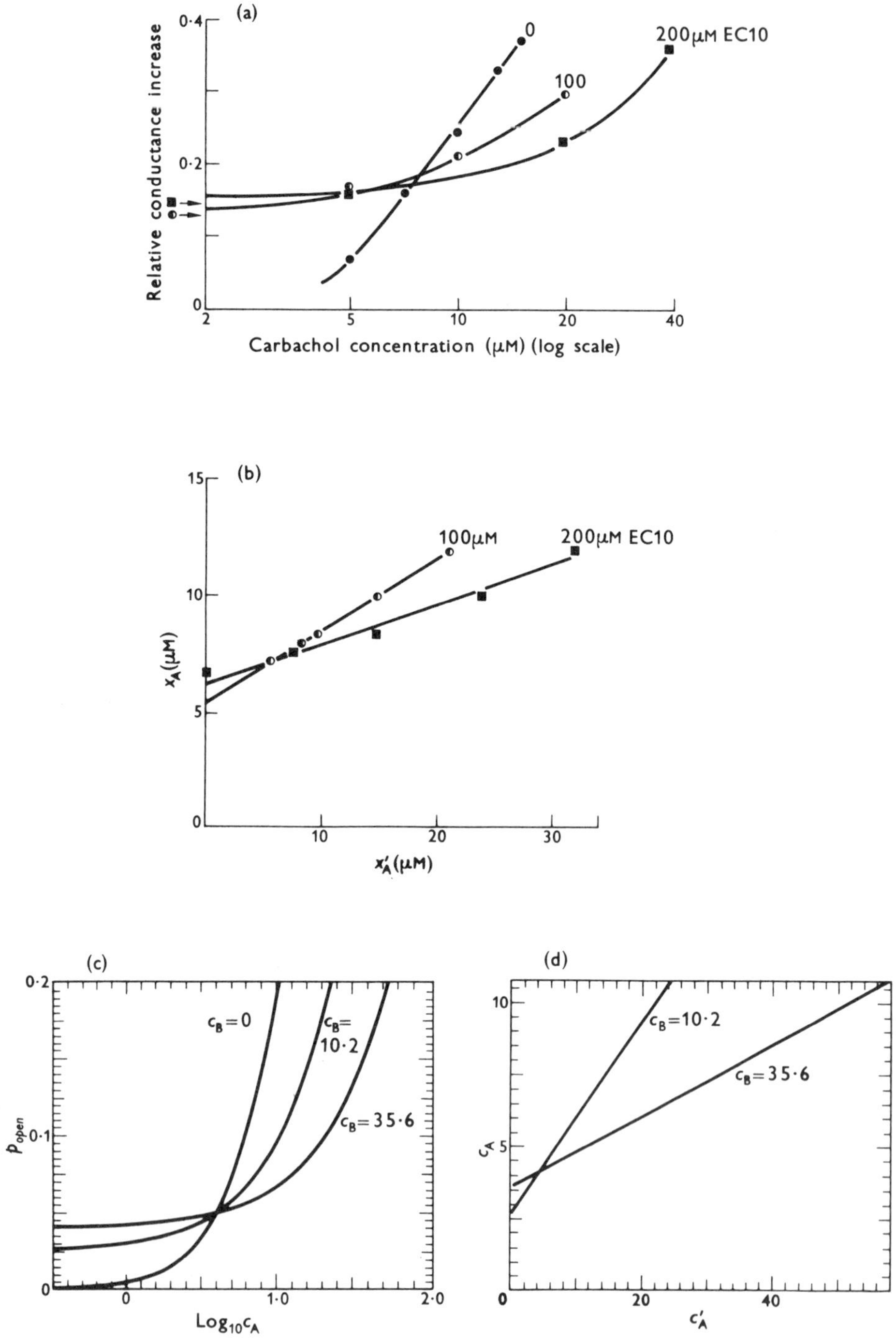
(a)
Relative conductance increase
0·4
0·2
0
0
100
200μM EC10
2
5
10
20
40
Carbachol concentration (μM) (log scale)
(b)
15
10
5
0
100μM
200μM EC10
$x_A$(μM)
10
20
30
$x'_A$(μM)
(c)
0·2
0·1
0
$p_{open}$
$c_B$=0
$c_B$= 10·2
$c_B$=35·6
0
1·0
2·0
$Log_{10}c_A$
(d)
10
5
0
$c_A$
$c_B$=10·2
$c_B$=35·6
20
40
$c'_A$

correspond to equal values of $p_{open}$, it is found that the relation between $x_A$ and $x'_A$ is given by

$$x_A = x'_A\left[\frac{1}{1+\dfrac{x_B}{K_{BT}}\left(\dfrac{1-M_A/M_B}{1-M_A}\right)}\right]+\left[\frac{K_{AR}\dfrac{x_B}{K_{BT}}\left(\dfrac{1/M_B-1}{1-M_A}\right)}{1+\dfrac{x_B}{K_{BT}}\left(\dfrac{1-M_A/M_B}{1-M_A}\right)}\right] \tag{21}$$

which is again a straight line as illustrated in Fig. 7d. And application of equation (20) to get an estimate of the equilibrium constant gives simply

$$K_{est} = K_{BT}\left(\frac{1-M_A}{1-M_A/M_B}\right) \tag{22}$$

This is very like the classical result, and with the similar assumption that the agonist, A, is much more efficacious than the partial agonist, that is, that A is more selective for the R conformation, so $M_A \ll M_B$, it is seen that $K_{est}=K_{BT}$. It should be noticed that, because values of $M_A$ cannot be accurately estimated (see p. 163), it is by no means certain that the factor $(1-M_A)/(1-M_A/M_B)$ is negligible.

Thus, the cooperative models yield similar predictions to the classical model, and making similar approximations, the former models all yield an estimate of the equilibrium constant for interaction of the partial agonist for the T conformation, which is the conformation associated with the shut channel.

Comparison of the classical and cooperative models shows that the ratio of efficacies in the classical model, $e_A/e_B$, is replaced, on the cooperative models, by

$$\frac{1/M_A-1}{1/M_B-1} \tag{23}$$

as discussed in Section IV, and footnote on pp. 156–7.

---

FIG. 7. Interaction method for partial agonists. (a), Interaction between carbachol (CCh) and two concentrations of decamethylene-*bis*(ethyldimethylammonium) (EC10) at the voltage-clamped frog neuromuscular junction (Rang, unpublished). The responses produced by EC10 alone are marked on the ordinate. (b), Plot of equieffective concentrations of CCh with ($x'_A$) and without ($x_A$) EC10, from Fig. 7(a). (c), Independent model, $n=4$, $L=5\cdot6$ (so, $p_{open}(0)=0\cdot5\times10^{-3}$). Full agonist has $M=0\cdot001$ (so, $p_{open}(\infty)=0\cdot98$). Partial agonist has $M=0\cdot2$ (so, $p_{open}(\infty)=0\cdot05$). All lines cross just as in the classical theory, at a point the ordinate of which is the maximum response of which the partial agonist is capable, that is, $p_{open}(\infty)=0\cdot05$ in this example. The normalized concentrations, $c_B$, of partial agonist supposed present, which are marked on the curves, are such that in the absence of the full agonist they will open 2·5% and 4% of the channels (that is, 50% and 80% of the maximum response that the partial agonist is capable of producing). (d), Plot of equieffective concentrations as in Fig. 7b. The lines are straight as in the classical theory, and intercept the ordinate above the origin. Either of these lines gives a good estimate of $K_T$ (from equations (19) and (22)) because, in this example, $(1-M_A)/(1-M_A/M_B)=0\cdot996$, nearly unity.

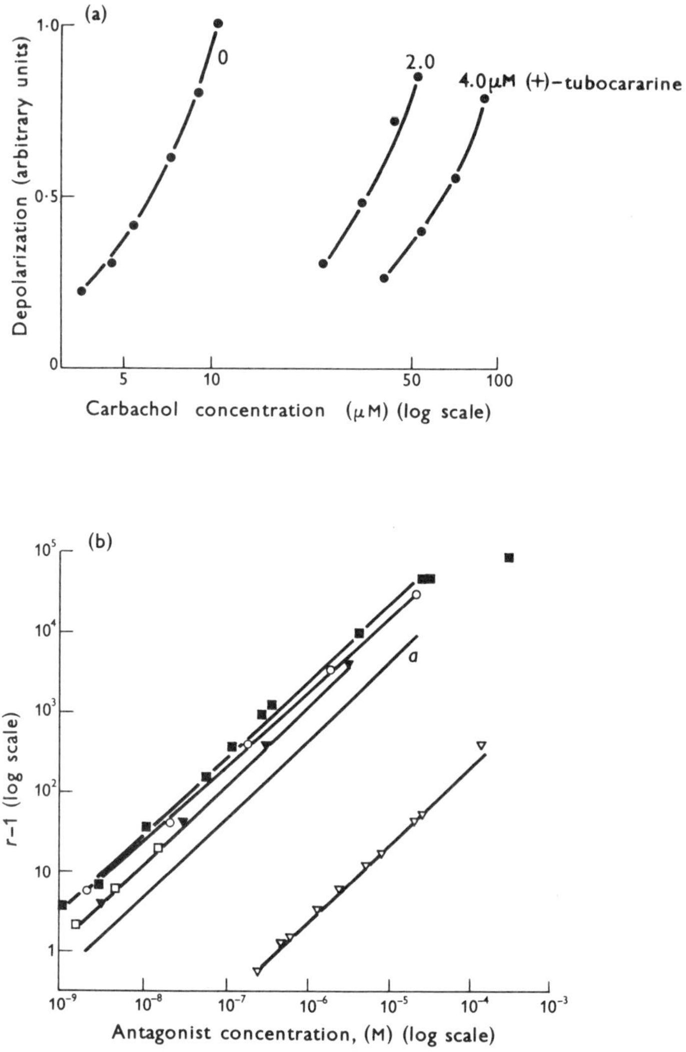


FIG. 8. Experimental results with antagonists. (a), An example of parallel shift of effect–log concentration curves by an antagonist. Depolarization (arbitrary units) of the frog neuromuscular junction by carbachol. (+)-Tubocurarine concentration: left curve, 0; middle curve, $2\times10^{-6}$ M; right curve, $4\times10^{-6}$ M. (From Jenkinson, 1960.) (b), Schild dose–ratio plots. Log $(r-1)$ is plotted against log $x_B$ (antagonist concentration). (■), Hyoscine as antagonist of acetylcholine on guinea-pig ileum (Paton, 1961). (○), Atropine as antagonist of carbachol on guinea-pig atria (Thron & Waud, 1968). (□), Mepyramine as antagonist of histamine on guinea-pig ileum (Paton, unpublished). (▼), Atropine as antagonist of acetylcholine on guinea-pig ileum (Arunlakshana & Schild, 1959). (*a*), Propranolol as antagonist of (−)-isoprenaline on guinea-pig atria (Blinks, 1967). (▽), (+)-Tubocurarine as antagonist of acetylcholine on frog toe muscle (Jenkinson, 1960). In each case the slope is close to 1·0. Data replotted from the papers indicated. From Rang & Ritter (1971), by courtesy of the authors and Oslo University Press.

*Antagonists*

It has frequently been observed (see Fig. 8) that in the presence of a competitive antagonist, the log concentration–response curve is shifted in a parallel fashion to the right by a distance, defined as log $r$, where the dose ratio, $r$, is $x'_A/x_A$, the relative concentrations of agonist (A) producing the same response after and before adding the agonist (B). According to the classical theory of drug antagonism (Arunlakshana & Schild, 1959)

$$r = 1 + x_B/K_B \tag{24}$$

a result which may appropriately be called the Schild equation. This predicts that $r$ is constant, regardless of the response level chosen, which is consistent with the observed parallelism. It also predicts that a plot of log $(r-1)$ against log $x_B$ should be a straight line with unit slope. This prediction has been repeatedly confirmed with considerable accuracy, over a large range of concentrations, and for many drugs. Some of these results are shown in Fig. 8. The equilibrium constant can be estimated from the intercept of this plot, log $K_B$, or with one value of $r$, from

$$K_{est} = \frac{x_B}{r-1} \tag{25}$$

which, from (24), gives $K_B$.

The relation between $x_A$ and $x'_A$, for all cooperative models of the class defined by equation (5), is given by (21). An ideal competitive antagonist, that had no other effect than to exclude agonist, would have equal affinities for both R and T states ($M_B = 1$) so that it would not disturb the $R \rightleftharpoons T$ equilibrium. When $M_B = 1$ is put into (21), we obtain

$$\frac{x'_A}{x_A} \equiv r = 1 + \frac{x_B}{K_{BT}} \tag{26}$$

which is just the same as the Schild equation (24), and shows that, as for partial agonists, we obtain (for example, from equation 25) the equilibrium constant of the antagonist (B) for the T conformation, $K_{BT}$.

The cooperative models include the possibility that the antagonist will not merely fail to open channels, but it may actually close whatever channels are open in the resting state, namely, we could have $M_B > 1$. From equation (21) we obtain, in general

$$\frac{x'_A}{x_A} = r = \frac{x_B}{K_{BT}} \left[ \left( \frac{1 - M_A/M_B}{1 - M_A} \right) + \left( \frac{1 - 1/M_B}{1 - M_A} \right) \frac{K_{AR}}{x_A} \right] + 1 \tag{27}$$

where $x_A$ is the concentration of agonist that produces, when given alone, the standard response level at which the dose ratios are measured. The appearance of this quantity on the right-hand side shows that the shift of the response–log concentration curve will not be exactly parallel when the antagonist prefers the shut (T) conformation ($M_B > 1$). Correspondingly, the estimate of the equilibrium constant from (25) is, in general,

$$K_{est} = K_{BT}\left[\frac{(1-M_A)}{(1-M_A/M_B)+(1-1/M_B)\,K_{AR}/x_A}\right] \quad (28)$$

which is only exactly $K_{BT}$ when $M_B = 1$.

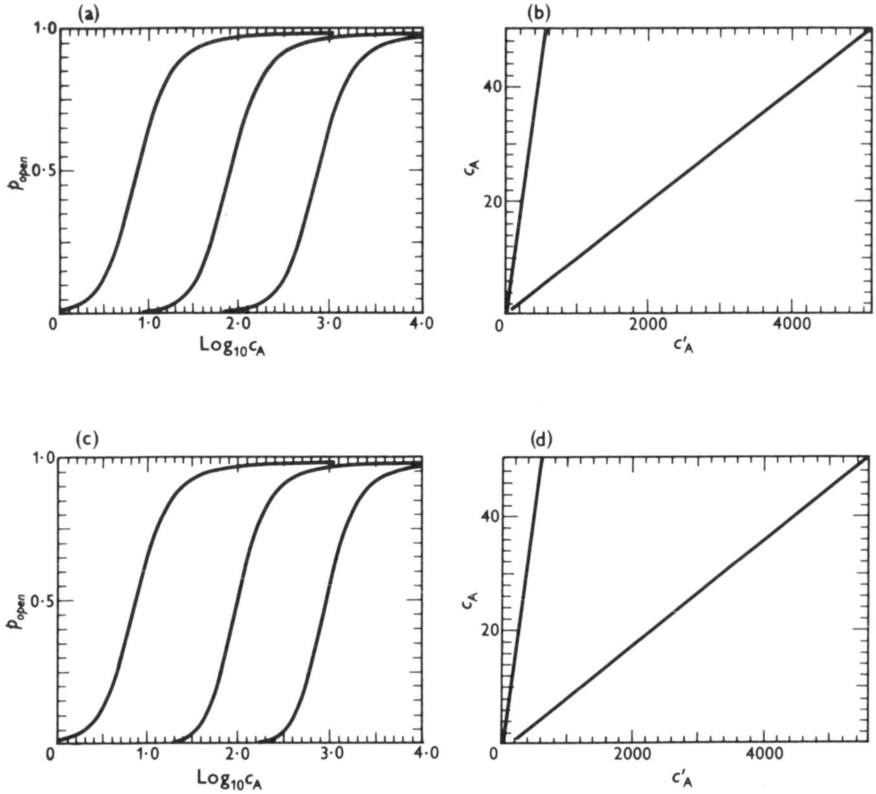


FIG. 9. Theoretical predictions for antagonists. MWC model, $n=4$, $L=1000$, so $p_{open}(0)=0{\cdot}001$. Agonist (A) has $M_A=0{\cdot}067$, so $p_{open}(\infty)=0{\cdot}98$. (a), Parallel shift of effect–log concentration curves by an antagonist (B) with $M_B=1{\cdot}0$, in concentrations producing dose ratios of 11 and 101 ($c_{BR}=10$ and 100). The dose ratio method gives $K_{BT}$ exactly (equation 26). (b), Plot of $c_A$ against $c'_A$ corresponding to Fig. 9a. Both lines are straight, and go through the origin showing that the dose ratio $r=x'_A/x_A$ is a constant, independent of $x_A$, i.e. that the shift is parallel in Fig. 9a. (c), Shift of effect–log concentration curves by an antagonist with preferential affinity for the shut conformation, $M_B=100$. The shift is not quite parallel. Although the nonparallelism does not look striking, the equilibrium constant estimated from the dose ratio at the bottom end of the curves is $0{\cdot}67\ K_{BT}$ whereas measuring the dose ratio at the top gives $0{\cdot}88\ K_{BT}$ (from equation 28). (d), Plot of $c_A$ against $c'_A$ corresponding to Fig. 9c. The fact that the lines do not go exactly through the origin reflects the nonparallelism in Fig. 9c, that is, the dependence of $r$ on $x_A$. The slope of either of these lines, if concentration rather than normalized concentration were used, would give the equilibrium constant as $K_{BT}(1-M_A)/(1-M_A/M_B)=0{\cdot}93\ K_{BT}$.

However, equation (27) *does* predict that the plot of log $(r-1)$ against log $x_B$, illustrated in Figs. 8 and 9, will still be linear with unit slope even if $M_B > 1$, provided that all dose ratios are measured at the same response level, so that $x_A$ is constant. In fact, the degree of nonparallelism predicted when $M_B > 1$ is small, as illustrated in Fig. 9. This is true especially, as equations (27) and (28) show, if $x_A \gg K_{AR}$, which is the case for many plausible parameter values (see Fig. 9, for example). Experimentally the straight dose-ratio plots with unit slope, shown in Fig. 8b, are much better documented than *precise* parallelism.

It is interesting that even if $M_B > 1$ then, from equation (21), the plot of $x_A$ against $x'_A$ should still be exactly straight, and the slope of this plot should give, using equation (20), the result

$$K_{est} = K_{BT}\left(\frac{1-M_A}{1-M_A/M_B}\right)$$

just as for a partial agonist. This result is the same as equation (22) and shows that this method will give $K_{BT}$ as long as a sufficiently powerful agonist is used, (that is, $M_A \ll M_B$). It is illustrated in Fig. 9 that, although the $x_A$ versus $x'_A$ plot should always be straight, it only goes exactly through the origin when $M_B = 1$, so only in this case is $r = x'_A/x_A$ a constant. Equation (21) and Figs. 7 and 9 show that when $M_B < 1$ (partial agonist) the line passes above the origin, and when $M_B > 1$ (antagonist) it passes below the origin.

## *VI. Comparison of full agonists with partial agonists*

The equilibrium constants, and relative efficacies, of partial agonists can also be estimated by comparing the doses of full agonist ($x_A$) and partial agonist ($x_B$) that produce the same response when each drug is given on its own (Barlow, Scott & Stephenson, 1967; Waud, 1969). Fig. 10 shows typical experimental results. In this case the classical theory predicts that a double reciprocal plot of $1/x_A$ against $1/x_B$ will be straight and, as shown in Fig. 10, this is observed. The equilibrium constant can be estimated as

$$K_{est} = \frac{slope}{intercept} \tag{29}$$

from this plot, and on the classical theory, this gives $K/(1-e_B/e_A)$, exactly as for the interaction method. And, again exactly as before, all the cooperative models of the form of equation (5) predict linear plots (see Fig. 10), and the quantity estimated by (29) is $K_{BT}(1-M_A)/(1-M_A/M_B)$, as in equation (22).

It should be stressed that double reciprocal plots are shown here only because they have been widely used by other authors. Such plots are usually a poor way of estimating parameters, especially if the experimental results are variable (see, for example, Colquhoun, 1971). The properties of estimates made by means of the usual unweighted double reciprocal plot are not known in detail for the present sort of experiment, but past experience in simpler situations certainly suggests that properly weighted fitting, as described by Parker & Waud (1971), should be used.

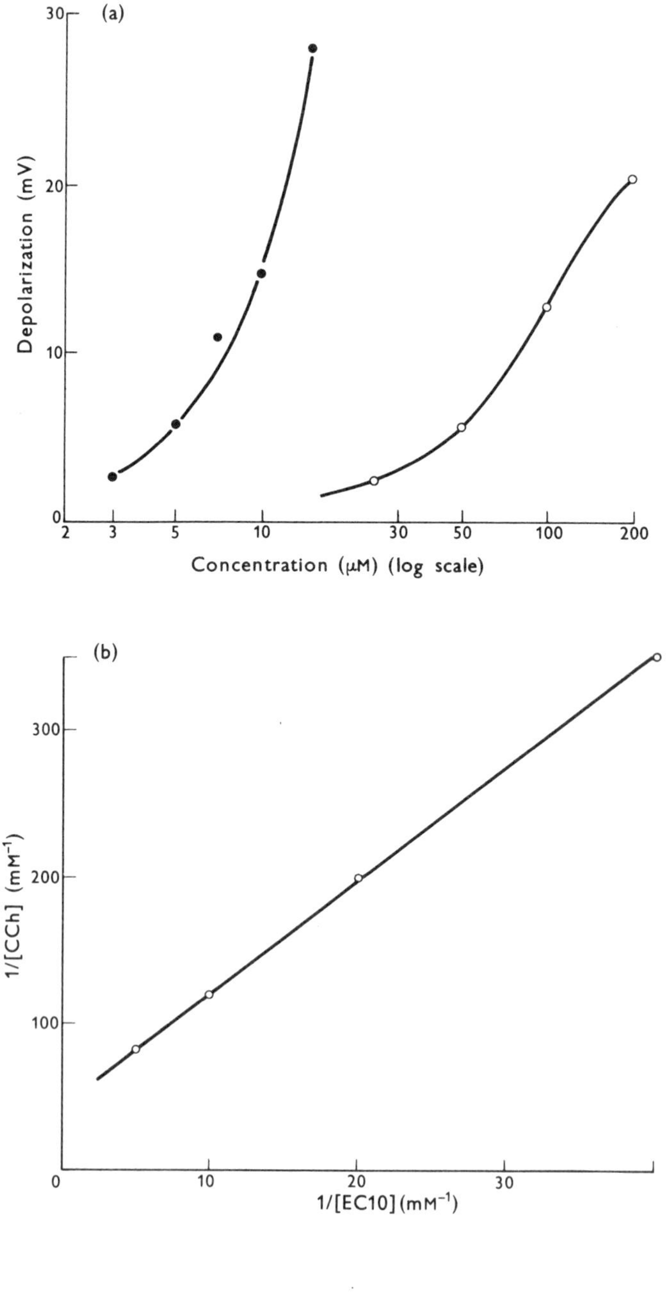

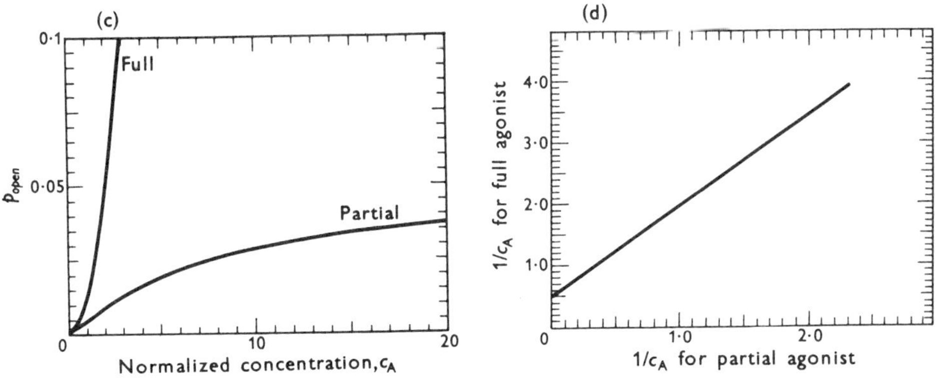


FIG. 10. Comparison method for partial agonists. (a), Concentration–effect curves for the depolarization produced at the frog neuromuscular junction by carbachol (CCh), (●); and decamethylene-*bis*(ethyldimethylammonium) (EC10), (○). (Rang, unpublished.) (b), Double reciprocal plot of equieffective concentrations of CCh and EC10, determined in the experiment shown in Fig. 10a. (Rang, unpublished.) (c), MWC model $n=4$, $L=1000$. Effect–concentration curves for two agonists given separately. Full agonist (A) has $M_A=0\cdot067$, so $p_{open}(\infty)=0\cdot98$. Partial agonist (B) has $M_B=0\cdot371$, so $p_{open}(\infty)=0\cdot05$. (d), Double reciprocal plot of equieffective concentrations, $1/c_A$ against $1/c_B$, corresponding to Fig. 10c. This gives an estimated equilibrium constant of $K_{BT}(1-M_A)/(1-M_A/M_B)=1\cdot14\ K_{BT}$, from equation (29).

## *VII. The use of irreversible antagonists to determine the affinities and relative efficacies of agonists*

This method, used by Waud (1963), Furchgott (1966), Mackay (1966), and Stephenson (1966), is the only available method for investigation of powerful agonists. Unfortunately, experiments done by this method are not performed under equilibrium conditions and are not described by equations of the form of equation (5). No such simple conclusions as those in earlier sections seem possible at the moment. However, the discussion below certainly shows no obvious inconsistency, either qualitative or quantitative, between the experimental observations and cooperative models.

### *Classical model*

The concentrations of agonist that produce the same response before ($x_A$) and after ($x'_A$) exposure to an irreversible antagonist are measured. The classical model predicts that a double reciprocal plot of $1/x_A$ agonist $1/x'_A$ will be straight. From this plot

$$K_{est}=\frac{slope\ -1}{intercept} \tag{30}$$

provides an estimate of the equilibrium constant, $K_A$, for the agonist, and $1/slope$ = fraction of receptors not blocked. Experimental results are shown in Fig. 11.

*Independent model*

The simplest assumption is that the irreversible antagonist will permanently inactivate a certain fraction of channels, leaving the rest unchanged. This would happen, for example, if it occupied one or more of the $n$ receptor sites associated with each channel. If the fraction of *sites* not occupied by the irreversible antagonist is $p_{OB}$ then the fraction of open channels is equation (9) multiplied by $p_{OB}^n$ (which is the fraction of channels remaining functional). This model does not predict linear double reciprocal plots in general, but numerical calculations show that in many cases the deviation is small. In particular, when $x_A \gg K_{AR}$ over the range of measurement, the plot will be straight. This condition is met when $L$ is large enough, values of $L$ in the guessed range, above $1000^{1/n}$ (see p. 163) usually giving reasonable

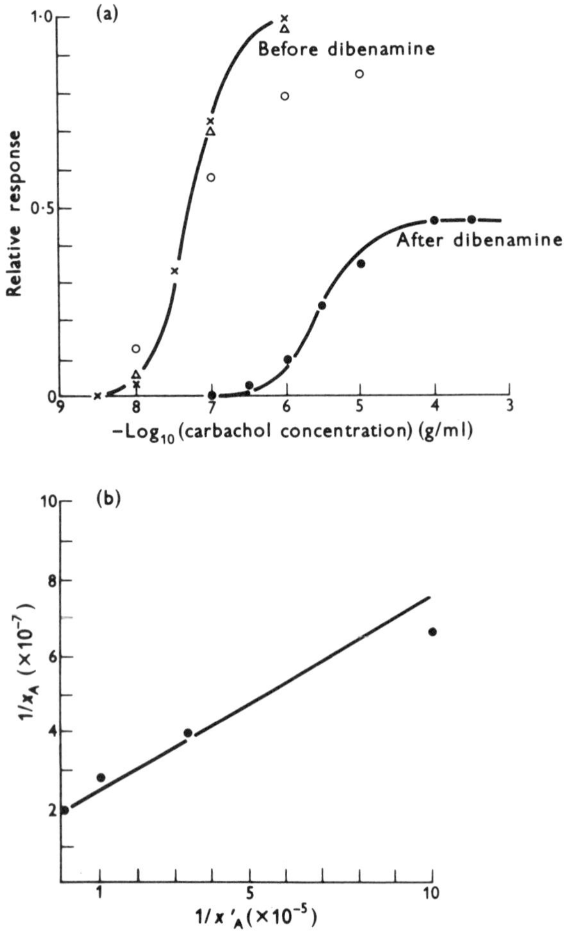

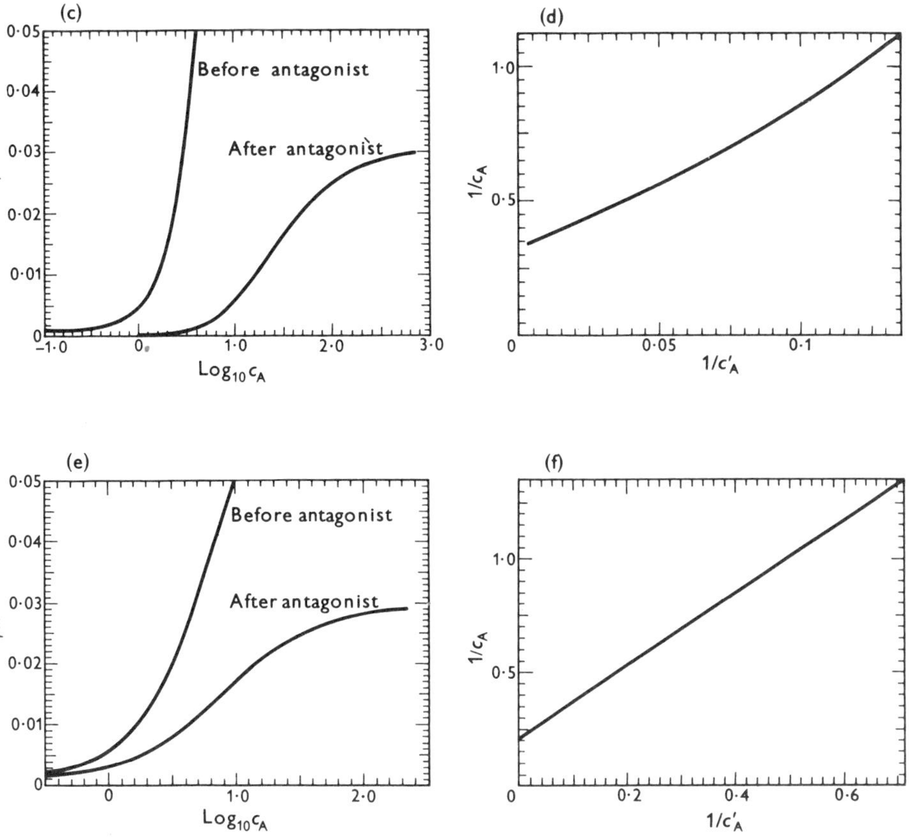


FIG. 11. Irreversible antagonist method. (a), Response of rabbit stomach smooth muscle to carbachol before and after dibenamine treatment. (Redrawn from Furchgott & Bursztyn (1967).) (b), Double reciprocal plot of equieffective concentrations of carbachol before and after dibenamine, $1/x_A$ against $1/x'_A$, from Fig. 11a. (c), Independent model $n=4$, $L=5 \cdot 6$, for a full agonist with $M_A=0 \cdot 00136$; that is, $p_{open}(\infty)=0 \cdot 98$. Fraction of binding sites not irreversibly blocked, $p_{OB}=1 \cdot 0$, $0 \cdot 422$. (d), Double reciprocal plot corresponding to Fig. 11c. This plot gives an estimate of the equilibrium constant for the agonist of $9 \cdot 7\, K_{AR}$, compared with $K_{AT}=730\, K_{AR}$ and $K_{AR}(1+L)/(1+LM)=6 \cdot 6\, K_{AR}$ (see equation (31)). $1/slope=0 \cdot 24$ compared with $p_{OB}=0 \cdot 42$. In this example equation (31) is only a rough approximation. (e), MWC model (equation (32)), $n=4$, $L=1000$, for a partial agonist with $M_A=0 \cdot 308$, that is, $p_{open}(\infty)=0 \cdot 1$. Fraction of binding sites not irreversibly blocked, $p_{OB}=1 \cdot 0$, $0 \cdot 614$. (f), Double reciprocal plot corresponding to Fig. 11e. This gives an estimated equilibrium constant of $0 \cdot 92\, K_{AT}$, close to the equilibrium constant for the shut conformation. The reciprocal of the slope is $0 \cdot 62$, close to $p_{OB}$.

lines, as shown in Fig. 11. When this condition holds, equation (30) estimates approximately

$$K_R \left( \frac{1+L}{1+LM_A} \right) \tag{31}$$

For partial agonists this quantity is close to $K_T$ (that is, $K_R/M$), which is roughly consistent with experimental results as discussed in Section VIII. This happens mostly because for quite a large range of partial agonists, the value of $K_T$ cannot be grossly different from the value of $LK_R$, that is, $LM$ is of the order of unity. For more potent agonists, equation (31) suggests that the method will provide an approximate estimate of $LK_R$, rather than $K_T$ (cf. p. 159).

*Monod–Wyman–Changeux model*

There is no good experimental basis for predicting the effect of an irreversible inhibitor. One assumption would be to suppose that a certain fraction of the oligomers was completely blocked, the remainder being normal. Most of the calculated examples give rather nonlinear double reciprocal plots in this case. Another plausible approach is to suppose that the antagonist is randomly bound to individual sites where it has no other effect but to exclude the agonist, so that a tetramer, for example, would be effectively converted to a mixture of tetramers, trimers, dimers, monomers and completely blocked tetramers. In this case

$$p_R = \sum_{i=0}^{n} \frac{\binom{n}{i} p_B^i \, p_{OB}^{n-i}}{1 + L\left(\dfrac{1+\sum Mc}{1+\sum c}\right)^{n-i}} \qquad (32)$$

where $p_{OB} = 1 - p_B$ is the fraction of binding *sites* not occupied by the irreversible inhibitor. Again, this does not, in general, give straight double reciprocal plots. However, if the conditions are such that the agonist concentrations, $c_A'$, used in the presence of the antagonist, would open only a small fraction of channels even in the *absence* of antagonist, then the plots will be approximately straight, as in Fig. 11. This condition must be true for almost all partial agonists (for which even $p_{open}(\infty) \ll 1$), and numerical calculations suggest that it may well be true for many full agonists too, but ignorance of realistic $M$ values for full agonists prevents more precise conclusions. When this approximation is valid, equation (30) gives quite a close approximation to $K_T$, and 1/*slope* estimates $p_{OB}$, as with the classical model. An example is shown in Fig. 11.

*Furchgott's method*

Furchgott & Bursztyn (1967) used an irreversible inhibitor to reduce the response of a partial agonist to near zero, while leaving a measurable response to a full agonist. The partial agonist then behaved like an antagonist, producing a parallel shift to the right of the log concentration–response curve for the full agonist. The equilibrium constant for the partial agonist was calculated from the shift (that is, the dose ratio) in the conventional way,

by means of the Schild equation (equations 24 and 25). Some experimental results obtained by this method are shown in Table 1. This method is simple to analyse because the receptor blockade by the irreversible antagonist is the same before and after the addition of the partial agonist, so the equations discussed earlier in this section conform with equation (5). Consequently, the dose ratio produced by the partial agonist would be expected to have the same form as before, that given in equation (27), where A stands for the full and B for the partial agonist. Clearly, the lines before and after B will become parallel when enough irreversible inhibitor has been bound to make $x_A \gg (1 - 1/M_B)$ over the range of measurement, so that $r$ is independent of $x_A$. And in this case equation (28) shows that this method should estimate $K_{BT}(1 - M_A)/(1 - M_A/M_B)$, exactly like the methods of Sections V and VI.

### *VIII. Conclusions concerning the interpretation of experiments*

Three facts that must be considered when thinking of alternatives to the classical model are (1) when the classical theory predicts a straight line, an approximately straight line has usually been observed; (2) several authors (Furchgott & Bursztyn, 1967; Waud, 1969; Parker, 1972; Rang, unpublished) have found that several methods for determining the equilibrium constants for partial agonists all give approximately (within a factor of 2 or so) the same result (some of these results are shown in Table 1); and (3) in the case of, for example, atropine (Paton & Rang, 1965) and tetrodotoxin (Colquhoun & Ritchie, 1972a; Colquhoun, Henderson & Ritchie, 1972), the affinity measured by binding to intact cells agrees with that found by various indirect null methods.

If any of the wide class of two-state models discussed in Section III were a

TABLE 1. *Estimates of equilibrium constants for cholinergic agonists*

| Drug | Method | K | |
|---|---|---|---|
| $MeN^+Et_3$ (frog *rectus*) | Interaction ($Me_4N^+$)<br>Comparison ($Me_4N^+$) | 4·07 mM<br>2·75 mM | Barlow, Scott & Stephenson (1967) |
| Pilocarpine (rabbit stomach) | Irrev. (DBN)<br>CCh antag. (DBN) | 1·42 μM<br>1·28 μM | Furchgott & Bursztyn (1967) |
| Heptyl-TMA (guinea-pig ileum) | Comparison (CCh)<br>Irrev. (DBN)<br>CCh antag. (DBN) | 71 μM<br>105 μM<br>32 μM | Waud (1969) |
| Decamethonium (frog neuromuscular junction) | Interaction (CCh)<br>Comparison (CCh)<br>Irrev. (DNM) | 54 μM<br>48·7 μM<br>39·4 μM | Rang (unpublished) |

Methods: *Interaction*, interaction with the stated full agonist (Section V). *Comparison*, comparison with the stated full agonist (Section VI). *Irrev.*, use of the stated irreversible antagonist (Section VII). *CCh antag.*, Furchgott's method with the stated irreversible antagonist (Section VII). CCh, Carbachol; DBN, dibenamine; DNM, dinaphthyldecamethonium mustard.

good approximation to the true explanation for the observed cooperativity, it would suggest the following conclusions.

The agreement with classical theory is expected to be very good for antagonists. And good agreement is expected between the equilibrium constants of antagonists found by binding and by the Schild method. Both should give approximations to $K_T$ (see p. 153 and Section V). The observed linearity and unit slope of the Schild plot (Fig. 8), is, however, predicted even when the shift of response–log concentration curves is not exactly parallel, and if this happens a plot of $x_A$ against $x'_A$ would be more appropriate, as discussed in Section V. This would give $K_{BT}(1-M_A)/(1-M_A/M_B)$, which is close to $K_{BT}$ if the full agonist (A) is potent ($M_A \ll 1$) *or* if the antagonist (B) has a similar affinity for both open and shut conformation ($M_B$ near 1).

For partial agonists (B), both interaction (Section V) and comparison (Section VI) with a full agonist (A) estimate the same quantity, $K_{BT}(1-M_A)/(1-M_A/M_B)$, and the same quantity would be expected using Furchgott's method (Section VII) also. This too should be close to $K_T$, though the term $(1-M_A)/(1-M_A/M_B)$* may not be completely negligible. For the example in Fig. 10 the error would be about 14%. The estimate of $K_T$ is biased by the same factor using all three methods (as in the classical case), so agreement between the methods does not indicate lack of bias.

The methods using irreversible antagonists are more difficult (except for Furchgott's method). The considerations in Section VII make it very probable that the equilibrium constant estimated by the use of irreversible antagonists would also be about $K_T$ for *partial* agonists. This, and the predicted approximate linearity of the plots, shown in Fig. 11, certainly explain the experimental agreement between this method and the others, shown in Table 1. However, for powerful agonists the discussion in Section VII makes it unlikely that this method estimates $K_T$. Unfortunately, in this case, no other method is known to check the values obtained. In Section VII it is suggested that the quantity estimated for a very potent agonist is about $LK_{AR}$ for the independent model.

I am grateful to Professor H. P. Rang for many discussions on the topics discussed in this article.

*Note added in proof*

Thron (1973, *Mol. Pharmac.*, **9**, 1) has recently published a comparison of the classical and MWC models which independently arrives at some of the results discussed in this paper. The main difference lies in the treatment of irreversible antagonists.

In contrast to Thron's result, which is similar to equation (31) above, the results in Section VII suggest that, for the MWC model, the irreversible

* If $1/M-1$ were taken as an analogue of efficacy (pp. 156, 157, 169), this factor would be the same as that occurring in the classical theory, $1/(1-e_B/e_A)$, (pp. 167, 173).

antagonist method should give $K_T$ approximately for a *partial* agonist, as should other methods, thus explaining the experimental agreement between methods for partial agonists: but for agonists of high efficacy the present treatment suggests that there is at present not enough knowledge to interpret with any certainty the irreversible antagonist method in terms of cooperative models.

## REFERENCES

Ariens, E. J. (1964), Editor. *Molecular Pharmacology.* New York: Academic Press.
Arunlakshana, O. & Schild, H. O. (1959). *Br. J. Pharmac.*, **14**, 48.
Barlow, R. B., Scott, N. C. & Stephenson, R. P. (1967). *Br. J. Pharmac.*, **31**, 188.
Blinks, J. R. (1967). *Ann. N.Y. Acad. Sci.*, **139**, 673.
Brown, W. E. L. & Hill, A. V. (1923). *Proc. R. Soc.*, B, **94**, 294.
Changeux, J.-P. & Podleski, T. (1968). *Proc. natn. Acad. Sci., U.S.A.*, **59**, 944.
Changeux, J.-P., Thiéry, J., Tung, Y. & Kittel, C. (1967). *Proc. natn. Acad. Sci., U.S.A.*, **57**, 335.
Clark, A. J. (1933). *Mode of Action of Drugs on Cells.* London: Arnold.
Clark, A. J. (1937). *Handbuch Exp. Pharmak.*, **4**, 1937.
Colquhoun, D. (1968). *Proc. R. Soc.*, B, **170**, 135.
Colquhoun, D. (1971). *Lectures on Biostatistics.* Oxford: Clarendon Press; London, New York: Oxford U.P.
Colquhoun, D. & Ritchie, J. M. (1972a). *J. Physiol., Lond.*, **221**, 533.
Colquhoun, D. & Ritchie, J. M. (1972b). *Mol. Pharmac.*, **8**, 285.
Colquhoun, D., Henderson, R. & Ritchie, J. M. (1972). *J. Physiol., Lond.*, **227**, 95.
Edelstein, S. J. (1971). *Nature, Lond.*, **230**, 224.
Feltz, A. (1971). *J. Physiol., Lond.*, **216**, 391.
Feltz, A. & Mallart, A. (1971). *J. Physiol., Lond.*, **218**, 101.
Furchgott, R. F. (1964). *A. Rev. Pharmac.*, **4**, 21.
Furchgott, R. F. (1966). *Adv. Drug Res.*, **3**, 21.
Furchgott, R. F. & Bursztyn, P. (1967). *Ann. N.Y. Acad. Sci.*, **144**, 882.
Gaddum, J. H. (1937). *J. Physiol., Lond.*, **89**, 7P.
Gaddum, J. H., Hameed, K. A., Hathway, D. E. & Stephens, F. F. (1955). *Q. Jl exp. Physiol.*, **40**, 49.
Hewitt, J. A., Kilmartin, J. V., Ten Eyck, L. F. & Perutz, M. F. (1972). *Proc. natn. Acad. Sci., U.S.A.*, **69**, 203.
Hill, A. V. (1909). *J. Physiol., Lond.*, **39**, 361.
Hill, T. L. & Chen, Yi-Der (1971). *Proc. natn. Acad. Sci., U.S.A.*, **68**, 1711.
Hodgkin, A. L. & Huxley, A. F. (1952). *J. Physiol., Lond.*, **117**, 500.
Jenkinson, D. H. (1960). *J. Physiol., Lond.*, **152**, 309.
Karlin, A. (1967). *J. Theor. Biol.*, **16**, 306.
Kasai, M. & Changeux, J.-P. (1971a). *J. Memb. Biol.*, **6**, 1.
Kasai, M. & Changeux, J.-P. (1971b). *J. Memb. Biol.*, **6**, 58.
Katz, B. & Thesleff, S. (1957). *J. Physiol., Lond.*, **138**, 63.
Koester, J. & Nastuk, W. L. (1970). *Fedn Proc.*, **290**, 716.
Langley, J. N. (1905). *J. Physiol., Lond.*, **33**, 374.
Langmuir, I. (1918). *J. Am. chem. Soc.*, **40**, 1361.
Mackay, D. (1966). *Adv. Drug Res.*, **3**, 1.
Manalis, R. S. & Werman, R. (1969). *Physiologist*, **12**, 292.
Minton, A. P. (1971). *Nature, Lond.*, **232**, 145.
Monod, J., Wyman, J. & Changeux, J.-P. (1965). *J. Mol. Biol.*, **12**, 88.
Ogata, R. T. & McConnell, H. M. (1972). *Proc. natn. Acad. Sci., U.S.A.*, **69**, 335.
Parker, R. B. (1972). *J. Pharmac.*, **180**, 62.
Parker, R. B. & Waud, D. R. (1971). *J. Pharmac.*, **177**, 1.
Paton, W. D. M. (1961). *Proc. R. Soc.*, B, **154**, 21.
Paton, W. D. M. & Rang, H. P. (1965). *Proc. R. Soc.*, B, **163**, 1.
Perutz, M. F. (1970). *Nature, Lond.*, **228**, 726.

Podleski, T. & Changeux, J.-P. (1970). In: *Fundamental Concepts in Drug-Receptor Interaction.* London & New York: Academic Press.
Rang, H. P. (1966). *Proc. R. Soc.*, B, **164**, 488.
Rang, H. P. (1971). *Nature, Lond.*, **231**, 91.
Rang, H. P. (1973). *Bull. Neurosci. Res. Prog.*, in press.
Rang, H. P. & Ritter, J. M. (1970a). *Mol. Pharmac.*, **6**, 357.
Rang, H. P. & Ritter, J. M. (1970b). *Mol. Pharmac.*, **6**, 383.
Schild, H. O. (1949). *Br. J. Pharmac.*, **4**, 227.
Stephenson, R. P. (1956). *Br. J. Pharmac.*, **11**, 379.
Stephenson, R. P. (1966). *Proc. 3rd Int. Pharmac. Congress*, Sao Paulo, **1**.
Stephenson, R. P. & Ginsborg, B. L. (1969). *Nature, Lond.*, **222**, 790.
Takeuchi, A. & Takeuchi, N. (1967). *J. Physiol., Lond.*, **191**, 575.
Takeuchi, A. & Takeuchi, N. (1969). *J. Physiol., Lond.*, **205**, 377.
Thron, C. D. & Waud, D. R. (1968). *J. Pharmac.*, **160**, 91.
van Rossum, J. M. (1966). *Adv. Drug Res.*, **3**, 189.
Waud, D. R. (1963). Thesis: University of Oxford.
Waud, D. R. (1968). *Pharmac. Rev.*, **20**, 49.
Waud, D. R. (1969). *J. Pharmac.*, **170**, 117.
Werman, R. & Brookes, N. (1969). *Fedn Proc.*, **28**, 831.

## DISCUSSION

*Worcel (Paris)*

The Langmuir equation in the case of a reaction order greater than one predicts a sigmoid rather than a hyperbolic saturation curve. Although this interpretation demands integral values for the Hill coefficient, would you invariably exclude it as an explanation of sigmoid concentration–effect curves?

*Colquhoun (Yale)*

The reaction *order* (as opposed to molecularity) is essentially an empirical quantity, so it merely describes the observations and does not explain them. In order to find any sort of explanation one must postulate some sort of physical mechanism and see how its predictions agree with experiment. There does not seem to be any strong evidence that Hill slopes are usually integers, and even when they are, the observation would be compatible with a number of different mechanisms. One such mechanism would be the sor first postulated by A. V. Hill for haemoglobin, which is implied in you question. But this has not turned out to be physically correct in othe systems such as haemoglobin, and it is not very plausible physically because implies an infinite interaction energy between subunits.

# THE USE OF AFFINITY LABELS IN THE IDENTIFICATION OF RECEPTORS

S. J. SINGER, A. RUOHO AND H. KIEFER*

*Department of Biology, University of California at San Diego, La Jolla, California, USA*

J. LINDSTROM AND E. S. LENNOX

*The Salk Institute, La Jolla, California, USA*

Most drug and hormone receptors that are membrane bound are in the category of 'integral' membrane proteins (Singer, 1971; Singer & Nicolson, 1972); that is, they are not readily solubilized from the membranes, and require detergents or other hydrophobic bond-breaking agents to release them. After release of the receptor from the membrane, the physiological functions by which the receptor activity is recognized are usually lost, and even the capacity of the receptor to bind its specific drug or hormone may be destroyed or radically modified. In order to identify any such receptor, therefore, it would be useful to label it *in situ* with a high degree of specificity, and then use the label to follow the receptor during isolation. An approach that holds promise to provide a general method for such specific labelling is *affinity labelling* (Wofsy, Metzger & Singer, 1962; Singer, 1967; Baker, 1967; Shaw, 1970). In this method, a reagent is designed which combines specifically and reversibly with the active site of the receptor, and then, by virtue of a reactive group on the reagent, reacts to form a covalent bond with some suitably disposed amino-acid residue(s) in the active site. The specificity of labelling is achieved because the initial reversible binding of the reagent to the site in question increases the local concentration of the reagent in the site compared to that in the free solution.

The application of the method to the identification of receptors, and the special problems that might be encountered, have been discussed elsewhere (Singer, 1970). The method has already been investigated with certain receptor systems as long ago as 1949 (Nickerson & Gump, 1949) for the adrenergic receptor, and more recently by Gill & Rang (1966), Belleau &

* Also at Basel Institute for Immunology, Basel, Switzerland.

Tani (1966), Changeux, Podleski & Wofsy (1967), and Kiefer, Lindstrom, Lennox & Singer (1970) for cholinergic receptors and other acetylcholine-binding sites. These studies, however, have generally not yet resulted in a successful isolation of the receptor. On the other hand, Hill (1971) has provided evidence that he has identified antigen-specific receptors on the membranes of lymphoid cells of guinea-pigs sensitized to give delayed-type hypersensitivity, using a diazonium affinity labelling reagent. Fewtrell & Rang (this symposium, p. 211), continuing the studies of Gill & Rang (1966), have similarly used affinity labelling nitrogen mustards in an attempt to identify the muscarinic receptor protein on the membranes of guinea-pig smooth muscle preparations. Also a special variant of affinity labelling has been developed for the cholinergic receptor of the eel electroplax by Karlin and his colleagues (this symposium, p. 193). In the last case, it appears that the method has been used successfully to identify the receptor protein; however, the special devices that were employed are not likely to be of general applicability.

A major problem for the success of the method is to achieve the required high degree of specificity of affinity labelling. With the usual affinity labelling reagents, containing a moderately reactive chemical group X (Fig. 1, top), nonspecific labelling outside the active site in question will occur at finite rates. Although individual nonspecific reactions may occur relatively slowly, the sum of these nonspecific reactions may cumulatively be very large, and quantitatively may obscure the specific affinity labelling reactions in the receptor site (Singer, 1970). This is particularly a problem if the receptor protein in question is only a very small fraction of the total protein of the membrane preparation.

An important variant of affinity labelling which in principle is capable of high degrees of specificity, is *photo-affinity labelling*. In this method (Fig. 1, bottom) a reagent is used which can combine specifically and reversibly with the active site, and which contains a photolysable group P. P is unreactive in the dark, but when photolysed, is converted to an extremely reactive intermediate P*; if certain conditions are satisfied, P* may then react to form a covalent bond, with residue(s) in the active site before the reagent dissociates from the site. In other words, under such circumstances, $k_{P^*2} > k_{-P^*3}$ (Fig. 1, bottom). As was pointed out by Kiefer *et al.* (1970), these conditions could lead to a very high degree of specificity of labelling of the active sites in question; any reagent molecules which underwent photolysis in free solution would be expected to react with the solvent or with an added scavenger, and nonspecific reactions with the membrane proteins might thus be greatly reduced.

Photolysable reagents were introduced into protein chemistry by Westheimer and his colleagues (Singh, Thornton & Westheimer, 1962; Shafer, Baronowsky, Laursen, Finn & Westheimer, 1966; Vaughan & Westheimer, 1969). They used diazoacyl reagents which upon photolysis are converted

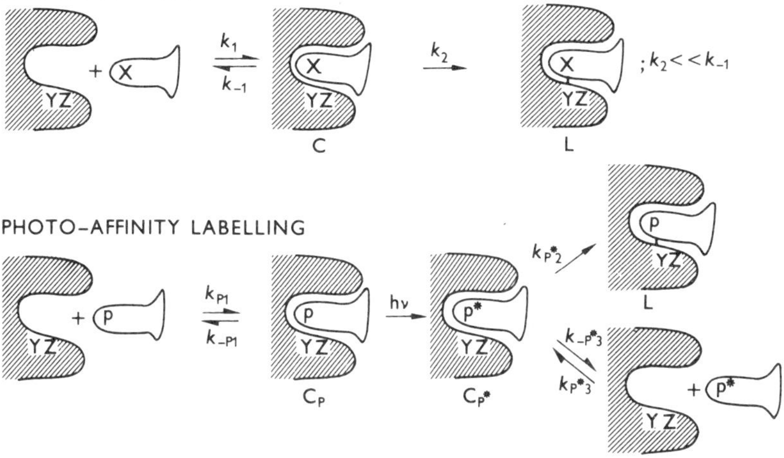


FIG. 1. A schematic view of the mechanisms of ordinary affinity labelling (top) and photo-affinity labelling (bottom). In affinity labelling, the functional group X on the reagent is a group of ordinary chemical reactivity. In photo-affinity labelling, the group P is chemically unreactive, but can be photolysed to a highly reactive intermediate P*. Depending on the relative values of $k_{P^*2}$ and $k_{-P^*3}$, P* reacts to form a covalent bond with residue YZ in the site, or it dissociates from the site without reacting. L is the labelled protein, the C's are the appropriate reversible complexes.

to very reactive carbenes (equation (1a)). Such a reagent has been used in the photo-affinity labelling of pure antibodies by Converse & Richards (1969). More recently, Fleet, Knowles & Porter (1969) have used aryl azides, which upon photolysis are converted to nitrenes (equation (1b)).

$$(1)\quad \begin{array}{ll} \text{(a)} & \mathrm{R{-}C({=}O){-}C(H){=}\overset{\oplus}{N}{=}\overset{\ominus}{N}} \xrightarrow{h\nu} \underset{\text{(carbene)}}{\mathrm{R{-}C({=}O){-}\ddot{C}H}} + N_2 \\ \text{(b)} & \mathrm{R{-}N{=}\overset{\oplus}{N}{=}\overset{\ominus}{N}} \xrightarrow{h\nu} \underset{\text{(nitrene)}}{\mathrm{R{-}\ddot{N}:}} + N_2 \end{array}$$

Carbenes and nitrenes are extremely reactive radicals; they can even insert into C–H bonds. Thus they should exhibit a very broad range of reactivity, and be capable of reacting with any appropriately proximal residue in the active site.

In our laboratories, we undertook to study the photo-affinity labelling of acetylcholine-binding proteins using the particular aryl azides HK-83 and HK-68 shown on page 186.

Our initial studies have been reported (Kiefer *et al.*, 1970). They showed that the acetylcholinesterase (AChE) activity of intact human erythrocyte membranes, and the acetylcholine receptor (AChR) activity of the frog sartorius

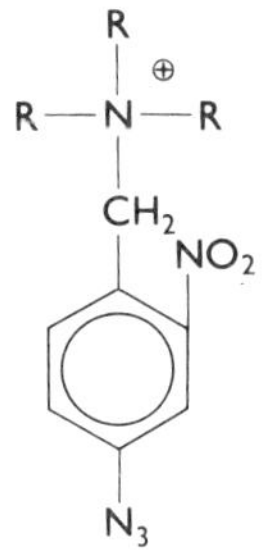

HK-83 : R = $CH_3$

HK-68 : R = $C_2H_5$

muscle, could be irreversibly inactivated by photolysis in the presence of HK-83 or HK-68. We have since obtained very similar results with these reagents and both the AChE and the AChR of the eel electroplax (J. Lindstrom & A. Ruoho, unpublished results), using the microsac preparation of electroplax excitable membranes of Kasai & Changeux (1971). These activities were largely retained, however, under any of the following conditions: (1) in the presence of the aryl azides, but without photolysis; (2) photolysis of the systems in the absence of the aryl azides; (3) photolysis in the presence of aryl azides *and* an excess of specific active site inhibitors (protectors); or (4) prior photolysis of the aryl azides, followed by the addition of the photolysed solution to the membrane preparation. These results therefore demonstrated that the inactivation which was produced required photolysis; the inactivation was specific since it could be blocked by protectors of the active sites; and the photoreactive species were short-lived. All of these results fit the mechanism proposed for photo-affinity labelling, and we therefore prepared [$^3$H] HK-83 at a specific activity of about 2 Ci/mmol (Kiefer & Singer, unpublished) for the purpose of labelling, detecting, and isolating AChR proteins. Most of our recent studies have dealt, however, with the AChE of the erythrocyte membrane, as a model system for the AChR. The ability to specifically inactivate AChE with diisopropylfluorophosphate (DFP) (Cohen & Warringa, 1953) has been a useful quantitative guide to our photo-affinity labelling experiments.

A detailed account of these experiments is in preparation and will be presented elsewhere. A few selected results which are essential to the following discussion are presented in Table 1. Using similar procedures to those described by Kiefer *et al.* (1970), we found that photolysis at 365 nm for 90 s of a suspension of human erythrocyte membranes ($\sim$1 mg membrane protein/ml) in the presence of $1 \times 10^{-5}$ M [$^3$H] HK-83 (specific activity 250 mCi/mmol) led to an irreversible loss of 75% of the original AChE activity. This inactivation could be completely prevented by the presence of $1 \times 10^{-5}$ M HK-37, a reversible protector which is bound to AChE with an equilibrium dissociation constant of $4{\cdot}7 \times 10^{-10}$ M (Kiefer *et al.*, 1970). The amounts of $^3$H irreversibly bound to the membranes in these two experiments were, however, indistinguishable. Furthermore, the amounts were two orders of magnitude larger than expected from the amount of [$^3$H] DFP bound in separate experiments. Clearly, a considerable amount of nonspecific modification of the membrane occurred upon photolysis. The nonspecific reaction might be due to nitrene formed by the photolysis of unbound HK-83 in free solution; the nitrene so formed might react only slowly with water, and therefore would react preferentially and nonspecifically with protein. We therefore added substances (scavengers) to the solution to react with any free nitrene and after preliminary successful experiments with proteins such as ribonuclease and bovine serum albumin, we found that *p*-aminobenzoate (PAB) was satisfactory for our purposes. PAB at $10^{-2}$ M does not absorb light significantly at 365 nm, nor has it any inhibitory effect on AChE activity. Added to the mixture of erythrocyte membranes and HK-83, PAB did reduce by 10-fold the amount of $^3$H which was irreversibly bound upon photolysis (Table 1). (The exact nature of the reaction product of PAB and nitrene

TABLE 1. *Scavenging of photo-affinity labelling of red blood cell acetylcholinesterase*

| Azide M | Protector M | Scavenger M | % remaining activity | c.p.m./OD |
|---|---|---|---|---|
| $10^{-5}$ | 0 | 0 | 24 | 27 200 |
| $10^{-5}$ | $10^{-5}$ | 0 | 100 | 26 650 |
| $10^{-5}$ | 0 | $10^{-2}$ | 95 | 2 500 |
| $10^{-5}$ | $10^{-5}$ | $10^{-2}$ | 100 | 2 800 |

is not known.) However, the *presence of PAB also prevented the inactivation of the AChE.* We have repeated this set of results many times, and have obtained similar results with the protein scavengers.

If the photo-affinity labelling and inactivation of AChE occurred by the expected mechanism (Fig. 1, bottom), and the P* that formed within the active site reacted before it could dissociate from the site, PAB should have had no effect on the specific irreversible inactivation that was produced in the absence of PAB. We have found no satisfactory trivial explanation of our results. Neither PAB, nor the product(s) of its photolytic reaction with HK-83, are competitive inhibitors of AChE; hence, one cannot explain the scavenging results as due to an increased displacement of HK-83 from unreacted AChE sites during the photolysis experiments in PAB-containing solutions. At least two possibilities exist: either (1) HK-83 is not photolysed at a significant rate when bound to the AChE site (perhaps because of energy transfer from HK-83 to some chromophore in or near the active site), but only when it is in free solution; or (2) HK-83 is photolysed in both the enzyme-bound and free states, but the nitrene formed within the site does not react rapidly enough in the active site, and generally first dissociates from the site (that is, $k_{-P^*3} \gg k_{P^*2}$, Fig. 1). We have been unable to decide definitively which of these two explanations is correct. We have carried out photolysis experiments in the frozen state, in the hope that if HK-83 were converted to the nitrene while bound to the AChE active site, and the dissociation of the nitrene from the site was retarded in the frozen state, nonscavengeable inactivation might have been observed. These experiments suffered from complications that cannot be detailed here, but the results of photolysis in the frozen state were not clearly different from those in solution at 25° C. Thus, we have no evidence that photolysis of HK-83 does occur while it is bound in the AChE site.

In any event, the scavenging results establish that although affinity labelling occurs in this case, it is not truly photo-affinity labelling, but is *ordinary* affinity labelling (Fig. 1, top) with a (more than usually reactive) reagent that is produced by photolysis. Whether the inactivation is in fact produced by reaction with the nitrene itself, or with a short-lived intermediate derived from the nitrene, is not known.

This conclusion for this one system has led us to ask whether in other investigators' experiments true photo-affinity labelling has actually ever been effected, or whether more generally inactivation occurred by the ordinary affinity labelling mechanism. Others have not used scavengers in their photo-affinity labelling experiments, so only indirect evidence is available on this point. It is significant, however, that in the work of Press, Fleet & Fisher (1971), which extended the earlier study of Fleet *et al.* (1969), it was reported that the compound 4-azido-2-nitrophenyl-lysine (NAP-lysine) was apparently a successful photo-affinity labelling reagent for one batch of pure antibodies directed to the NAP group, but was much less effective with a second batch of anti-NAP antibodies. The two batches of antibodies were otherwise indistinguishable. Such different results are not to be expected if the nitrene formed upon photolysis of the NAP group was indiscriminate in its reactivity towards different amino-acid residues, and could even insert into C–H bonds. The nitrene ought to have inactivated both batches of antibodies, to an equivalent extent. These results of Press *et al.* (1971) are rather those to be expected if indeed ordinary affinity labelling was involved. (For an example of such results in ordinary affinity labelling, see Koyama, Grossberg & Pressman, 1968.) In other instances of photo-affinity labelling (Converse & Richards, 1969; Brunswick & Cooperman, 1971) not enough information is available to determine which mechanism was involved. However, in the former case, the carbene formed upon photolysis could have undergone a Wolff rearrangement to a ketene, which could function as a highly reactive but ordinary affinity labelling reagent. The appropriate use of a scavenger, as is described in this report, is a simple way to determine whether photo- or ordinary affinity labelling is involved in any one case, and is recommended as a general adjunct of photo-affinity labelling experiments.

Our findings also raise a different problem. In photo-affinity labelling experiments, specific active site protectors are used to show that any inactivation produced in the absence of the protector is site specific (as we have used HK-37 in our experiments, Table 1). However, it must be shown that the protector is not acting as a scavenger of P*; if it scavenges P*, the inactivation produced by photolysis in the presence of the protector may thereby appear artifactually reduced. In our case, HK-37 did not act as a scavenger under the conditions of the experiments, since the amount of $^3H$ bound to the erythrocyte membranes was the same with or without the protector present (Table 1).

Our results suggest, therefore, that the apparent virtues of photo-affinity labelling may not yet have been fully realized in practice. In order for true photo-affinity labelling to occur, the condition that $k_{P^*2} \gg k_{-P^*3}$ (Fig. 1) must be satisfied. We need to know a great deal more about the chemistry of photolysable reagents, and whether, and under what conditions, they can be photolysed while reversibly bound in a protein active site. If such photolysis can indeed be effected, information about the spectroscopy and reactivity of the carbenes and nitrenes produced upon their photolysis is needed in order to design reagents with appropriately large values of $k_{P^*2}$.

In the last few years, several informative investigations of aryl azides and aryl nitrenes have been carried out. Nitrenes can be formed either in a singlet excited state, or a triplet ground state. It is only in the former state that the nitrene can undergo electrophilic insertion reactions. In the triplet state, the nitrene cannot insert; it can only abstract protons or recombine with other radicals. Flash photolysis of several aryl azides in hydrocarbon solvents, and absorption spectroscopic measurements of the nitrene produced, have shown that the latter were essentially exclusively formed in the triplet state (Reiser, Willets, Terry, Williams & Marley, 1968). The rates with which these nitrenes abstracted protons from the hydrocarbon solvent were relatively slow. If the 'solvent' was a relatively rigid polystyrene matrix, the half-time of the abstraction reaction could be as long as 0·5 s. If similar properties characterize HK-83 and HK-68, and their nitrenes are formed in the triplet ground state, our photo-affinity labelling results can be readily understood. True photo-affinity labelling with aryl azides may require that their nitrenes be formed in the singlet excited state.

The consequences of these spectroscopic findings will be further explored. It also appears that since carbenes are much more reactive than triplet state aryl nitrenes, and the rearrangements which acyl carbenes undergo can be suitably minimized (Brunswick & Cooperman, 1971), appropriate diazo compounds will prove more suitable as photo-affinity labelling reagents than aryl azides. It also follows that, other things being equal, the more strongly the nitrene is *reversibly* bound in the complex $C_{P^*}$ (Fig. 1, bottom), the smaller will be $k_{-P^*3}$, and the more likely will true photo-affinity labelling occur. Therefore, the affinity of the reagent for the site is a factor to be considered in its design.

While the first flush of optimism about the likely success of photo-affinity labelling may have to be temporarily tempered, and much work remains to be done, there is still good reason to hope that it will ultimately provide a highly specific and general method for the identification, characterization, and isolation of membrane-bound receptors.

## REFERENCES


BAKER, B. R. (1967). *Design of Active-Site Directed Irreversible Enzyme Inhibitors.* New York: John Wiley and Sons.

BELLEAU, B. & TANI, H. (1966). *Mol. Pharmac.*, **2**, 411.

BRUNSWICK, D. J. & COOPERMAN, B. S. (1971). *Proc. natn. Acad. Sci., U.S.A.*, **68**, 1801.

CHANGEUX, J.-P., PODLESKI, T. & WOFSY, L. (1967). *Proc. natn. Acad. Sci., U.S.A.*, **58**, 2063.

COHEN, J. A. & WARRINGA, M. G. P. J. (1953). *Biochem. biophys. Acta*, **11**, 52.

CONVERSE, C. A. & RICHARDS, F. F. (1969). *Biochemistry*, **8**, 4431.

FEWTRELL, C. M. S. & RANG, H. P. (1973). This symposium.

FLEET, G. W. J., KNOWLES, J. R. & PORTER, R. R. (1969). *Nature, Lond.*, **224**, 511.

GILL, E. W. & RANG, H. P. (1966). *Mol. Pharmac.*, **2**, 284.

HILL, W. C. (1971). *J. Immunol.*, **106**, 414.

KARLIN, A., COWBURN, D. A. & REITER, M. J. (1973). This symposium.

KASAI, M. & CHANGEUX, J.-P. (1971). *J. Memb. Biol.*, **6**, 1, 24, 58.

KIEFER, H., LINDSTROM, J., LENNOX, E. S. & SINGER, S. J. (1970). *Proc. natn. Acad. Sci., U.S.A.*, **67**, 1688.

KOYAMA, J., GROSSBERG, A. L. & PRESSMAN, D. (1968). *Biochemistry*, **7**, 1935.

NICKERSON, M. & GUMP, W. S. (1949). *J. Pharmac. exp. Ther.*, **97**, 25.

PRESS, E. M., FLEET, G. W. J. & FISHER, C. E. (1971). In: *Progress in Immunology*, ed. Amos, B., p. 233. New York: Academic Press.

REISER, A., WILLETS, F. W., TERRY, G. C., WILLIAMS, V. & MARLEY, R. (1968). *Trans. Faraday Soc.*, **64**, 3265.

SHAFER, J., BARONOWSKY, P., LAURSEN, R., FINN, F. & WESTHEIMER, F. H. (1966). *J. Biol. Chem.*, **241**, 421.

SHAW, E. (1970). *Physiol. Revs.*, **50**, 244.

SINGER, S. J. (1967). *Advances in Protein Chem.*, **22**, 1.

SINGER, S. J. (1970). In: Ciba Foundation Symposium on *Molecular Properties of Drug Receptors*, ed. Porter, R. & O'Connor, M., p. 229. London: J. A. Churchill.

SINGER, S. J. (1971). In: *Structure and Function of Biological Membranes*, ed. Rothfield, L. I., p. 145. New York: Academic Press.

SINGER, S. J. & NICOLSON, G. L. (1972). *Science*, **175**, 720.

SINGH, A., THORNTON, E. R. & WESTHEIMER, F. H. (1962). *J. Biol. Chem.*, **237**, PC 3006.

VAUGHAN, R. J. & WESTHEIMER, F. H. (1969). *J. Am. chem. Soc.*, **91**, 217.

WOFSY, L., METZGER, H. & SINGER, S. J. (1962). *Biochemistry*, **1**, 1031.


## DISCUSSION

*Barnard* (*New York*)

You pose the interesting question as to whether, when a specific ligand molecule is bound in a protein active centre, photo-activation of a reactive group on the ligand may be *prevented* by the local environment. I wonder how this relates to the earlier observations of Westheimer and colleagues (Shafer, Baronowsky, Laursen, Finn & Westheimer, 1966) on such a photo-activation, which, if I recall correctly, was in the α-chymotrypsin active site?

*Singer (San Diego)*

You are correct that in the particular case you refer to, which involved a diazoacyl ligand that was *covalently* bound to the active site of chymotrypsin, photolysis to the corresponding carbene did apparently occur within the site. Whether this can be generalized to other types of photo-affinity labelling reagents, however, remains to be established.

# MOLECULAR PROPERTIES OF THE ACETYLCHOLINE RECEPTOR

A. KARLIN, D. A. COWBURN AND M. J. REITER

*Department of Neurology, College of Physicians and Surgeons, Columbia University, New York, N.Y. 10032, USA*

Covalent modification of the acetylcholine receptor enables the function of the receptor to be related to its chemical structure. An important by-product is a chemical specification of the receptor by which it may be identified in isolation. Site-directed reactions with affinity reagents (cf. Singer, Ruoho, Kiefer, Lindstrom & Lennox, this symposium) relate function to the chemical structure in the immediate vicinity of the binding site for acetylcholine and are a potential means for mapping the 'active site'. A sketchy picture of the acetylcholine receptor has emerged from the effects of both affinity and nonaffinity reagents on the functions of single cells (electroplax) from the electric tissue of *Electrophorus electricus*. Some of these results have been reproduced using muscle cells from other species (see below). This picture contains a relatively unreactive sulphydryl (SH) group some distance from the negative subsite and a relatively easily reduced disulphide (S–S) group in the near vicinity of the negative subsite. The negative subsite is the postulated locus of ion-pair formation between the receptor and the quaternary ammonium group of cholinergic ligands. Some of the reactions inferred from the physiological results have been more directly demonstrated by means of a radioactive quaternary ammonium maleimide derivative applied to intact electroplax and to membrane fragments isolated from electric tissue. Labelled components have been solubilized and separated by gel electrophoresis, and these results add to the above picture that the receptor or a subunit of the receptor is a polypeptide chain of molecular weight 42 000. We will review the evidence for these various features and discuss some possible implications for the mechanism of action of depolarizing substances.

## *SH groups*

The evidence for reactive SH groups on the receptor is not strong and is based on the effects of mercurials on the electroplax. It was found that incubation for 5 min with 0·5 mM *p*-chloromercuribenzoate (PCMB) strongly inhibits the response to acetylcholine and its congeners but causes little change in the resting potential, action potential, or sodium pump activity (Karlin & Bartels, 1966). The inhibition is reversed by thiols but not by washing. Mercuric ion is a very potent depolarizer of the electroplax, acting rapidly (5 min) at 60 μM. Mercuric ion at 10 μM causes a slow depolarization and inhibits the carbachol response by 40%. None of the effects of mercuric ion are reversed by washing or with added thiols.

A number of other mercurials have been tested, including some with a quaternary ammonium group, and generally a gradual depolarization results at a concentration equal to or at most twice as great as the concentration resulting in 50% inhibition of the carbachol response (unpublished). The depolarization and the inhibition are not reversible by thiols. For example, the quaternary ammonium mercurial 4-(*p*-trimethylammoniumphenylazo)-2-chloromercuriphenol (TAMP; Bloemmen, Joniau & Lontie, 1967), at 20 μM (5 min) blocks the carbachol response by 90% and also causes a slow depolarization (Silman & Karlin, unpublished). Neither effect is reversed by thiols, or prevented by the presence of 10 μM (+)-tubocurarine. A negatively charged mercurial, 4-(*p*-sulphophenylazo)-2-chloromercuriphenol (SAMP), similar to the preceding but with a sulphonate group instead of the trimethylammonium group (Joniau, Bloemmen & Lontie, 1966), at 100 μM (5 min), causes a rapid depolarization. Two other quaternary ammonium mercurials, *p*-chloromercuriphenyltrimethylammonium and *p*-chloromercuribenzyltrimethylammonium at 100 μM (5 min) also irreversibly depolarize the electroplax (Karlin & Chang, unpublished). The potencies of the quaternary ammonium mercurials are not sufficiently different from those of the negatively charged mercurials (for example, SAMP, PCMB) to support the notion that there is a free SH group in the close vicinity of the negative subsite.

In contrast to the mercurials, alkylating and acylating agents do not block the response to carbachol or themselves cause a depolarization. Compounds such as N-ethylmaleimide (NEM) and iodoacetamide eventually block active sodium transport with no apparent effect on the receptor (Karlin & Bartels, 1966). Quaternary ammonium alkylating and acylating agents such as 4-(*N*-maleimido)-α-benzyltrimethylammonium (MBTA) (Karlin, 1969) and the nitrophenyl ester of *p*-carboxyphenyltrimethylammonium (NPTMB) (Silman & Karlin, 1969) are *reversible* competitive inhibitors of the receptor, and bromoacetylcholine (BAC) (Silman & Karlin, 1969) is a *reversible* activator. These reagents react covalently only after the receptor has been reduced with dithiothreitol (DTT).

Disulphides such as 5,5′-dithio-*bis*(2-nitrobenzoate) (DTNB) (Karlin & Bartels, 1966) and dithiobischoline ($(ChS)_2$) (Bartels, Deal, Karlin & Mautner, 1970) rapidly form mixed disulphides with available SH groups but have no effect on the carbachol response of the intact electroplax. $(ChS)_2$, which ordinarily acts as a reversible competitive inhibitor like hexamethonium, would be expected to react rapidly with a free SH group in the vicinity of the negative subsite if such were present, but this only occurs following reduction of the receptor by dithiothreitol (see below). That DTNB reacts with available SH groups is demonstrated by the result that more than 95% of the groups on the surface of the electroplax available to react with high concentrations of MBTA are blocked by prior reaction with DTNB. Bath application of DTNB fails to depolarize or to block the carbachol response not only in electroplax but also in frog rectus abdominis (Mittag & Tormay, 1970; Karlin & Cunningham, unpublished), frog sartorius (Lindstrom, Kiefer, Lennox & Singer, in press; del Castillo, personal communication), and chick biventer cervicis (Rang & Ritter, 1971). Ferricyanide is also without effect on the electroplax. These results of bath application of potential oxidizing agents of SH groups are contrary to the results of del Castillo, Escobar & Gijon (1971), who find that such oxidizing agents applied by microelectro-osmosis to frog sartorius endplates variably depolarize and/or inhibit carbachol. These latter effects are transient, suggesting that covalent oxidation reactions may not be involved.

In summary, within the limits of the specificity of organic mercurials for SH groups, it appears that there may be at least one hindered SH group in the receptor which can react with mercurials but not readily with akylating, acylating, or oxidizing agents (cf. for example, Katz & Mommaerts, 1962; Fraenkel-Conrat, 1959). The SH group(s) do not appear to be *affinity* labelled by quaternary ammonium alkylating, acylating, or oxidizing agents or by quaternary ammonium mercurials, even though the latter appear to react, and thus an SH group is not likely to be within the acetylcholine-binding site or its near vicinity.

### *S–S groups*

Dithiothreitol, a potent S–S reducing agent (Cleland, 1964), added to the electroplax at low concentrations (0·2–1 mM) for 10 min, has profound effects on the response of the cell to cholinergic agents (Table 1). The depolarizing responses to monoquaternary activators (Karlin & Bartels, 1966) and to succinylcholine are decreased by reduction; conversely, the response to decamethonium is increased (Karlin, 1969), and hexamethonium, ordinarily an inhibitor, depolarizes the reduced electroplax (Karlin & Winnik, 1968). The physiological effects of dithiothreitol are quite specific; there is no effect on the resting potential, the action potential, or on active sodium transport. All the physiological effects of dithiothreitol are reversed by application of agents, such as DTNB, capable of reoxidizing dithiols to disulphides. If, however, a thiol alkylating agent is applied after reduction and before oxidation, the reversal is prevented. It appears therefore that there is at least one disulphide bond whose reduction alters the specificity of the receptor. This disulphide appears to have only a structural function. It is not reduced and reoxidized during an activity cycle; in the absence of prior treatment

TABLE 1. *Effect of dithiothreitol and of subsequent alkylation on the response of the electroplax to cholinergic ligands*

| Compound | Potency relative to acetylcholine | Change in response after DTT % | Change in response after DTT, NEM % |
|---|---|---|---|
| Acetylcholine | 1 | −80 | −96 |
| Butyltrimethylammonium | 0·3 | −75 | |
| Carbachol | 0·1 | −81 | −92 |
| Tetramethylammonium | 0·001 | −55 | −70 |
| (+)-Acetyl-β-methylcholine | 0 | 0 | |
| Decamethonium | 1 | +44 | −94 |
| Hexamethonium | 0 | depolarizes 14 mV | 0 mV |
| Dithiobischoline $(ChS)_2$ | 0 | depolarizes | |

Reference, Karlin (1969).

with dithiothreitol, there is no alkylation by NEM in the presence of carbachol or by BAC, itself a depolarizing agent. The change in the concentration–effect curve for carbachol due to dithiothreitol-reduction is characterized by a 4-fold increase in the half-maximal concentration and a decrease in the Hill coefficient from 1·8 to 1·1 (Karlin, 1967a).

The reducible S–S group appears to be close to the negative subsite. The evidence for this is that alkylating agents possessing a quaternary ammonium group react with the reduced receptor up to 3 orders of magnitude faster than comparable uncharged reagents. Three types of affinity reaction have been demonstrated: affinity reduction, affinity reoxidation, and affinity alkylation. From the stereochemistry of these reactions it is calculated that the reducible S–S group is approximately 1 nm from the negative subsite (Karlin, 1969).

A number of affinity alkylating and acylating reagents have been tested on the electroplax both before and after application of dithiothreitol (Table 2). In the maleimide series (first five compounds in Table 2), the quaternary ammonium derivatives block the reversal by DTNB of the physiological effects of dithiothreitol at least 1000 times faster than uncharged NEM (first compound) or 4-(*N*′-maleimido)-*N*,*N*-dimethylaniline (second compound) also uncharged at pH 7. MBTA (fifth compound) apparently reacts with the reduced receptor 4700 times faster than does NEM; however, MBTA also reacts with cysteine in solution 4·3 times faster than NEM, so that the enhancement in rate due to affinity for the site is approximately 1100-fold (Karlin, 1969). The physiological evidence implies that MBTA reacts preferentially with the reduced receptor, and this is supported by labelling experiments with [$^3$H] MBTA and [$^{14}$C] NEM (see below). Following reaction of the quaternary ammonium maleimides with the reduced electroplax, the response to carbachol is blocked. In addition, two of these compounds produce small, irreversible depolarizations upon reaction. In the absence of prior treatment of the electroplax with dithiothreitol, all three

TABLE 2. *The effects of alkylating agents on the untreated and dithiothreitol-treated electroplax*

| Compound | Length (nm) | Untreated | Dithiothreitol-treated | | Reference |
|---|---|---|---|---|---|
| | | | Conc. blocking DTNB reversal by 50% nM | Max. irreversible depolarization mV | |
| 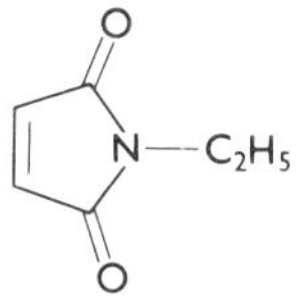 | | No immediate effect at $< 250\ \mu M$ | 20 000 | 0 | Karlin & Bartels (1966) |
| 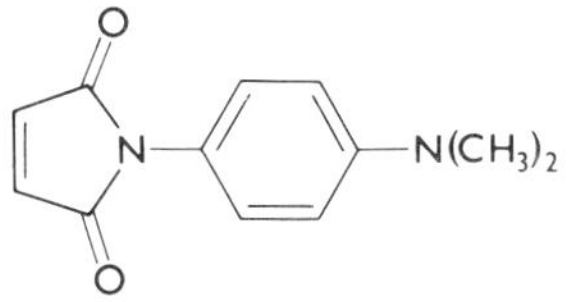 | | No effect | 20 000 | 0 | Karlin & Winnik (1968) |
| 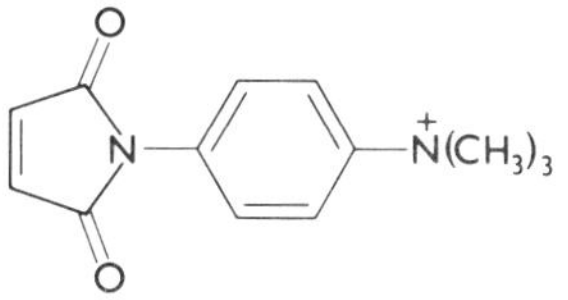 | 0·83 | Reversible inhibitor, $K_I = 80\ \mu M$ | 8 | 1 | Karlin & Winnik (1968) |
| 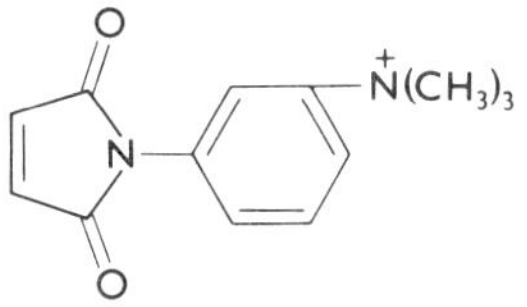 | 0·78 | Reversible inhibitor | 12 | 2 | Karlin (1969) |
| 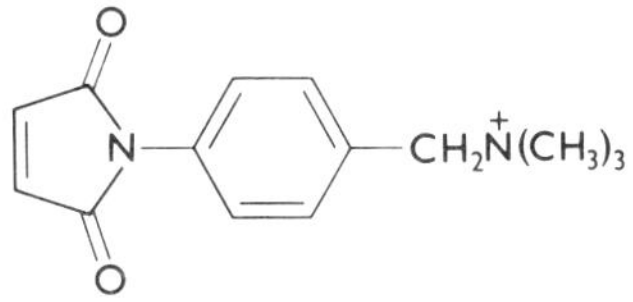 | 0·90 | Reversible inhibitor ($K_I = 80\ \mu M$) | 4 | 0 | Karlin (1969) |
| $BrCH_2.COO.CH_2CH_2\overset{+}{N}(CH_3)_3$ | 0·66 | Reversible activator ($K_A \simeq 10\ \mu M$) | | > 30 | Silman & Karlin (1969) |
| 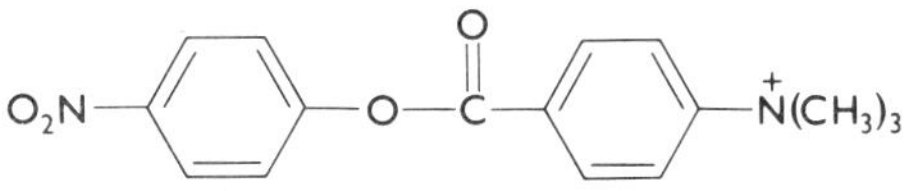 | 0·67 | Reversible inhibitor ($K_I = 6\ \mu M$) | | > 30 | Silman & Karlin (1969) |
| 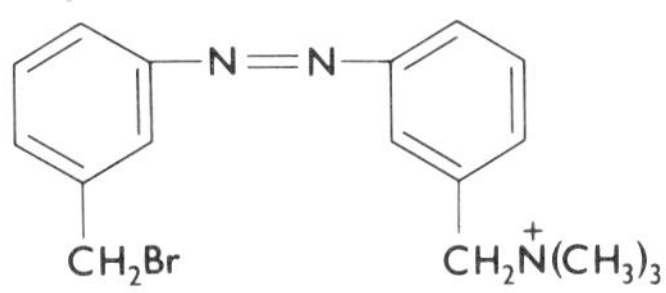 | 0·6–1·0 | Reversible partial agonist | | 10–20 | Bartels, Wasserman & Erlanger (1971) |

$K_A$ and $K_I$ values are apparent equilibrium constants for activators and inhibitors. The length of the molecule is the maximum distance between the reactive carbon atom and quaternary ammonium group, except in the case of the last compound (see text).

quaternary ammonium maleimides act as completely reversible competitive inhibitors of the receptor. [$^3$H] MBTA can be shown to react with pre-existing membrane SH groups of the unreduced electroplax; but these reactions do not affect the physiological functions monitored and apparently involve components other than the receptor.

Two other compounds, BAC (sixth compound) and NPTMB (seventh compound), cause a depolarization after dithiothreitol which is not reversed by washing but is temporarily reversed in the presence of high concentrations of reversible competitive inhibitors such as (+)-tubocurarine. Upon removal of the competitive inhibitor the depolarization reappears. These results are interpreted as being due to the covalent attachment of a quaternary ammonium moiety to an SH group (formed by reduction) at the periphery of the acetylcholine-binding site and the reversible association of the quaternary ammonium group itself with the negative subsite. The moiety can rotate around its covalent point of attachment into or out of the site and is thus displaceable from the site by competitive inhibitors. Before the cell has been exposed to dithiothreitol, BAC is a completely reversible activator and NPTMB is a completely reversible competitive inhibitor. Another reactive compound, 3-(α-bromomethyl)3′-[α-(trimethylammonium)methyl] azobenzene bromide (QBr, eighth compound) has similar properties to NPTMB (Bartels, Wasserman & Erlanger, 1971).

The degree of activation by a covalently attached quaternary ammonium moiety appears to vary inversely with its length (Karlin, 1969). The approximate centre-to-centre distances from the quaternary nitrogen to the reactive carbon for these compounds are given in Table 2. Among the maleimides, a decrease in this distance corresponds to an increase in the maximum depolarization, and this trend continues with NPTMB, BAC, and QBr. The attached moieties of the latter two have a range of possible conformations; and the maximum distance is given for BAC and the extremes for QBr. These results suggest that in the active state the acetylcholine-binding-site is in a shortened conformation relative to its conformation in the inactive state; that is, the region of the S–S group, which may include a hydrophobic subsite, is closer in the active state to the negative subsite (Karlin, 1969). In the resting, inactive state of the receptor one of the SH groups formed by reduction, and probably the parent S–S group also, is approximately 1 nm from the negative subsite, where the SH group can be most efficiently affinity-alkylated by MBTA.

The reoxidation of the reduced receptor can also be considerably enhanced by affinity of the oxidizing agent for the negative subsite (Table 3). The mechanisms of reoxidation of the receptor dithiol to a disulphide are not the same for all the agents. The disulphide compounds (DTNB and $(ChS)_2$) act most probably through a mixed disulphide intermediate. The mechanism of the action of cysteine and of cholinethiol is not known. It has been shown that monothiols catalyse the air oxidation of dithiols (Cleland, 1964). Both

TABLE 3. *Reversal of effects of dithiothreitol on the electroplax*

| Compound | Effective concentration applied ~10 min μM | Reference |
|---|---|---|
| $K_3Fe(CN)_6$ | 1000 | Karlin & Bartels (1966) |
| 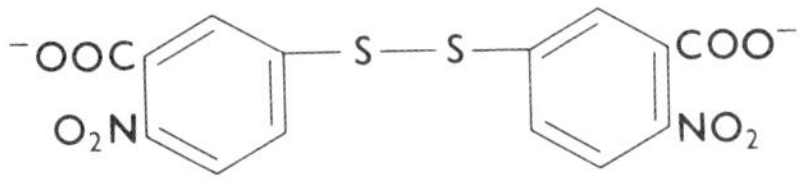 | 1000 | Karlin & Bartels (1966) |
| $^{-}OOCCHCH_2SH$ (with $^{+}NH_3$ on CH) | 5000 | Karlin & Bartels (1966) |
| $(CH_3)_3\overset{+}{N}CH_2CH_2SH$ | 1 | Bartels, Deal, Karlin & Mautner (1970) |
| $(CH_3)_3\overset{+}{N}CH_2CH_2S$—$SCH_2CH_2\overset{+}{N}(CH_3)_3$ | 0·2 | Bartels, Deal, Karlin & Mautner (1970) |

cysteine and cholinethiol catalyse the air oxidation of dithiothreitol. It is possible that they act through a sulphenic acid intermediate. Cysteine at 50 mM reduces the receptor. It is clear from a comparison of the concentrations capable of completely reversing the effects of dithiothreitol that the quaternary ammonium group imparts a 1000-fold advantage to cholinethiol compared with cysteine and a 5000-fold advantage to $(ChS)_2$ compared with DTNB. If not preceded by dithiothreitol, $(ChS)_2$ acts as a reversible competitive inhibitor like hexamethonium.

The reduction reaction also apparently can be site-directed by addition of a quaternary ammonium group (Table 4). Preliminary results with three derivatives of dithiothreitol and one of lipoic acid indicate that attachment of a quaternary ammonium group results in a 100- to 1000-fold increase in the rate of reduction. There are, however, two difficulties with these derivatives. Firstly, they are difficult to reduce and maintain reduced, so that they are added as a mixture of dithiol and disulphide forms. The disulphide forms, however, have only reversible (noncovalent) effects on the electroplax. Secondly, the covalent effects ascribable to the reduced forms are not completely reversed by DTNB, suggesting that to some extent the reaction with the receptor stops at the mixed disulphide stage. This is supported by the result that dithiothreitol followed by DTNB does reverse fully the effects of these derivatives, suggesting that dithiothreitol completes the reduction, and eliminates the mixed disulphide.

TABLE 4. *Affinity reducing agents*

| Compound | Concentration applied 10 min (red./ox.) μM | Inhibition of carb. response % | Residual inhibition after DTNB % |
|---|---|---|---|
| 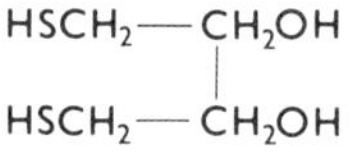 | 190/10 | 75 | 0 |
| 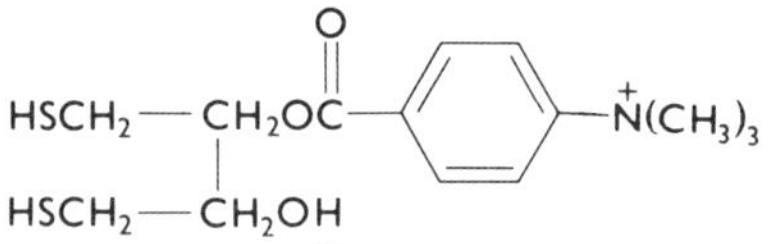 | 10/10 | 95 | 30 |
| 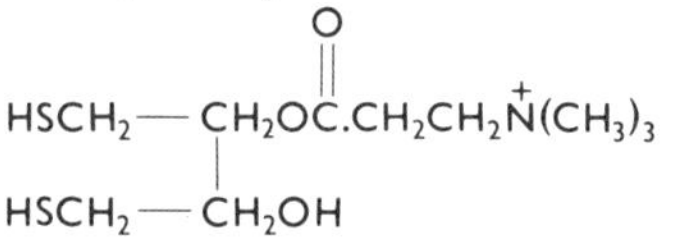 | 5/5 | 80 | 35 |
| 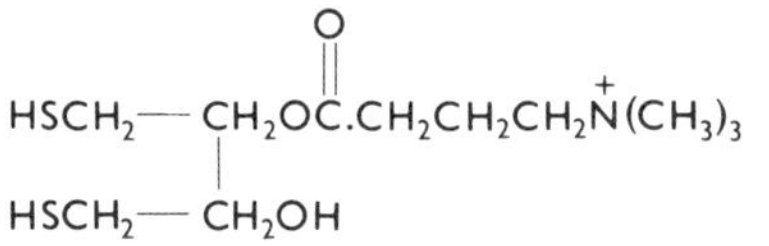 | 4/1 | 95 | 30 |
| $CH_2SH.CH_2.CH_2SH.(CH_2)_4.COO^-$ | 1500/500 | 65 | 15 |
| 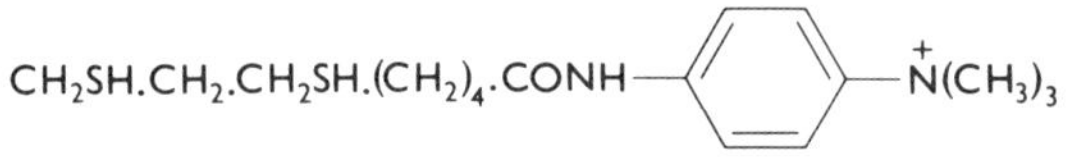 | 2/3 | 85 | 60 |

Reference, Karlin, Chang & Cowburn (unpublished).
The estimated concentrations of reduced and of oxidized forms in the solution applied to the electrop[lax] are given.

The effects of reduction by dithiothreitol on the electroplax have been reproduced on other tissues (Table 5), suggesting that an easily reducible S–S group close to the acetylcholine-binding-site is a common property of the nicotinic-type acetylcholine receptor. None of the reagents mentioned have any effect on the activity of acetylcholinesterase under conditions that strongly alter the properties of the receptor (Karlin, 1967b; and unpublished).

### *Receptor assay by affinity-labelling*

The much greater rate of alkylation of the reduced receptor in the electroplax by MBTA than by NEM appears to be due mainly to the affinity of MBTA for the receptor and to a much lesser extent to the difference in intrinsic reactivity (Karlin, 1969). Assuming that NEM reacts with the SH group(s) in the vicinity of the binding site of the reduced receptor at approximately the same rate that it reacts with other SH groups in the membrane, we expect that MBTA will react with an SH group close to the receptor site

TABLE 5. *Effects of dithiothreitol on 'nicotinic' receptors*

| Preparation | Inhibit response to monoquat. compounds | Enhance response to bisquat. compounds | Reversed by oxidation | Reversal blocked by alkylation | Affinity alkylation |
|---|---|---|---|---|---|
| *Eel electroplax* | | | | | |
| Karlin and co-workers (1966, 1968, 1969) | + | + | + | + | + |
| Podleski, Meunier & Changeux (1969) | + | + | | | |
| *Frog rectus abdominis* | | | | | |
| Karlin & Cunningham (unpublished) | + | | + | + | |
| Mittag & Tormay (1970) | + | | + | | + |
| *Frog sartorius* | | | | | |
| Lindstrom, Kiefer, Lennox & Singer (unpublished; cited by Singer, 1970) | + | | + | + | − |
| del Castillo, Escobar & Gijon (1971) (microelectrophoresis) | + (transient) | | (transient depolarization) | | |
| *Chick biventer cervicis* | | | | | |
| Rang & Ritter (1969, 1971) | + | + | + | + | + |
| *Rat skeletal muscle* (denervated) | | | | | |
| Albuquerque, Sokoll, Sonesson & Thesleff (1968) | + | | | | |

(+), Indicates a positive effect.

approximately 1100 times faster than with all other SH groups (see p. 196). Despite this high specificity, MBTA would also be expected to react with other SH groups, which may be present in great excess. Criteria based on physiological observations for distinguishing alkylation of the specific sites from nonspecific alkylation are as follows. (1) The specific reaction should be eliminated by prior treatment of the reduced receptor with the affinity-oxidizing agent, $(ChS)_2$, at a concentration shown to reverse completely the effects of reduction. (2) The specific reaction should be retarded in the presence of hexamethonium. (3) The extent of specific reaction should show saturation, and half-saturation should occur at approximately the same concentration as in comparable physiological experiments. These criteria are fulfilled in studies of the binding of [$^3$H] MBTA on dithiothreitol-treated electroplax (Karlin, Prives, Deal & Winnik, 1970, 1971). The asymptotic limit of the specific, saturating component of the labelling is approximately 10 pmol/g of electroplax and 2 pmol/mg protein. Half-saturation is at 16 nM [$^3$H] MBTA, compared with 4 nM determined physiologically from block of the reversal of reduction. The number of acetylcholinesterase sites determined directly is 7 times the number of receptor sites. These results refer to intact, single cells (electroplax) dissected from the organ of Sachs.

The question of whether the specific, saturating portion of the labelling of intact electroplax represents a single component was approached by the solubilization of labelled electroplax and the separation of protein components into molecular weight classes by polyacrylamide gel electrophoresis in the presence of sodium dodecyl sulphate (SDS) (Reiter, Cowburn, Prives & Karlin, 1972). A single major peak of $^3$H-activity, corresponding to a polypeptide of molecular weight 42 000, is obtained. This peak is considerably diminished in extracts of electroplax which have been labelled either after specific reoxidation of the receptor SH groups by $(ChS)_2$ or in the presence of hexamethonium. In addition, a low concentration ($\sim 0{\cdot}2$ $\mu$M) of cobra toxin from *Naja naja siamensis*, which blocks the receptor in the electroplax irreversibly (Lester, 1971; Prives, Reiter, Cowburn & Karlin, 1972), also blocks a portion of the labelling by [$^3$H] MBTA, and the gels of extracts of electroplax labelled after exposure to $0{\cdot}2$ $\mu$M cobra toxin also show diminished $^3$H-activity in the region of the major peak. Thus, a component of molecular weight 42 000 is protected against labelling by three diverse agents, an affinity oxidizing agent, a small reversible blocking agent, and a large irreversible blocking agent. The polypeptide nature of this labelled component is supported by the consistency of the molecular weight estimates obtained at three different gel concentrations when co-linearity with protein standards is assumed.

One further criterion of specificity of labelling is the inferred relative rates of reaction of MBTA and of NEM with the reduced receptor. Electroplax were reduced and then alkylated with a mixture of [$^3$H] MBTA and [$^{14}$C] NEM, and the SDS-extracts were subjected to gel electrophoresis (Reiter *et al.*, 1972). A single peak in the ratio of $^3$H to $^{14}$C is obtained, which corresponds to the major peak in $^3$H-activity. This peak in the ratio is completely eliminated by treatment of the electroplax with $(ChS)_2$ prior to alkylation. By several criteria, therefore, the major peak contains labelled acetylcholine receptor, and by comparison with polypeptide molecular weight standards, either the receptor or a receptor subunit is a polypeptide of molecular weight 42 000 (cf. Changeux, Meunier, Olsen & Weber, this symposium).

A membrane fraction from the electric tissue of the main organ of *Electrophorus* was labelled with [$^3$H] MBTA and [$^{14}$C] NEM under conditions very similar to those used with intact electroplax (Karlin, Cowburn & Reiter, in preparation). The SDS-extract was subjected to gel electrophoresis. A major peak of $^3$H-activity and of $^3$H : $^{14}$C ratio is obtained which is nearly eliminated by prior addition of cobra toxin or $(ChS)_2$ (Fig. 1) or by the presence of carbachol or hexamethonium during labelling. These agents have no effect on the [$^{14}$C] NEM labelling. The mobility of the major peak again corresponds to that of a polypeptide of molecular weight 42 000. In the

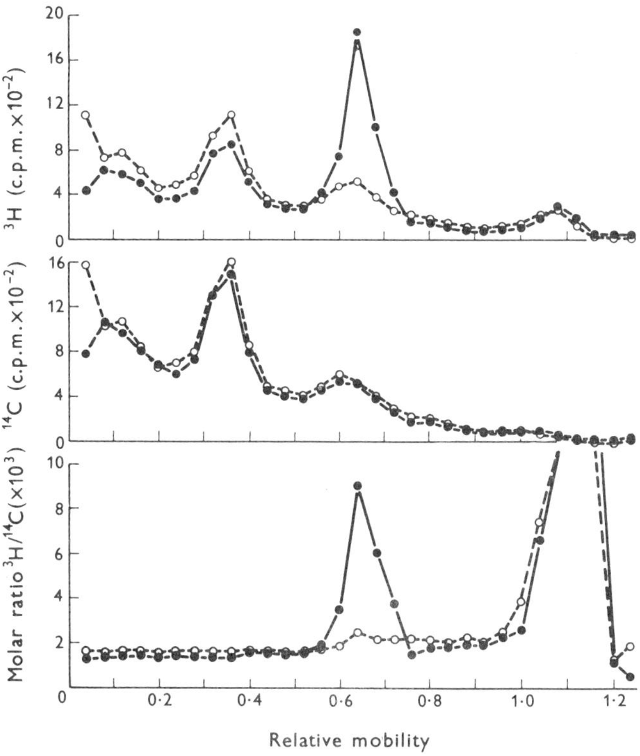


FIG. 1. The electrophoretic distribution on acrylamide gel of $^3$H (c.p.m.), $^{14}$C (c.p.m.), and $^3$H : $^{14}$C ratio (mol[$^3$H] MBTA/mol[$^{14}$C] NEM) in extracts of membrane fragments double-labelled with [$^3$H] MBTA and [$^{14}$C] NEM. The membrane fragments were prepared from main organ electric tissue by a modification of a previously described procedure (Karlin, 1965) and contained 37% of the acetylcholinesterase and 13% of the protein of the total homogenate. Approximately 20 mg of membrane protein was suspended in 8 ml eel Ringer solution and treated sequentially with reagents as indicated, with thorough washing after each incubation by repeated sedimentation and resuspension in eel Ringer solution. The sequences are: (●——●), 0·2 mM dithiothreitol (pH 8·0), 10 min; 12 nM [$^3$H] MBTA + 9·6 μM [$^{14}$C] NEM (pH 7·1), 2 min; and (○----○), 0·2 mM dithiothreitol (pH 8·0), 10 min; 0·5 μM $(ChS)_2$ (pH 7·1), 5 min; 12 nM [$^3$H] MBTA + 9·6 M [$^{14}$C] NEM (pH 7·1), 2 min. The dithiothreitol reaction was stopped by lowering the pH temporarily to 6·8, and that with the alkylating agents by adding an excess of β-mercaptoethanol. All reagents were in eel Ringer solution at the indicated pH. The final pellets were extracted for 2 h at 50° with 2% SDS + 5 mM dithiothreitol + 10 mM Tris-acetate (pH 8·0), solubilizing 98% of the radioactivity. Aliquots of the extracts were electrophoresed on 7·5% acrylamide gel, in 1% SDS + 2 mM dithiothreitol + 100 mM Tris-acetate (pH 8·0). Fractions for counting were prepared and the data treated as previously described (Reiter *et al.*, 1972).

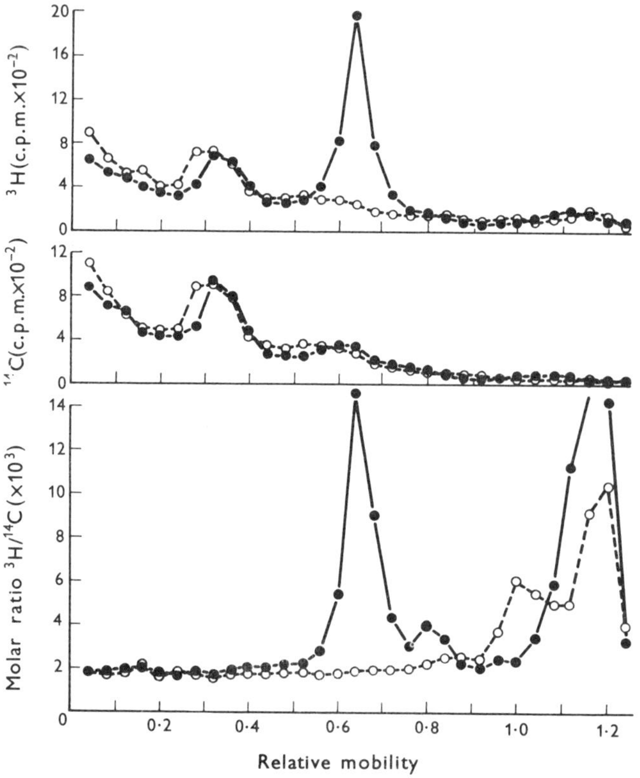


FIG. 2. The electrophoretic distribution of extracts of membrane fragments either treated with dithiothreitol (●——●) or not treated with dithiothreitol (○----○) prior to labelling with [$^3$H] MBTA + [$^{14}$C] NEM as in Fig.1.

absence of prior reduction by dithiothreitol, there is little $^3$H-activity in the region of the major peak and no elevation in the $^3$H : $^{14}$C ratio (Fig. 2).* An estimate of the density of receptor sites in this fraction, obtained by extrapolation to saturating conditions, is 3 pmol/mg of membrane protein or 9 pmol/g of original tissue.

The use of double-labelling with an affinity and a nonaffinity label followed by gel electrophoresis in SDS appears to be a reliable, well-founded chemical assay for the acetylcholine receptor, though it is cumbersome for routine use on large numbers of fractions. It may be applied to the isolation of receptor in two ways: to the isolation of prelabelled receptor, feasible because the label is covalently attached, and to the assay of unlabelled receptor at each stage of purification. The latter is likely to be successful only if the native conformation of the receptor is retained at least in the vicinity of the binding site,

* The elevation of the $^3$H : $^{14}$C ratio at the end of the gels is due to a small quantity of $^3$H-activity which runs ahead of the bromophenol blue marker.

for the preferential labelling depends on the matching of the geometry of the affinity label to the geometry of the site.

*Some implications*

The receptor mediates a change in the permeability of the postsynaptic membrane to sodium and potassium ions. There are two questions of immediate interest. (1) Does the receptor participate directly or indirectly in the translocation of these cations? (2) Is translocation via a carrier or a channel? We cannot yet answer the first question, but the information may be available for an answer to the second.

During the peak of the e.p.s.p. or of a response to carbachol in the electroplax (organ of Sachs), as much as 100 $mA/cm^2$ of inward $Na^+$ current passes through the innervated membrane (Ruiz-Manresa & Grundfest, 1971). The average electroplax used in affinity labelling experiments weighs 35 mg and contains $2 \times 10^{11}$ receptor sites (Karlin *et al.*, 1971). The area of a plane of the same outline as the innervated face of such a cell is 0·33 $cm^2$. Such a cell can conduct 33 mA of inward $Na^+$ current or $2 \times 10^{17}$ $Na^+$ ions per s during an e.p.s.p. The flux associated with each receptor site is thus $10^6$ cations per s per site. The question is whether a carrier mechanism could reasonably account for such a flux. It has been shown that rhodopsin (molecular weight 40 000) rotates relatively freely in the rod outer segment disc membrane (Brown, 1972; Cone, 1972). The axis of rotation is perpendicular to the plane of the membrane. The relaxation time is estimated to be 20 $\mu$s and approximately 10 relaxation times are required for a complete rotation; hence, rhodopsin completes $10^3$–$10^4$ cycles per s (Cone, 1972). A carrier of comparable size rotating around an axis *in the plane of the membrane* would undoubtedly rotate more slowly. Even without allowing for this, the rate of rotation of rhodopsin is too slow by 2–3 orders of magnitude to carry the required flux of $10^6$ cations per s. The carrier mechanism thus seems unlikely, and we must assume that the activation of the receptor results in the opening of cation conducting channels.

Can a channel mechanism account for the required flux? In the electroplax, the maximum peak synaptic conductance observed during activation was approximately 0·6 $mho/cm^2$ (Ruiz-Manresa & Grundfest, 1971). Using again 0·33 $cm^2$ outline area and $2 \times 10^{11}$ receptor sites per cell, we obtain an upper value of $10^{-12}$ mho per receptor site during activation. In an artificial bimolecular lipid membrane, the unit conductance of the gramicidin A channel (Tosteson, Andreoli, Tiffenberg & Cook, 1968; Goodall, 1970; Krasne, Eisenman & Szabo, 1971; Urry, 1971) in 0·2 M NaCl medium is $10^{-11}$ mho (Hladky & Haydon, 1970), or 10 times that required for the receptor in the electroplax. On the other hand, Katz & Miledi (1971) estimate the single channel conductance in the frog muscle endplate during activation to be approximately $10^{-10}$ mho, so that the acetylcholine-activated channel may have to be more efficient than the gramicidin A channel.

The estimate of Katz & Miledi (1971) is of the instantaneous conductance of an open channel, while ours, based on a measurement of membrane conductance due to a large number of channels, is closer to a time-average of the conductance of a single channel. A possible implication of the difference by a factor of two orders of magnitude is that even during occupation of the receptor with acetylcholine, the associated channel(s) might be open only 1 % of the time.

## *A model*

The various observations and tentative conclusions can be combined in a model (Fig. 3), hopefully heuristic. The receptor is represented as a dimer, the minimal oligomer accounting for a Hill coefficient of the concentration–effect curve close to 2 (Karlin, 1967a; Changeux & Podleski, 1968). The molecular weight of the dimer would be 84 000, and at a density of 1·4 g/cm³ would have the volume of a right cylinder 5 nm × 5 nm. This is represented as transversing the lipid bilayer (for example, Branton, 1969; Wilkins, Blaurock & Engelman, 1971; Steck, Fairbanks & Wallach, 1971; Bretscher, 1971; Singer & Nicolson, 1972). Since acetylcholine does not act on the

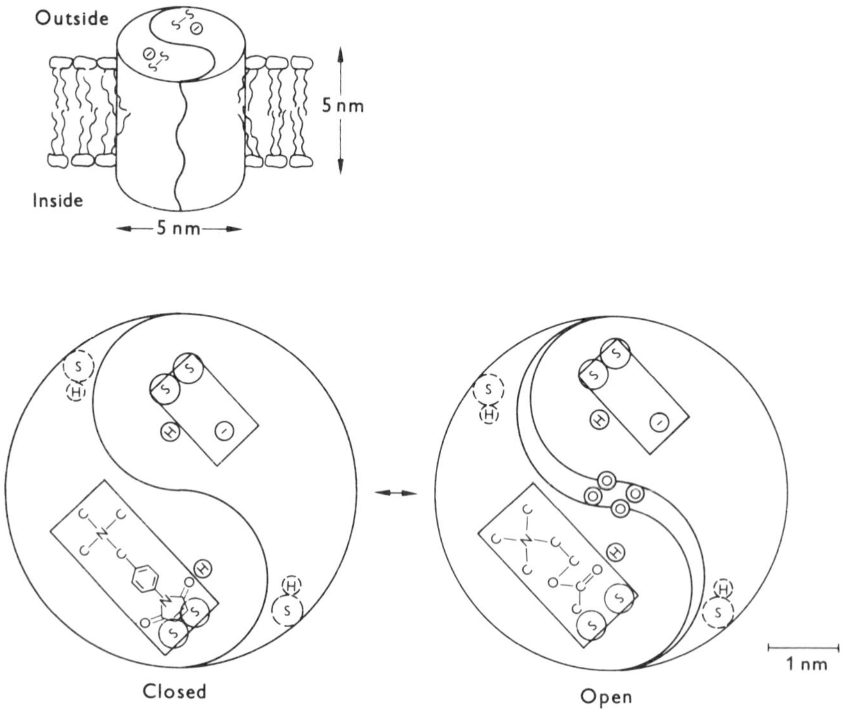


FIG. 3. Dimer model of the receptor. See text for details.

inside of the membrane (del Castillo & Katz, 1955), we represent both binding sites facing outward; thus, the dimer has a dyad axis of symmetry perpendicular to the plane of the membrane and is asymmetrical across the plane of the membrane.

The binding site for acetylcholine is represented as a slot in the outer 'surface' of each protomer. Close to one end of the slot is the negative subsite and overlapping the other end is the reducible disulphide group. The region in the vicinity of the disulphide is considered to be involved in hydrophobic interaction with ligands. Explicitly included is a hydrogen-bond donor site, the possible importance of which in the binding of many cholinergic ligands has been emphasized by Beers & Reich (1970). Some non-hydrogen bonding cholinergic ligands, however, are as potent activators as acetylcholine itself. It was surmised that an essential aspect of 'the transition from inactive to active state involves a conformational change around the quaternary ammonium–negative subsite ion-pair and a linked decrease in the distance between the negative subsite and the hydrophobic subsite, stabilized in potent activators by a bridge of the correct length positively interacting at both subsites' (Karlin, 1969). The two conformations are represented (active = open), each with one site occupied. The site in the inactive conformation is shown occupied by MBTA acting as a competitive inhibitor but also being well positioned to affinity-alkylate one of the SH groups, were the S–S group reduced. The site in the active conformation is shown occupied by acetylcholine, and the length of the site is decreased by 0·3 nm, corresponding roughly to the difference between the length of the covalently attached moiety of MBTA and those of BAC or NPTMB (Table 2). An unreactive SH group has been placed some distance from the negative subsite. The channel, assumed to be a pathway of readily exchangeable coordination sites for sodium and potassium ions, is shown lying on the axis between the subunits. The binding of acetylcholine, it is suggested, is translated into a relative shift of the subunits which generates the channel in the interface.

The work was supported by grants from U.S.P.H.S., from N.S.F. and from the New York Heart Association, Inc.

## REFERENCES

ALBUQUERQUE, E. X., SOKOLL, M. D., SONESSON, B. & THESLEFF, S. (1968). *Eur. J. Pharmac.*, **4**, 40.

BARTELS, E., DEAL, W., KARLIN, A. & MAUTNER, H. G. (1970). *Biochem. biophys. Acta*, **203**, 568.

BARTELS, E., WASSERMANN, N. H. & ERLANGER, B. F. (1971). *Proc. natn. Acad. Sci., U.S.A.*, **68**, 1820.

BEERS, W. H. & REICH, E. (1970). *Nature, Lond.*, **228**, 917.

BLOEMMEN, J., JONIAU, M. & LONTIE, R. (1967). *Arch. Int. Physiol. Biochim.*, **75**, 552.

BRANTON, D. (1969). *Ann. Rev. Plant Physiol.*, **20**, 209.

BRETSCHER, M. S. (1971). *Nature, New Biol., Lond.*, **231**, 229.

BROWN, P. K. (1972). *Nature, New Biol., Lond.*, **236**, 35.

CHANGEUX, J.-P., MEUNIER, J.-C., OLSEN, R. & WEBER, M. (1973). This symposium.

CHANGEUX, J.-P. & PODLESKI, T. R. (1968). *Proc. natn. Acad. Sci., U.S.A.*, **59**, 944.
CLELAND, W. W. (1964). *Biochemistry*, **3**, 480.
CONE, R. (1972). *Nature, New Biol., Lond.*, **236**, 39.
DEL CASTILLO, J., ESCOBAR, I. & GIJON, E. (1971). *Int. J. Neurosci.*, **1**, 199.
DEL CASTILLO, J. & KATZ, B. (1955). *J. Physiol., Lond.*, **128**, 157.
FRAENKEL-CONRAT, H. (1959). In: *Sulfur in Proteins*, ed. Benesch, R., p. 339. New York: Academic Press.
GOODALL, M. C. (1970). *Biochim. biophys. Acta*, **219**, 470.
HLADKY, S. B. & HAYDON, D. A. (1970). *Nature, Lond.*, **225**, 451.
JONIAU, M., BLOEMMEN, J. & LONTIE, R. (1966). *Arch. Int. Physiol. Biochim.*, **74**, 727.
KARLIN, A. (1965). *J. cell. Biol.*, **25**, 159.
KARLIN, A. (1967a). *J. Theor. Biol.*, **16**, 306.
KARLIN, A. (1967b). *Biochim. biophys. Acta*, **139**, 358.
KARLIN, A. (1969). *J. gen. Physiol.*, **54**, 245s.
KARLIN, A. & BARTELS, E. (1966). *Biochim. biophys. Acta*, **126**, 525.
KARLIN, A., PRIVES, J., DEAL, W. & WINNIK, M. (1970). In: Ciba Foundation Symposium on *Molecular Properties of Drug Receptors*, p. 247. London: Churchill.
KARLIN, A., PRIVES, J., DEAL, W. & WINNIK, M. (1971). *J. Mol. Biol.*, **61**, 175.
KARLIN, A. & WINNIK, M. (1968). *Proc. natn. Acad. Sci., U.S.A.*, **60**, 668.
KATZ, B. & MILEDI, R. (1971). *Nature, New Biol., Lond.*, **232**, 124.
KATZ, A. M. & MOMMAERTS, F. H. N. (1962). *Biochim. biophys. Acta*, **65**, 82.
KRASNE, S., EISENMAN, G. & SZABO, G. (1971). *Science, N.Y.*, **174**, 412.
LESTER, H. A. (1971). *J. gen. Physiol.*, **57**, 255.
LINDSTROM, J., KIEFER, H., LENNOX, E. S. & SINGER, S. J. *J. Memb. Biol.*, in press.
MITTAG, T. W. & TORMAY, A. (1970). *Fedn Proc.*, **29**, 547abs.
PODLESKI, T., MEUNIER, J.-C. & CHANGEUX, J.-P. (1969). *Proc. natn. Acad. Sci., U.S.A.*, **63**, 1239.
PRIVES, J. M., REITER, M. J., COWBURN, D. A. & KARLIN, A. (1972). *Mol. Pharmac.*, **8**, 786.
RANG, H. P. & RITTER, J. M. (1969). *Br. J. Pharmac.*, **37**, 538P.
RANG, H. P. & RITTER, J. M. (1971). *Mol. Pharmac.*, **7**, 620.
REITER, M. J., COWBURN, D. A., PRIVES, J. M. & KARLIN, A. (1972). *Proc. natn. Acad. Sci., U.S.A.*, **69**, 1168.
RUIZ-MANRESA, F. & GRUNDFEST, H. (1971). *J. gen. Physiol.*, **57**, 71.
SILMAN, I. & KARLIN, A. (1969). *Science, N.Y.*, **164**, 1420.
SINGER, S. J. (1970). Discussion in Ciba Symposium on *Molecular Properties of Drug Receptors*, p. 40. London: Churchill.
SINGER, S. J. & NICOLSON, G. L. (1972). *Science, N.Y.*, **175**, 720.
SINGER, S. J., RUOHO, A., KIEFER, H., LINDSTROM, J. & LENNOX, E. S. (1973). This symposium.
STECK, T. L., FAIRBANKS, G. & WALLACH, D. F. H. (1971). *Biochemistry*, **10**, 2617.
TOSTESON, D. C., ANDREOLI, T. E., TIFFENBERG, M. & COOK, P. (1968). *J. gen. Physiol.*, **51**, 373s.
URRY, D. W. (1971). *Proc. natn. Acad. Sci., U.S.A.*, **68**, 672.
WILKINS, M. H. F., BLAUROCK, A. E. & ENGELMAN, D. M. (1971). *Nature, New Biol., Lond.*, **230**, 72.

## DISCUSSION

*Barnard (New York)*

Would you comment on the relation between your results on the effects of reducing agents on receptor properties and those of del Castillo and his co-workers (del Castillo, Escobar & Gijon, 1971), who conclude that the cholinergic receptor has a free SH group, and is stabilized when the SH group is oxidized to the S–S form, for example by reaction with *o*-iodosobenzoate.

*Karlin (New York)*

As I have emphasized, affinity reagents which would be expected to react with such an SH group if it were in the binding site, have no effect on the unreduced receptor in a number of different cells. Furthermore, the reversibility within milliseconds of the effects seen by del Castillo and his co-workers applying oxidizing agents or mercurials by microelectro-osmosis requires either that the effects are due to noncovalent reactions or that there is some as yet unknown system on the external side of the postsynaptic membrane, with access to the receptor, which can rapidly and repeatedly reduce disulphide bonds and also displace mercurials from their extremely strong complex with SH groups ($K \simeq 10^{-20}$). It seems likely that the effects seen by del Castillo and co-workers are not due to *covalent* reactions with the receptor.

# THE LABELLING OF CHOLINERGIC RECEPTORS IN SMOOTH MUSCLE

C. M. S. FEWTRELL AND H. P. RANG*

*Department of Pharmacology, University of Oxford, Oxford OX1 3QT, England*

## *Introduction*

It was found some years ago (Paton & Rang, 1965) that the longitudinal smooth muscle layer of guinea-pig small intestine binds radioactive atropine. When the uptake of atropine was studied as a function of concentration, three components were discernible; one component, which accounted for most of the binding at low atropine concentrations, appeared to saturate at a level of about 180 pmol/g wet weight, and its equilibrium constant ($1{\cdot}1 \times 10^{-9}$ M) was identical with the equilibrium constant for the binding of atropine to muscarinic receptors determined by measurements of pharmacological antagonism. Moreover, the binding of atropine was inhibited by low concentrations of drugs that antagonize the effects of acetylcholine in smooth muscle and unaffected by substances without any muscarinic blocking activity.

Thus, it seemed likely that atropine at low concentrations bound with reasonable specificity to the receptor sites, and that this approach might be used to extract the labelled receptor material from the tissue. Atropine itself, however, forms a freely reversible complex with the receptors, and if it is to be used as a label, it is essential that the receptor material should remain, throughout the preparative procedures, in a state in which the binding of atropine is unmodified. Preliminary experiments on the binding of labelled atropine to subcellular fragments of guinea-pig intestinal muscle (H. P. Rang, unpublished) showed that even quite gentle procedures tended to reduce binding substantially, and it seemed unlikely that any substantial purification of the binding material could be achieved without loss of its affinity for atropine. It appears (see below) that the muscarinic acetylcholine receptor material in smooth muscle may be a good deal more labile than the receptor

* Present address of authors: Department of Physiology and Biochemistry, University of Southampton, Southampton SO9 3TU, England.

proteins that have been extracted from electric tissue (Miledi, Molinoff & Potter, 1971; Changeux, Meunier & Huchet, 1971; De Robertis, Lunt & La Torre, 1971) and from striated muscle (Miledi & Potter, 1971) where the binding activity is retained even after solubilization of the material by treatment with detergents.

For isolation of the receptor from smooth muscle, there appeared to be great advantages in using a label that would bind covalently to the receptor site, making it unnecessary for the binding affinity to be retained throughout the preparative procedures. To this end, an alkylating derivative of the reversible atropine-like drug, benzilylcholine, was prepared (Fig. 1). This

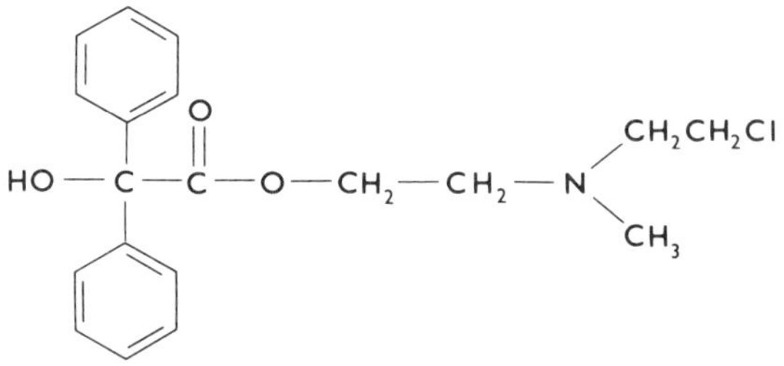


FIG. 1. Structure of benzilylcholine mustard.

substance, benzilylcholine mustard (BCM), was shown to be a potent, specific and irreversible antagonist at muscarinic receptors (Gill & Rang, 1966) and a suitable agent with which to attempt to label and isolate the receptors. Moran & Triggle (1970) have prepared a range of similar compounds, and have also reported on the binding of these compounds by various smooth muscle preparations. Their compounds form labile bonds with the receptors, so their blocking action is transient and the labelled material is washed out when the tissue is exposed to drug-free solution. They have compared the rates of washout of the label, and of recovery of the drug sensitivity of the tissue, as a means of checking on the specificity of the binding. In this study we have used radioactive BCM as a label, which does not wash out of the tissue at an appreciable rate, and have used as a guide to the specificity of BCM binding the ability of other muscarinic blocking agents to inhibit the binding of BCM.

### *The binding of BCM to smooth muscle*

Tritiated BCM, prepared from [$^3$H] benzilic acid at a specific activity of about 1 Ci/mmol, is strongly bound by strips of intestinal smooth muscle from the guinea-pig (Rang, 1967). As with atropine, however, the binding does not show clear properties of saturation, tending to increase indefinitely as the duration of exposure to BCM is increased, and as the bath concentration of BCM is increased (Fig. 2a). This is not really surprising, since BCM

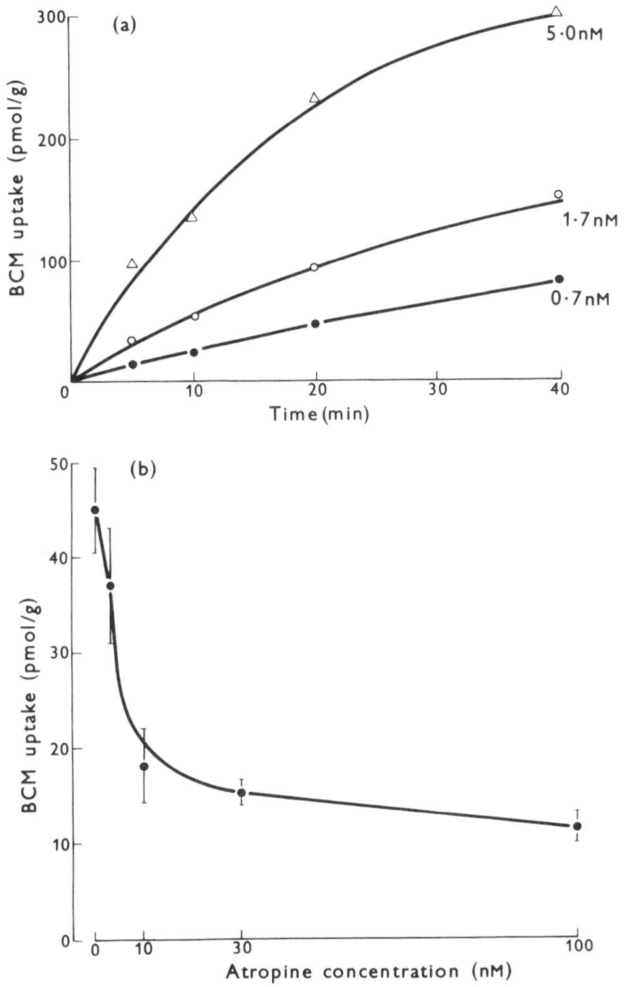


FIG. 2. BCM binding by intact longitudinal muscle. (a), Binding curves for different BCM concentrations. (b), Effect of atropine on the binding of BCM after five min exposure to $2{\cdot}4 \times 10^{-9}$ M BCM. The muscle strips were exposed to atropine for 20 min before the BCM was added. Bars show standard error.

forms a highly reactive ethyleniminium ion, and there are likely to be non-specific binding sites (for example, free carboxylate and sulphydryl groups) in much greater abundance than the receptors. Slow alkylation of these sites will thus result in a steady uptake of BCM on top of the more rapidly saturating receptor component.

In order to analyse the uptake of BCM quantitatively a series of experiments was carried out in which uptake as a function of time was measured at

BCM concentrations ranging from $7\times10^{-10}$ M to $7\times10^{-8}$ M. After being exposed to BCM the strips of muscle were washed in nonradioactive medium for 30 min in order to remove unbound radioactivity, and then counted.

Least squares curve-fitting of the experimental results using the *Pattern-search* procedure (Colquhoun, 1971) showed that the results were well fitted by an equation containing two exponential terms, of the form

$$Uptake = A(1-e^{-k_A xt}) + B(1-e^{-k_B xt})$$

where $x$ is the BCM concentration, and $t$ is time. This is consistent with the presence of two separate binding sites, with capacities A and B respectively, each saturating according to first order kinetics, the rate constants being $k_A$ and $k_B$ respectively. It was of interest to compare the calculated capacities and rate constants for these two sites with the values obtained for the binding of atropine (Paton & Rang, 1965) and with the rate constant calculated for the occlusion of muscarinic receptors by BCM in this tissue (Gill & Rang, 1966). The values are shown in Table 1. It can be seen that there is quite good agreement between the capacity of the high affinity site for atropine (180 pmol/g) and of the rapidly-saturating site for BCM (220 pmol/g). The rate constant ($2{\cdot}3\times10^5$ M$^{-1}$ s$^{-1}$) for the binding of BCM to this site is however considerably smaller than the rate constant for receptor occlusion ($1{\cdot}1\times10^6$ M$^{-1}$ s$^{-1}$). In this context it may be relevant that a similar *kinetic* discrepancy was found with atropine uptake, the binding occurring at a rate considerably smaller than the rate at which the antagonism

TABLE 1. *Comparison of parameters for the reaction of BCM and atropine with muscarinic receptors in guinea-pig ileum*

| | |
|---|---|
| **BCM** | |
| Binding site 1: | |
| Capacity (A) | 220 pmol/g |
| Rate constant ($k_A$) | $2{\cdot}3\times10^5$ M$^{-1}$ s$^{-1}$ |
| Binding site 2: | |
| Capacity (B) | 2540 pmol/g |
| Rate constant ($k_B$) | $2{\cdot}2\times10^3$ M$^{-1}$ s$^{-1}$ |
| Rate constant for receptor occlusion | $1{\cdot}1\times10^6$ M$^{-1}$ s$^{-1}$ |
| **Atropine** | |
| Binding site 1: | |
| Capacity | 180 pmol/g |
| Equilibrium constant | $1{\cdot}1\times10^{-9}$ M |
| Binding site 2: | |
| Capacity | 950 pmol/g |
| Equilibrium constant | $4{\cdot}5\times10^{-7}$ M |
| Equilibrium constant for receptor occlusion | $1{\cdot}1\times10^{-9}$ M |

develops (Paton & Rang, 1965). Waud (1968) has suggested that the discrepancy with atropine could be explicable in terms of the diffusional characteristics of the muscle, and a similar explanation might also apply in the case of BCM. At present it is not possible to resolve this discrepancy, but the inhibitory effect of other muscarinic antagonists on BCM binding strongly suggests that the high affinity site does in fact represent binding to the receptors. Fig. 2b shows the inhibitory effect of atropine on BCM binding, and it can be seen that 50% of the maximal attainable inhibition occurs at an atropine concentration of about $5 \times 10^{-9}$ M. The maximum inhibition is roughly 70%, and requires a concentration of about $3 \times 10^{-8}$ M. Results obtained with several other potential competing agents are shown in Table 2.

TABLE 2. *Inhibition of uptake of BCM by intact muscle*

| Inhibitor | Concentration (M) | % inhibition | Equilibrium constant for ACh antagonism (M) |
|---|---|---|---|
| Hyoscine | $10^{-8}$ | 37 | $3 \cdot 0 \times 10^{-10}$ |
| | $3 \cdot 5 \times 10^{-8}$ | 67 | |
| Atropine | $10^{-8}$ | 52 | $1 \cdot 1 \times 10^{-9}$ |
| | $10^{-7}$ | 73 | |
| Lachesine | $10^{-8}$ | 58 | $1 \cdot 5 \times 10^{-9}$ |
| | $10^{-7}$ | 78·5 | |
| Benzhexol | $7 \cdot 5 \times 10^{-8}$ | 51 | $2 \cdot 4 \times 10^{-9}$ |
| | $2 \cdot 5 \times 10^{-7}$ | 67 | |
| Tricyclamol | $10^{-8}$ | 39 | c. $2 \times 10^{-9}$ |
| | $10^{-7}$ | 65 | |
| Cocaine | $10^{-5}$ | 9 | c. $6 \times 10^{-5}$ |
| | $10^{-4}$ | 54 | |
| Physostigmine | $10^{-5}$ | 39 | ? |
| Mepyramine | $10^{-6}$ | 7·5 | $> 10^{-5}$ |
| | $10^{-5}$ | 30 | |
| Pentolinium | $10^{-5}$ | 8·0 | $> 10^{-5}$ |
| (+)-Tubocurarine | $3 \times 10^{-5}$ | 5·2 | $> 10^{-4}$ |

The muscles were incubated in the presence of 1·5–2·5 nM BCM and the inhibitor for 5 or 30 min, and the binding compared with control muscles incubated without any inhibitor.

There is a close correlation between the ability of a drug to block muscarinic receptors and its ability to block BCM uptake. With all of the muscarinic antagonists, a maximum inhibition of about 70–80% was reached at low concentrations, suggesting that 20–30% of the binding under these conditions may be to nonspecific sites. According to the calculated parameters for BCM binding (Table 1), the high affinity site should, in the conditions used in Fig. 2b (2·4 nM BCM for 5 min) take up 33 pmol/g, a figure that corresponds well with the maximum degree of inhibition obtained with atropine.

*Subcellular fractionation of smooth muscle*

Various differential centrifugation procedures were tried out on smooth muscle labelled with BCM in order to obtain maximum enrichment of the radioactive BCM, and the scheme shown in Fig. 3 was finally adopted. From four guinea-pigs, a total of 0·5–1 g (wet weight) of intestinal muscle was obtained. After incubation for 30 min with $2 \times 10^{-9}$ M [$^3$H] BCM, the muscle was washed in nonradioactive solution for 30 min, then finely chopped and homogenized in 0·3 M sucrose. The debris precipitated by the first low-speed centrifugation was usually rehomogenized and centrifuged once or twice more in order to extract as much radioactivity as possible from it. In most experiments, the resuspended debris was sonicated briefly, which further improved the extraction. Centrifugation of the low-speed supernatant at 10 000 *g* for 20 min precipitated a 'mitochondrial' pellet, and final centrifugation of the supernatant at 100 000 *g* for 60 min resulted in a 'microsomal' pellet and a supernatant containing soluble protein.

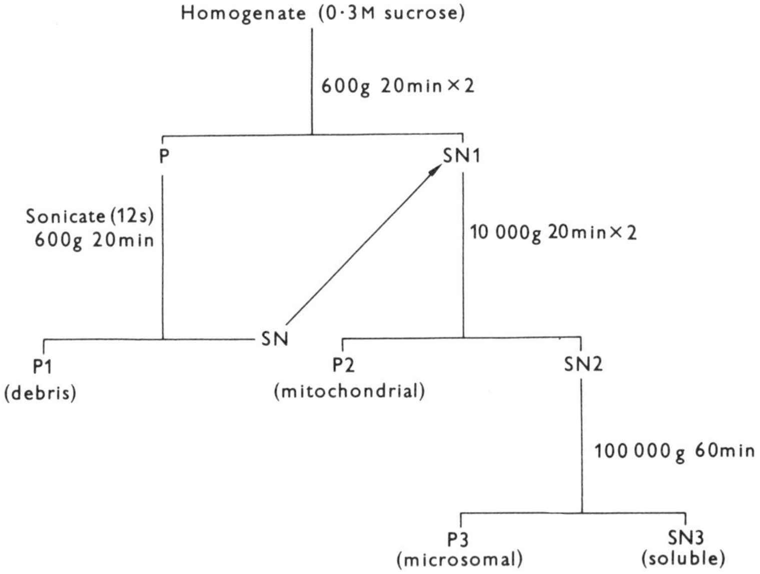


FIG. 3. Differential centrifugation scheme for longitudinal smooth muscle homogenates.

In more recent experiments the procedure has been modified by the use of a Polytron blender instead of a Potter homogenizer. Used at maximum speed for a total of 2 min, with a PT 10 head, the Polytron blender gave good recoveries of radioactivity in the microsomal fraction without the need for sonication.

*Distribution of radioactivity, protein and enzyme activities in subcellular fractions*

Protein concentration was measured by the Folin–Lowry procedure (Lowry, Rosebrough, Farr & Randall, 1951), cholinesterase activity by measuring the rate of acetylthiocholine hydrolysis (Ellman, Courtney, Andres & Featherstone, 1961) and 5′-nucleotidase activity by the method of Ipata (1967). This latter enzyme has been found to be associated almost exclusively with the cell membrane fraction in liver cells (Song & Bodansky, 1967) and its distribution in smooth muscle has been studied by Burger & Lowenstein (1970) and by Kidwai, Radcliffe & Daniel (1971).

The distribution of the various activities in the different subcellular fractions is shown in Fig. 4, in which the relative specific activity (that is, % activity in the fraction divided by % protein in the fraction) is plotted on the ordinate, against protein content on the abscissa. Thus the height of the column indicates the enrichment of activity in the fraction (a value of unity indicating that the activity/mg protein is the same in the fraction as in the whole tissue) and the area of the column indicates the total amount of activity in the fraction.

It can be seen that the pattern of distribution of radioactivity in the tissue closely parallels that of the two marker enzymes. In each case the highest relative specific activity (4–6) is found in the microsomal pellet. A variable amount of activity was precipitated with the cell debris (P1). This probably reflects the difficulty of homogenizing the tissue fully, rather than a separate component in the tissue. Of the activity not thrown down with the debris 59 % of the $^3H$, 42 % of the 5′-nucleotidase and 45 % of the cholinesterase was found in the microsomal pellet. The relatively large amount of cholinesterase in the soluble fraction (27 % of that not found in the debris) may result from the relative ease with which this enzyme is detached from the membrane. Thus, when the microsomal pellet was simply resuspended and centrifuged again, more than 20 % of the cholinesterase was found in the supernatant (see Table 3). Thus, the activities appearing in the final supernatant in Fig. 4 probably represent detachment of the active material from the microsomal fraction rather than activity associated with the soluble proteins of the cells.

*Density gradient centrifugation*

Suspensions of the microsomal fraction in 0·3 M sucrose were layered on to a linear density gradient in the range 0·5–1·5 M sucrose, and centrifuged for 16 h at 220 000 *g*, by which time equilibrium was assumed to have been reached. Radioactivity, cholinesterase and 5′-nucleotidase were all found in a single peak centred around 0·8 M sucrose. The protein was fairly evenly distributed throughout the gradient.

Thus, in both the differential centrifugation steps and on the density gradient, the radioactivity ran along with the cholinesterase and 5′-nucleotidase

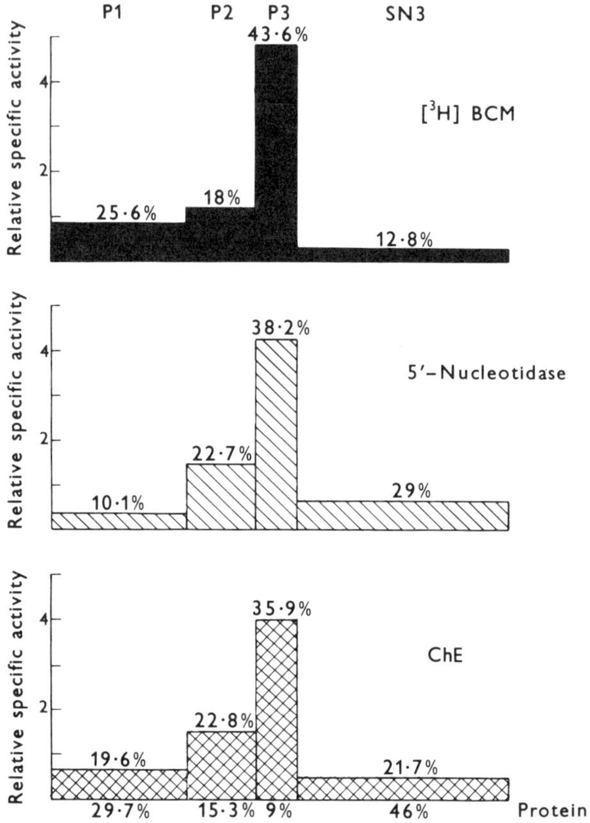


FIG. 4. Distribution of bound [$^3$H] BCM, 5′-nucleotidase, cholinesterase and protein in subcellular fractions obtained after differential centrifugation of labelled longitudinal smooth muscle homogenates. Relative specific activity = % activity/% protein for each fraction and is plotted against % protein. The figure above each box is the % activity in that fraction.

activities, so it is likely that all three are associated with the cell membrane fraction. Since the radioactive BCM in these experiments is converted to the quaternary ethyleniminium form before being applied to the tissue, it is unlikely that it would reach intracellular structures, and this is borne out by the cell fractionation studies.

### *The binding of BCM to microsomal particles*

It was of interest to compare the binding of BCM to the isolated microsomal fraction with the binding to the intact muscle. The experiments were carried out with a dilute suspension of microsomes in 140 mM NaCl solution buffered to pH 7·0 with 10 mM phosphate buffer. The protein concentration was about 20–25 μg/ml. This high dilution was used so that the free concentration of BCM in the medium was not substantially reduced as a result of BCM binding. After incubation for varying periods in the presence of BCM at 37° C, trichloroacetic acid was added in order to halt the binding reaction, and the resulting precipitate spun down and counted.

Fig. 5a shows the binding of BCM by microsomes. The overall pattern of the binding closely resembles that found with intact muscle in showing no clearly defined saturation. Moreover, the binding to microsomes is similarly inhibited by atropine (Fig. 5b), the maximal inhibition (about 85%) being obtained with atropine concentrations greater than $3 \times 10^{-8}$ M. Fifty per cent of the maximal inhibition was attained with about $3 \times 10^{-9}$ M atropine, which is very similar to the 50% inhibitory concentration for the intact muscle strips.

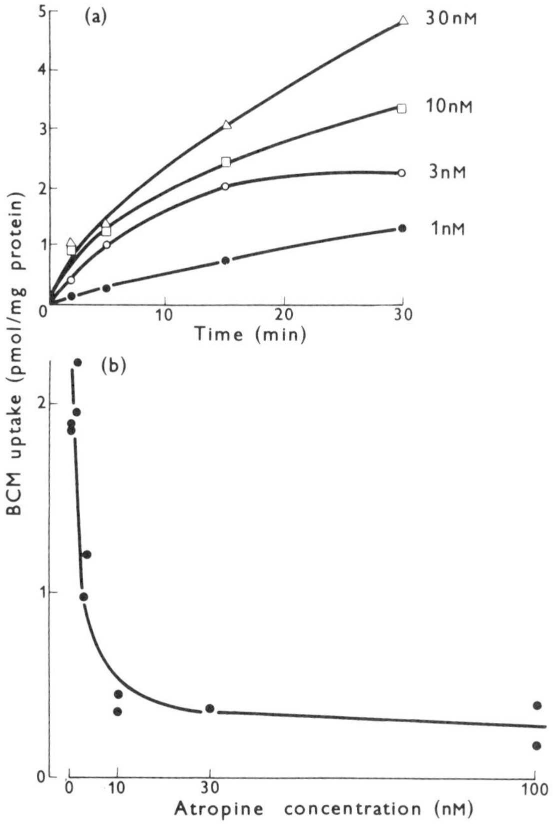


FIG. 5. BCM binding by the microsomal fraction obtained after differential centrifugation of homogenate of longitudinal smooth muscle. (a), Binding curves for different BCM concentrations. (b), Effect of atropine on the binding of BCM after 30 min exposure to $2 \times 10^{-9}$ M BCM. The microsomes were exposed to atropine for 20 min before the BCM was added.

Comparison of the binding curves in Figs. 2 and 5 shows that the two systems are in good qualitative agreement. Thus, after 30 min in the presence of $1{\cdot}8 \times 10^{-9}$ M [$^3$H] BCM, the microsomal binding amounts to just over 6 pmol/mg protein. Under the same conditions, intact muscle takes up about 130 pmol/g wet wt, or about 1·1 pmol/mg total protein. The specific radioactivity (expressed in relation to protein content) is increased by a factor of 4–6 in the microsomal preparation compared with the whole muscle, so the specific activity of microsomes prepared from labelled muscle (4·4–6·6 pmol/mg protein) is very similar to that found when the isolated microsomes are labelled with BCM. In all respects, therefore, the binding of BCM to the microsomes agrees well with the binding by the intact muscle, and this preparation should prove useful in further studying the properties of the receptors. Kasai & Changeux (1971a,b,c) have recently reported in detail on the properties of 'microsacs' formed from the innervated surface of eel electroplax cells. This preparation has been found to respond 'pharmacologically' by an increase in $Na^+$ permeability in the presence of cholinergic agonists as well as binding various drug molecules, and has proved valuable in testing the correlation between binding and effect with cholinergic agonists. It is hoped that similar studies can be carried out with the smooth muscle microsomal preparation.

### *Solubilization of bound [$^3$H] BCM by detergents*

In order to characterize the binding material, it was desirable to obtain it in a soluble form, and various detergents were tested for their ability to solubilize the radioactive material from the microsomes of muscles that had been labelled with [$^3$H] BCM.

Samples containing about 1 mg of microsomal protein were suspended in a mixture containing 160 mM NaCl, 10 mM phosphate buffer at pH 7·4, together with 1% detergent, and left overnight at room temperature before centrifuging for 1 h at 100 000 *g*. The supernatant was then removed, and assayed for radioactivity, protein, cholinesterase and 5′-nucleotidase. The final concentration of detergent in the enzyme assays was 0·03% for cholinesterase and 0·07% for 5′-nucleotidase.

The degree of solubilization of the various components is shown in Table 3. In all cases the radioactive material in solution could be precipitated by adding trichloroacetic acid, and there is no evidence of dissociation of the label from its binding sites in the presence of detergents.

N-lauroyl sarcosinate, sodium dodecyl sulphate and to a lesser extent deoxycholate solubilized the majority of the protein and radioactivity, but almost completely inactivated the enzymes. The non-ionic detergents Triton X-100, Lubrol PX and Lubrol WX on the other hand solubilized 50–70% of the radioactivity, and about 40% of the protein while the activity of both cholinesterase and 5′-nucleotidase was considerably increased by the deter-

TABLE 3. *Detergent solubilization of the microsomal fraction*

| Detergent | $^{3}H$ | Protein | % in supernatant Cholinesterase activity | 5′-Nucleotidase activity |
|---|---|---|---|---|
| Control extraction without detergent | 15·8 | 18·6 | 22·2 | 6·9 |
| Triton X-100 | 69·6 | 42·3 | 111·4 | 124 |
| Lubrol PX | 68·8 | 44·1 | 116 | 145 |
| Lubrol WX | 49·3 | 40 | 80·6 | 100 |
| N-Lauroyl sarcosinate | 88·5 | 97·7 | 0 | 31 |
| Deoxycholate | 60·8 | 63·3 | 5·6 | 6·9 |
| Sodium dodecyl sulphate | 88·5 | 84·6 | 0 | 0 |

Detergents were tested at 1% concentration and the extraction was carried on overnight at room temperature. Figures in the table show the percentages of the total material or activity which remained in the supernatant after the extract was centrifuged at 100 000 *g* for 1 h.

gents (yields of enzyme activity being up to 145% of those present in the original microsomal suspension). The enhancement of enzyme activity by these detergents could be due to an increase in the molecular activity of the enzymes or to an increase in the number of enzyme sites accessible to the substrate. This latter hypothesis has been shown to be the correct one in the case of sodium-potassium ATPase where incubation of microsomes with deoxycholate increased the enzyme activity and the ouabain-binding capacity of the preparation in a parallel fashion (Jørgensen & Skou, 1971).

### *Failure of solubilized protein to bind [³H] BCM*

In several experiments, microsomal preparations from unlabelled muscle have been treated with detergents, and the resulting extract diluted (to reduce the detergent concentration to about 0·01%). [³H] BCM was then added and the mixture kept at 37° C for 30 min before precipitation of the protein with trichloroacetic acid. In no case was any significant binding of BCM detected. Thus, it appears that solubilization of the binding material, even when carried out by treatment with detergents in which 5′-nucleotidase and cholinesterase were fully active, destroys its ability to bind BCM. This is in contrast to the results obtained with eel electroplax and other systems (Changeux, Meunier & Huchet, 1971; Miledi, Molinoff & Potter, 1971; Miledi & Potter, 1971) where the receptor protein retains its binding activity after solubilization with non-ionic detergents. Further work will be needed to discover the reason for this difference.

### *Gel filtration and electrophoresis*

The labelled microsomal pellet was dissolved in 1% sodium dodecyl sulphate (SDS) and run on a column of Sepharose 6B, equilibrated with

0·05 M phosphate buffer (pH 7) and 1% SDS. The radioactivity emerged in one main peak, though some higher molecular weight components were also present (Fig. 6). Calibration with marker proteins in the presence of 1% SDS suggested that the main peak had a molecular weight about 26 000.

This molecular weight estimate was confirmed by SDS polyacrylamide gel electrophoresis at neutral pH (Maizel, 1969). The SDS-solubilized microsomal pellet was run on 5% gels, and gave two peaks (in addition to a variable amount of radioactive material which failed to enter the gel) corresponding to molecular weights of 23 000 and 50 000 respectively. When the 26 000 mol. wt. peak from the Sepharose column was run on the polyacrylamide gel, it gave a radioactive peak corresponding to the 23 000 mol. wt. peak obtained with the unfractionated microsomal material.

With both of these fractionation procedures the microsomal proteins were fairly evenly distributed. Fig. 6 shows the protein elution pattern with the Sepharose column. On polyacrylamide gels 12–15 bands were seen when the gel was stained, but it was not possible to identify a particular protein band associated with the radioactive peak.

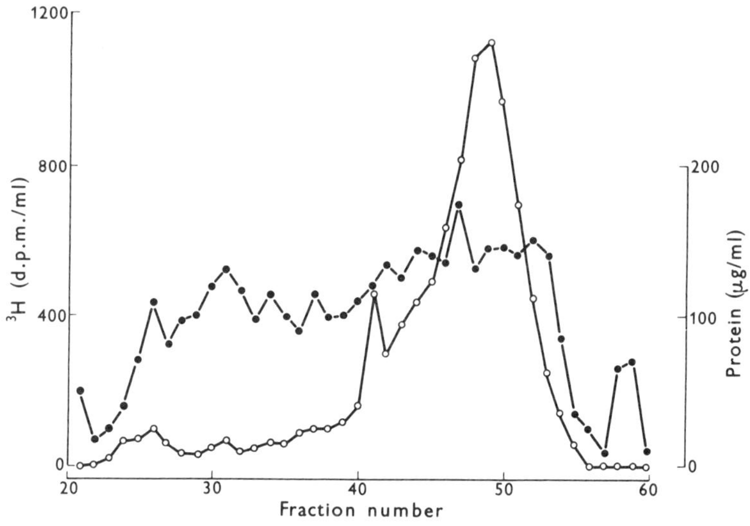


FIG. 6. Elution pattern obtained when a labelled microsomal pellet dissolved in 1% SDS was run on a column of Sepharose 6B equilibrated with 0·05 M phosphate buffer (pH 7) containing 1% SDS. (○——○), Radioactivity; (●——●), protein.

## *Discussion*

The number of BCM-binding sites that are susceptible to inhibition by reversible antagonists such as atropine appears to be 100–150 pmol/g wet weight, which is equivalent to approximately 200 sites per square micron of membrane. This figure is arrived at by allowing for an extracellular space equivalent to about 30% of the wet weight and using the value 1·5 μm for the volume: surface area ratio of the cells (obtained by Goodford & Leach, 1966, for guinea-pig taenia coli). The resting membrane conductance of the cells of guinea-pig taenia coli is approximately $2 \times 10^{-5}$ mho $cm^{-2}$ (Tomita, 1970), and longitudinal smooth muscle appears to be similar (Kuriyama, Osa & Toida, 1967). The results of Bolton (1972) suggest that carbachol can increase the membrane conductance approximately 100–500-fold, and Burgen & Spero (1968) found that the potassium permeability was increased by a maximum of 100-fold by carbachol and related drugs. The maximum increase in membrane conductance produced by carbachol must therefore be between $2 \times 10^{-3}$ and $10^{-2}$ mho $cm^{-2}$ and the conductance per site (density $2 \times 10^{10}$ $cm^{-2}$) is between $10^{-13}$ and $5 \times 10^{-13}$ mho. Estimates of the conductances of voltage-dependent ionic channels in excitable membranes (Hille, 1970) are about $2 \times 10^{-10}$ mho for the $Na^+$ channel and $10^{-13}$ mho for the $K^+$ channel, so this value seems quite plausible. It is however substantially greater than the conductance per decamethonium-binding site ($10^{-15}$ mho) calculated by Kasai & Changeux (1971) from simultaneous measurements of $Na^+$ efflux and decamethonium binding in vesicular membrane fragments from electroplax tissue.

The main difference which has so far emerged between the membrane constituent that binds BCM in smooth muscle and the binding protein for bungarotoxin in electroplax, is that the BCM binding is lost completely when the material is solubilized with non-ionic detergents, whereas the toxin-binding protein after solubilization shows properties similar to those of membrane fragments, (Changeux, Kasai, Huchet & Meunier, 1970). It also appears that the BCM-binding material is more firmly attached to the membrane, for treatment with deoxycholate or Triton extracted only 50–70% of the bound BCM, whereas Triton quantitatively extracted bound bungarotoxin from electroplax fragments (Miledi, Molinoff & Potter, 1971). Possibly the firmer attachment of the BCM-binding protein in the smooth muscle membrane makes it impossible to extract without disruption of its binding properties. It does not appear likely that the detergent *per se* causes the loss of binding activity, because the extracts were diluted 100-fold (bringing the detergent concentration down to 0·01%) before the binding was tested. Moreover, enzyme activities were preserved even in the presence of much higher detergent concentrations.

Electrophoresis on polyacrylamide gels, or gel filtration on Sepharose 6B of the SDS-solubilized material from smooth muscle gave radioactive peaks with molecular weights of 50 000 and 25 000, as well as a certain amount of higher molecular weight material which remained at the origin of the polyacrylamide gels. Similar studies on the cobra toxin-binding protein from eel electroplax (Meunier, Olsen, Menez, Morgat, Fromageot, Ronsseray, Boquet & Changeux, 1971) gave a molecular weight (on polyacrylamide gel electrophoresis) equal to about 50 000. In the presence of milder detergents, much larger subunits were found, which ran on Sepharose at the same rate as $\beta$-galactosidase which has a molecular weight of 540 000 (Meunier *et al.*, 1971; Raftery, Schmidt, Clark & Wolcott, 1971). Miledi, Molinoff & Potter (1971) obtained rather similar results on the toxin-binding proteins from *Torpedo* electric tissue. The subunit of the BCM-binding protein may thus be of similar size to that of the receptors in the electric tissue, but we have not yet studied the properties of the Triton-solubilized material from smooth muscle to see whether it, too, forms larger aggregates.

This work was supported by a grant from the Medical Research Council. C.M.S.F. is an M.R.C. Scholar.

REFERENCES

BOLTON, T. B. (1972). *J. Physiol., Lond.*, **220**, 647.
BURGEN, A. S. V. & SPERO, L. (1968). *Br. J. Pharmac.*, **34**, 99.
BURGER, R. M. & LOWENSTEIN, J. M. (1970). *J. biol. Chem.*, **245**, 6274.
CHANGEUX, J.-P., KASAI, M., HUCHET, M. & MEUNIER, J.-C. (1970). *C. R., Paris*, **270**, 2864.
CHANGEUX, J.-P., MEUNIER, J.-C. & HUCHET, M. (1971). *Mol. Pharmac.*, **7**, 538.
COLQUHOUN, D. (1971). *Lectures on Biostatistics*. Ch. 12, Oxford University Press.
DE ROBERTIS, E., LUNT, G. S. & LA TORRE, J. L. (1971). *Mol. Pharmac.*, **7**, 97.
ELLMAN, G. L., COURTNEY, K. D., ANDRES, V. & FEATHERSTONE, R. M. (1961). *Biochem. Pharmac.*, **7**, 88.
GILL, E. W. & RANG, H. P. (1966). *Mol. Pharmac.*, **2**, 284.
GOODFORD, P. J. & LEACH, E. H. (1966). *J. Physiol., Lond.*, **186**, 1.
HILLE, B. (1970). *Prog. Biophys. Mol. Biol.*, **21**, 1.
IPATA, P. L. (1967). *Analyt. Biochem.*, **20**, 30.
JØRGENSEN, P. L. & SKOU, J. C. (1971). *Biochim. biophys. Acta.*, **233**, 366.
KASAI, M. & CHANGEUX, J.-P. (1971a). *J. Memb. Biol.*, **6**, 1.
KASAI, M. & CHANGEUX, J.-P. (1971b). *J. Memb. Biol.*, **6**, 24.
KASAI, M. & CHANGEUX, J.-P. (1971c). *J. Memb. Biol.*, **6**, 58.
KIDWAI, A. M., RADCLIFFE, M. A. & DANIEL, E. E. (1971). *Biochim. biophys. Acta.*, **233**, 538.
KURIYAMA, H., OSA, T. & TOIDA, N. (1967). *J. Physiol., Lond.*, **191**, 239.
LOWRY, O. H., ROSEBROUGH, N. J., FARR, A. L. & RANDALL, R. J. (1951). *J. biol. Chem.*, **193**, 265.
MAIZEL, J. V. (1969). In: *Fundamental Techniques in Virology*, ed. Habel, K. & Salzman, N. P., p. 334. New York & London: Academic Press.
MEUNIER, J.-C., OLSEN, R., MENEZ, A., MORGAT, J. L., FROMAGEOT, P., RONSSERAY, A.-M., BOQUET, P. & CHANGEUX, J.-P. (1971). *C. R., Paris*, **273**, 595.
MILEDI, R., MOLINOFF, P. & POTTER, L. T. (1971). *Nature, Lond.*, **229**, 554.
MILEDI, R. & POTTER, L. T. (1971). *Nature, Lond.*, **233**, 599.
MORAN, J. F. & TRIGGLE, D. J. (1970). In: *Fundamental Concepts in Drug–Receptor Interactions*, ed. Danielli, J. F., Moran, J. F. & Triggle, D. J., p. 133. New York & London: Academic Press.
PATON, W. D. M. & RANG, H. P. (1965). *Proc. Roy. Soc.*, B., **163**, 1.
RAFTERY, M. A., SCHMIDT, J., CLARK, D. G. & WOLCOTT, R. G. (1971). *Biochem. biophys. Res. Commun.*, **45**, 1622.
RANG, H. P. (1967). *Ann. N.Y. Acad. Sci.*, **144**, 756.
SONG, C. S. & BODANSKY, O. (1967). *J. biol. Chem.*, **242**, 694.
TOMITA, T. (1970). In: *Smooth Muscle*, ed. Bülbring, E., Brading, A. F., Jones, A. W. & Tomita, T. London: Arnold.
WAUD, D. R. (1968). *Pharmac. Rev.*, **20**, 49.

# ACETYLCHOLINE RECEPTOR AND CHOLINESTERASE MOLECULES OF VERTEBRATE SKELETAL MUSCLES AND THEIR NERVE JUNCTIONS

E. A. BARNARD, T. H. CHIU, J. JEDRZEJCYZK, C. W. PORTER AND J. WIECKOWSKI

*Department of Biochemical Pharmacology, State University of New York, Buffalo, N.Y. 14214, USA*

## *1. Introduction*

If a pharmacologically active blocking agent of high specificity is introduced in radioactive form into a target tissue, it is possible by careful application of certain cellular autoradiographic techniques to determine the location of the receptor sites involved (Fig. 1a), and also their numbers (Barnard, 1970). This offers an approach to mapping the distribution and spatial relationships of the different functional components at a synaptic junction. It also permits the monitoring of attempted selective extractions of those components, for example, of the receptor from the junctions alone.

This simple idea cannot find realization in practice with any assurance of accuracy, unless the specific binding of the reagent employed is irreversible, or at least 'pseudo-irreversible' (Werkheiser, 1961), that is, forming a complex with a dissociation constant ($K_D$) so low (say $< 10^{-8}$ M) that the binding is not reversed in practice during the necessary processing. This processing must include the complete removal of all excess reagent that is merely adsorbed on, or dissolved in, tissue components. Autoradiography is very revealing in this respect, since after the usual pharmacological procedures for washout of a drug to recover responsiveness, it will generally be found (when the agent is used in radioactive form) that considerable radioactivity remains in the preparation, due to residual uptake at extraneous sites. Extractions (for liquid scintillation counting) of a muscle after such labelling and washout can, for the same reason, be highly misleading for receptor estimation, as will be illustrated below in the case of α-bungarotoxin. For an agent binding

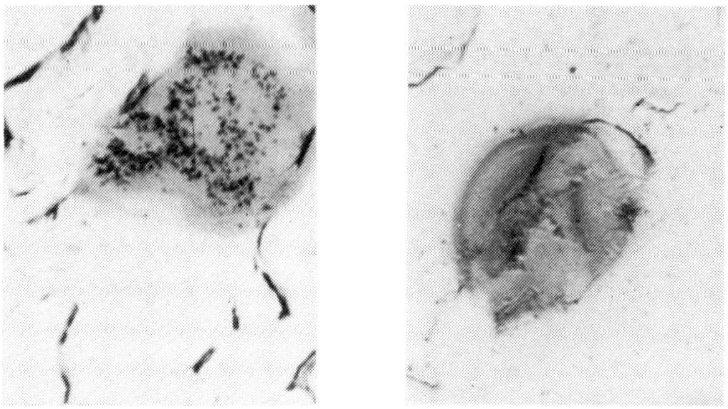


FIG. 1. Autoradiographs of mouse diaphragm muscle, showing an endplate (post-stained), with labelling due to [$^3$H] BuTX. (a), Muscle removed at death after intravenous injection of 1·5 $\mu$g/g [$^3$H] BuTX. Note labelling specific for the endplates. (b), Muscle removed at death after injection of 3 $\mu$g/g unlabelled BuTX, to block endplate sites, and treated *in vitro* with 10 $\mu$g/ml [$^3$H] BuTX (24° C, 2 h) followed by washing in Tyrode solution (24 h, 4° C, 10 changes, with continual stirring). Note the uptake at sites outside the endplates, not saturated by the unlabelled toxin blocking the endplates.

specifically and irreversibly or pseudo-irreversibly at a receptor site, one can employ a more effective washing procedure, namely, brief treatment with a large excess of the same agent in unlabelled form. This gives rapid exchange-out of isotope at all except the irreversible or pseudo-irreversible sites. With $^3$H-labelled $\alpha$-bungarotoxin (to be discussed below), we have found no detectable reversal of its specific binding at motor endplates upon washing (30 min) with a solution of the unlabelled toxin at 10 times the concentration used in the labelling reaction.

In contrast, (+)-tubocurarine (TC) complexes at the diaphragm endplate receptors with apparent $K_D = 4 \times 10^{-7}$ M (Kruckenberg and Bauer, 1971), but junctional block by TC in that preparation is removed by washing in aqueous medium, with $t_{1/2}$ for washout $\simeq 3$ min (after $10^{-6}$ M TC, at 37°). Hence, even with the rather firm binding of this and similar drugs, the exposures to aqueous media involved in normal autoradiographic processing entail a severe risk of loss or translocation of the label. Attempts to measure receptors by a form of autoradiography after application of labelled curariform or depolarizing drugs (Waser, 1967, 1970), may, therefore, meet with considerable difficulty or ambiguity. Diffusion errors can, in fact, be minimized by special autoradiographic techniques based on freezing (for example, as used by Creese & MacLagan (1970)). The latter study showed, however, that extensive extrajunctional sites exist in muscle for the binding of decamethonium.

Even when nonspecific adsorption is eliminated, a multiplicity of sites of apparently specific uptake often exists for a pharmacological agent: probably only one of these classes of binding site will be involved in a given form of receptor action. Thus, in the cholinergic (electroplax) system, several different classes of binding site for each of a series of specific antagonists have been deduced (Eldefrawi, Eldefrawi, Gilmour & O'Brien, 1971). The autoradiographic approach, at the light and electron microscope levels, can separate binding sites at the synapse from those at other locations.

### 2. *Measurement of cholinesterase molecules at an endplate*

To illustrate the methods used, we take the case of cholinesterases (ChE) at motor endplates. The reagent used (Ostrowski, Barnard, Stocka & Darzynkiewicz, 1963) is diisopropylfluorophosphate (DFP), well known to react covalently at the active centre residue in the 'serine-dependent esterases', which include all forms of ChE. When [$^3$H] DFP is applied to muscle, the lipophilic reagent penetrates completely, and labels all such esterases. Autoradiography (after washing with excess unlabelled DFP) then shows high concentrations of the silver grains over the endplate, and only very low levels in the muscle. This endplate labelling can be compared quantitatively, by grain density measurements in autoradiographs prepared under parallel conditions; the rate of uptake at the endplates alone was determined thus (Barnard & Wieckowski, 1970). This rate is rapid, with $t_{1/2}=3$ min at 1 $\mu$g/ml DFP (37° C), and is first-order, reaching a saturation value of endplate labelling that cannot be increased at higher reagent concentrations. Hence a distinct population of macromolecules readily reacting with DFP exists at the neuromuscular junction.

Assignment of these DFP-reactive sites to various enzymes has been made by the use of ligands specific for those active centres (Rogers, Darzynkiewicz, Salpeter, Ostrowski & Barnard, 1969; Barnard, Rymaszewska & Wieckowski, 1971a). Physostigmine, at $1 \times 10^{-5}$ M concentration or above, protects (in all mammalian skeletal muscles examined) about 70% of the endplate DFP-reactive sites, and these we class as ChE active centres of one type or another. The quaternary compound BW 284C51 is a highly selective inhibitor of AChE, at about $10^{-5}$ M concentration, and has also been used in the [$^3$H] DFP reaction bath to protect the AChE sites, which are thus measured (Rogers *et al.*, 1969). Pyridine 2-aldoxime methiodide (2-PAM) is a specific reactivator of DFP-inhibited AChE (Wilson, Ginsburg & Quan, 1958) and has also been used thus in the autoradiographic method (Rogers *et al.*, 1969). Use of the latter two methods has shown that only 35% of the DFP-reactive sites at the endplates in mouse or rat muscles comprises AChE (Table 1). In other species, however, this fraction may vary considerably (Barnard *et al.*, 1971a).

The [$^3$H] DFP autoradiographic method provides the *relative* densities of the ChE-type active centres at the endplates. Conversion to actual numbers of labelled molecules is difficult in the case of autoradiography with tritium, since this would involve assumptions about self-absorption and geometry of the specimen. On the other hand, the use in the same way of [$^{32}$P] DFP and $\beta$-track autoradiography gives the absolute numbers of reacted sites, without assumptions (Rogers *et al.*, 1969; Barnard, 1970). In this method, [$^{32}$P] DFP-labelled muscles are microdissected to yield single fibres, each bearing an intact nerve ending. These are immersed in nuclear emulsion, and after exposure for 1–2 days, development reveals the tracks due to the paths of individual $\beta$-particles (Fig. 2). The number of disintegrations per unit time due to $^{32}$P, in the endplate alone, is thus directly read, giving the absolute number of DFP molecules that have reacted there.

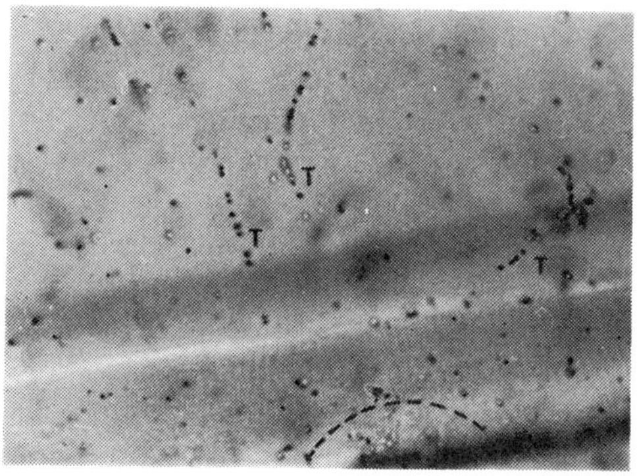


FIG. 2. Measurement of absolute number of labelled sites by $\beta$-track autoradiography. The microdissected fibre, from a muscle treated with [$^{32}$P] DFP (followed by exchange with DFP and washing), has been covered with nuclear emulsion and exposed 24 h. The endplate is unstained, but its location (marked approximately by broken boundary) is found by the attached nerve stump (not shown) and by phase contrast microscopy. Three $\beta$-tracks (T) are shown, each due to a single disintegration, and about 10 others from this endplate were present but not seen in this plane. One half of the tracks go upwards, and these are all countable by focusing. Each endplate is, therefore, a source of tracks radiating outwards, and the background of single grains does not interfere. The mean track count for 50 or more endplates is used to determine the absolute radioactivity per endplate.

In this way, the total numbers of ChE active centres per endplate have been determined in a variety of endplates from skeletal muscles of vertebrates. Some representative values are shown in Fig. 3. As an approximate rule, the number of ChE molecules at the junction increases with the muscle fibre cross-section, and is larger in white fibres than in the red or intermediate (Padykula & Gauthier, 1970) fibre types. We attribute this overall increase to an increase in the postsynaptic membrane area, due to larger junctions (Barnard *et al.*, 1971a). Since the percentage of AChE among these sites is known (Table 1), we obtain also the numbers of AChE active centres per endplate in each case.

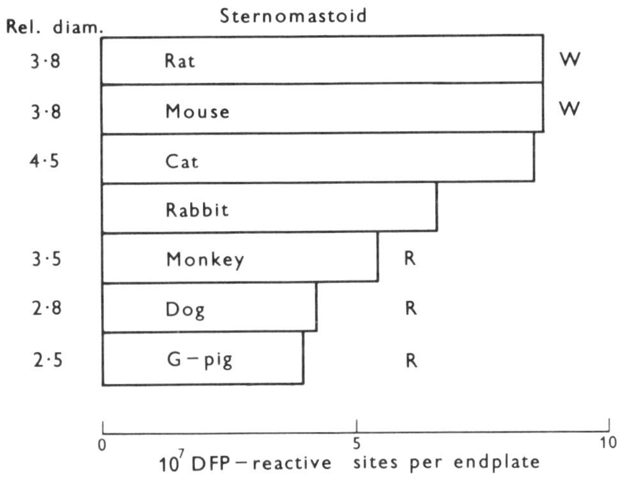


FIG. 3. Numbers of DFP-reactive sites per endplate in a single muscle type (sternomastoid) in a range of mammalian species. White (W) and red (R) fibres were present as shown. The relative mean diameter of the fibres is noted on the left-hand side.

TABLE 1. *Types of DFP-reactive sites at mouse and rat skeletal muscle endplates*

| Characteristic | ChE-type I | ChE-type II | ChE-type III | Non-ChE |
|---|---|---|---|---|
| (a) Physostigmine ($10^5$ M) binding | + | + | + | – |
| 2-PAM reactivation after DFP reaction | + | – | – | – |
| Ethopropazine ($3 \times 10^{-5}$ M) binding | – | + | – | – |
| BW 284C51 ($3 \times 10^{-5}$ M) binding | + | – | Partial | – |
| (b) Acetylthiocholine hydrolysis | + | ? | – | – |
| Butyrylthiocholine hydrolysis | – | + | – | – |
| Proportion* | 35% | 0–5% | ~30% | 30% |

For details of the binding measurements, made by protection from [$^3$H] DFP reaction (set (a)), see Barnard *et al.* (1971a). For set (b), the enzyme in microdissected sternomastoid (mouse) endplates was assayed by a microspectrophotometric method, with characterization of the component responsible by use, in parallel, of the treatments listed in (a) (J. Jedrzejczyk & E. A. Barnard, manuscript in preparation).

* Percentage of the total DFP-reactive sites at each endplate.

### 3. *Autoradiography of cholinergic receptors*

For similar measurements of receptor molecules we have employed α-bungarotoxin (BuTX; purified to homogeneity by chromatographic procedures from the venom of *Bungarus multicinctus*). There is strong evidence for the pharmacological specificity of this toxin for the nicotinic cholinergic receptor (Chang & Lee, 1963; Lee & Chang, 1966; Changeux, Kasai & Lee, 1970). Labelling was by $^3$H-acetylation (Ostrowski, Barnard, Sawicki, Chorzelski, Langner & Mikulski, 1970) under conditions that introduce not more than one acetyl group per toxin molecule. This derivative ([$^3$H] BuTX, having 0·4–0·9 acetyl groups per molecule, in different preparations used) was shown to have the same blocking potency as native BuTX, by demonstration of: (1) no change in the mean half-time for inhibition of the indirectly evoked twitch response in the mouse phrenic–diaphragm preparation under standard conditions, and (2) no change in equivalent uptake at endplates of [$^3$H] BuTX at different dilutions with unlabelled BuTX.

Application of [$^3$H] BuTX was either *in vivo* by lethal intravenous injection into mice, or *in vitro* by maintaining the excised muscle in stirred Tyrode solution containing [$^3$H] BuTX at 1–10 $\mu$g/ml, at 37° C. Washing was with 10 changes of Tyrode solution at room temperature, over 24 h, or, in certain cases, by an initial Tyrode wash, followed by treatment with unlabelled BuTX at 20 $\mu$g/ml, and Tyrode washes for 2 h. Autoradiography of muscle sections was by standard methods (Rogers *et al.*, 1969). In both mammalian and avian muscles, the autoradiographs obtained after application of [$^3$H] BuTX *in vivo* or at 1 $\mu$g/ml *in vitro* showed, after a few days exposure, distinct labelling at the motor endplates, and very little labelling elsewhere (Fig. 1a). This grain density represents the concentration of the specific BuTX-binding sites at the junctions.

By arresting the reaction with excess unlabelled BuTX, followed by Tyrode washes, a series of autoradiographs was prepared representing the extent of BuTX binding at the mouse diaphragm endplate after various times of reaction. The mean values for 200 endplate sections at each time were used thus to construct a rate curve (Fig. 4, curve *b*) for the specific endplate reaction (as distinct from the overall uptake of isotope by the muscle). This curve shows a first-order rate behaviour, with $t_{1/2}=4{\cdot}0$ min at 10 $\mu$g/ml [$^3$H] BuTX, at 37° C. For 2 $\mu$g/ml at 24°, $t_{1/2}=30$ min.

The key to using [$^3$H] BuTX to determine the absolute number of receptors at an endplate, even though tritium is involved, is the use in parallel of the reaction with $^{32}$P-labelled DFP, described above. This gives an internal standard for counting sites at the endplate, since we can also determine the relative extents of reaction (independently) of [$^3$H] DFP and of [$^3$H] BuTX. Specimens from the same muscle from an animal are treated separately, one part with [$^3$H] BuTX and another with [$^3$H] DFP, and after processing together the relative grain densities are compared. When corrected for the different specific isotopic activities of the two reagents, the results yield the ratio of the actual densities of the two types of active centre—receptor and ChE—at the individual endplate (Table 2). Using the absolute numbers determined by the $\beta$-track method for the ChE sites, we find at once the absolute numbers of BuTX-binding sites per endplate (Table 2, column 4).

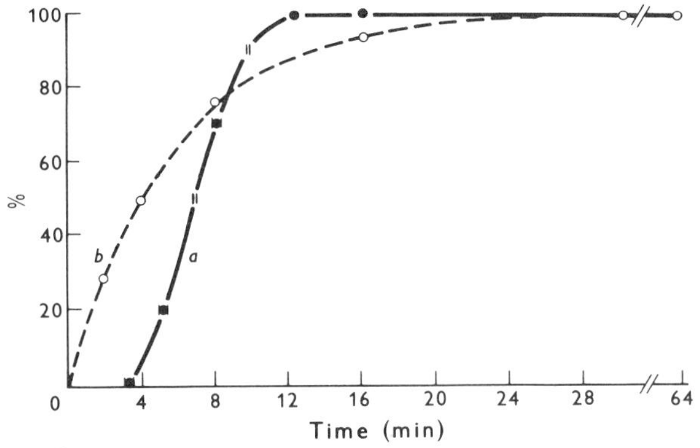


FIG. 4. Reaction of diaphragm endplate *in vitro* with [$^3$H] BuTX (10 $\mu$g/ml, 37° C). *a*, Inhibition (%) of twitch or tetanic (120 stimuli/s) response. Mean ±S.D. of the preparations from ten mice shown (S.D. omitted for values at 100%). *b*, Endplate labelling (each point is the mean for 100–200 fields over endplates), expressed as % of the maximum. Preparations from two mice each gave the same curve. (From Barnard *et al.*, 1971b.)

TABLE 2. *Ratio of α-bungarotoxin binding sites to DFP-reactive sites, and absolute numbers of receptors, in individual endplates*

| Species | Muscle | Ratio of sites* Toxin : DFP | Receptors per endplate† |
|---|---|---|---|
| Mouse | Diaphragm | 1·04 (10) | 3·0 (±0·4) × 10$^7$ |
| | | 1·09‡ (1) | |
| | Preblocked | 0§ (2) | |
| | Sternomastoid | 0·92 (2) | 8·7 (±0·3) × 10$^7$ |
| | | 0·93‡ (1) | |
| Rat | Diaphragm | 0·8 (1) | 5·3 (±0·3) × 10$^7$ |
| Chicken | Post. latissimus dorsi | | |
| (12 weeks) | (fast twitch fibres) | 1·00 (16) | 3·0 × 10$^7$ |
| (8 days) | | 0·99 (4) | |
| (12 weeks) | Biventer | | |
| | (slow twitch fibres) | 0·98 (2) | 2·7 × 10$^7$ |
| Frog | | | |
| (*Rana pipiens*) | Sartorius | ~1‖ | ~3 × 10$^7$ |

* The ratio was determined using the mean of autoradiographic measurements on 100–900 fields over labelled endplates, in each case. Number of animals used is in parentheses. Conditions of [$^3$H] BuTX labelling, *in vitro*, as used in Fig. 4. † Standard error of the mean is shown in parentheses, when > 50 fibres were taken for the $\beta$-track measurements which were used, together with the ratio shown, in determining the receptor number. ‡ The number of toxin-binding sites was measured on this specimen after *in vivo* labelling (3 $\mu$g [$^3$H] BuTX per g body weight, intravenously) followed by further attempted saturation by the *in vitro* treatment with [$^3$H] BuTX. § 3 $\mu$g/g BuTX (unlabelled) given intravenously, then the usual *in vitro* labelling treatment with toxin. No toxin labelling in these endplates, above muscle background level, was found. ‖ Approximate comparison, only, of silver grain densities is possible in frog endplates, due to their morphology.

The binding of BuTX to its sites *at the endplate*, measured thus, reaches a plateau figure which cannot be increased: this is seen in the time course for *in vitro* uptake of [$^3$H] BuTX (Fig. 4, curve *b*), and by the lack of further uptake at those sites after a further exposure *in vitro* following *in vivo* reaction (Table 2, values marked ‡ and §). In view of this, and since the reaction at these sites abolishes the impulse transmission (Fig. 4, curve *a*), we conclude that the sites measured are, in fact, the cholinergic receptor sites at each endplate. We see (Table 2) that the number of these receptor active centres at the junction is not constant, but, again, increases with fibre size. It is also easy to show that treatment with DFP (unlabelled) does not reduce the extent of a subsequent reaction with [$^3$H] BuTX; and conversely, treatment with BuTX (unlabelled) does not affect the [$^3$H] DFP reaction (Barnard, Wieckowski & Chiu, 1971b). Hence, the two types of active centre involved are different and independent.

### *4. The density of receptor molecules at the synaptic membranes*

Electron microscope (EM) extensions of this labelled inhibitor method have been made, using similar specimens (suitably processed subsequently) and examining the silver grain distribution in the EM in relation to ultrastructure (Budd, 1970). [$^3$H] DFP-reacted endplates of the mouse sternomastoid muscle have been analysed thus by Salpeter (1969). Those studies have shown that there is a concentration of these DFP-reactive sites (taken to be ChE active centres) in the postjunctional fold zone. In that zone they cannot be resolved, at the accessible resolutions, between the pre- and postjunctional membranes or the cleft between them. If they are related to the postsynaptic membrane, these ChE active centres occur at a surface density of 12 000 per $\mu m^2$ of that membrane (or about 10 500 per $\mu m^2$ of both membranes, if the presynaptic membrane is also taken into account (Salpeter, 1969). Since the same number of BuTX-binding sites as ChE sites is present at each endplate (Table 2), the same mean density would apply to the ACh receptor active centres. It is interesting that about the same value—roughly $10^4$ receptors per $\mu m^2$ of membrane—has been found using $^{131}$I-labelled BuTX, together with extraction techniques, for electroplax (Miledi, Molinoff & Potter, 1971). In muscle, Miledi & Potter (1971) found about $10^5$ receptors per $\mu m^2$, calculated for the total synaptic membrane at the frog sartorius endplate.

We have now investigated this question in a more direct manner. EM autoradiographs were prepared from mouse diaphragm muscle specimens, after labelling *in vivo* to saturation at the endplates with [$^3$H] BuTX (Fig. 5). Silver grains were found to be associated with the postjunctional fold area (Fig. 6), while the labelling elsewhere was negligible, including that at the highly accessible muscle cell membranes (Fig. 5). The limits of resolution of EM autoradiography in the conditions used (localization to about $\pm 80$ nm) do not permit us to state that the labelling is purely on the postsynaptic

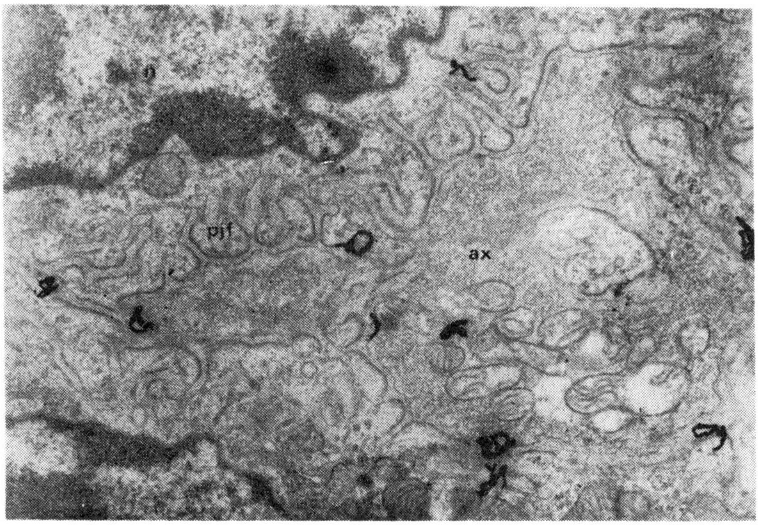


FIG. 5. Electron microscope autoradiograph of a section through a mouse diaphragm endplate, labelled with [$^3$H] BuTX. Note that the grains lie over the postjunctional folds or within the limits of scattered radiation from the folds. Axon, ax; postjunctional folds, pjf; nucleus, n. ($\times$ 30 000).

muscle membrane, and not in the cleft. Since, however, all physiological evidence in the ACh receptor system can only be understood if the receptors are in or attached to the membranes, in the analysis we have made the measurements of grain numbers with respect to the postsynaptic membrane, which location fits the distribution actually observed (Fig. 6). An alternative plot, assuming that all of the sites are on the presynaptic membrane, does not fit the densities, although a small percentage of the sites could be there without change in the observed results. Therefore, by measuring the profiles of the postsynaptic membranes in the autoradiographs, the surface density of labelling was computed, this being a mean of 10 800/$\mu$m$^2$ of postsynaptic membrane. The presynaptic membranes in the mouse diaphragm endplate were found to have on the average one-fifth of the area of the postsynaptic membranes, so that any change in this density value due to some receptor sites being on the former membrane would be minor. Within experimental error, the value found is equal to the density of DFP-reactive sites found at mouse sternomastoid endplate membranes by Salpeter (1969), supporting the deductions outlined above.

### 5. *Extrajunctional binding sites of α-bungarotoxin*

If extraneous binding sites in skeletal muscle exist for BuTX outside the ACh receptors at the endplate, even at low concentrations (not interfering

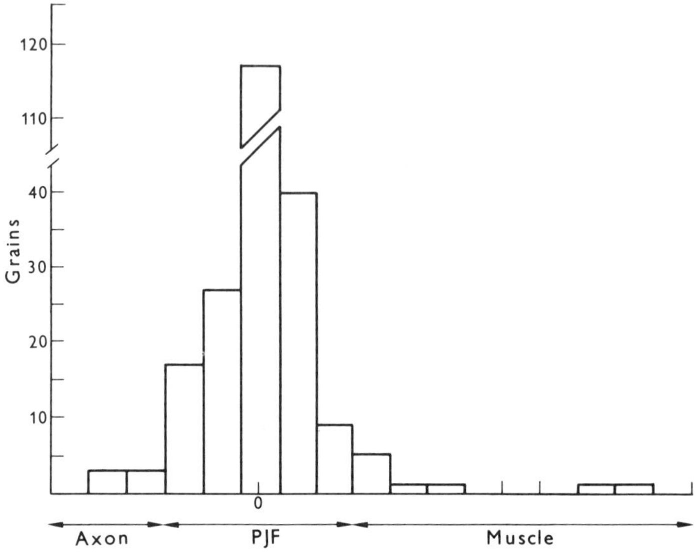


FIG. 6. Histogram showing the grain distribution in the EM autoradiograph, relative to the postjunctional membrane. (Based on 225 grains.) Postjunctional fold zone, PJF. Width of bar corresponds to 200 nm.

with endplate autoradiography), these may become significant in extractions of the labelled material, due to the vast volume of the muscle relative to the endplates. This effect has, in fact, been observed, and is very pronounced in frog muscles.

After treatment with [$^3$H] BuTX at 10 $\mu$g/ml, followed by 24 h washing at 4° C, frog sartorius fibres show marked labelling in patches over the muscle, in addition to the concentration at the endplates (Fig. 7). While there are

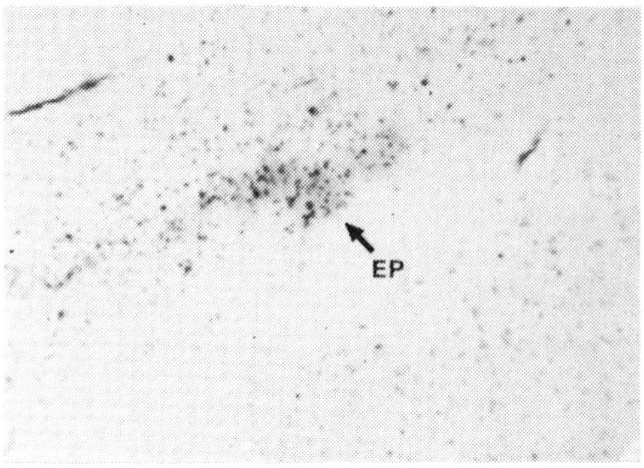


FIG. 7. Autoradiograph of frog sartorius muscle labelled *in vitro* with [$^3$H] BuTX (1 $\mu$g/ml). One endplate (EP, lightly stained) is seen, with labelling outside it, as well as associated with it.

known to be ACh-sensitive sites in frog muscle outside the endplate proper (Katz & Miledi, 1964), these have been recognized in patches on the muscle surface near the endplates (Feltz & Mallart, 1971). These exhibit marked seasonal variations, and can extend from each endplate to the next, which corresponds to our observations (made on *Rana pipiens*, in winter) with [$^3$H] BuTX. The BuTX-binding sites are seen, however, to occur both in the membrane and in the interior of the thick fibres, by autoradiography of sections through these. Similar extrajunctional uptake was observed after treatment with [$^3$H] BuTX at 1 $\mu$g/ml (3 h, 20° C) and the 24-h washing procedure, but the grain density then was lower than that of Fig. 7. In frog sartorius muscles treated precisely thus (using $^{131}$I-labelled BuTX), Miledi & Potter (1971) found a total uptake corresponding to about $10^9$ receptor molecules per endplate. The figure found by autoradiography at this endplate is about $3 \times 10^7$ (Table 2). The difference of 33-fold is far outside the experimental errors, but can be explained by the abundance of extrajunctional BuTX-binding sites in these species. These sites are obviously more extensive than the sensitive sites located by surface mapping of the fibre with an ACh micropipette (Katz & Miledi, 1964), and extend far into the fibre. If they are all, nevertheless, in extrajunctional regions of the fibres that are clustered near the nerve arborizations, then there is no inconsistency with the observation of Miledi & Potter (1971) that 20% of the labelled frog muscle that is endplate-free had only 2% of the total radioactivity.

Similar extrajunctional binding sites can also be found in mouse and rat muscles when [$^3$H] BuTX is applied at 10 $\mu$g/ml, with washing for 24 h (as illustrated in the experiment of Fig. 1b), although their abundance is much less than in the frog muscle. When [$^3$H] BuTX is applied instead at 1 $\mu$g/ml, with identical processing, this extrajunctional labelling in the muscle is negligibly low, although endplate labelling reaches the same plateau value as previously. If the labelling is performed (as in the studies of Barnard *et al.*, 1971b) by lethal intravenous injection of [$^3$H] BuTX (1·5 $\mu$g/g of body weight, in mice), the labelling is also quite specific to the endplates (Fig. 1a and Table 3 (experiment 1)). When mouse muscle labelled thus *in vivo* is excised and further exposed to [$^3$H] BuTX (10 $\mu$g/ml) *in vitro*, the endplate labelling is *not* increased (Table 3), although the muscle background labelling now becomes significant. Extrajunctionally bound [$^3$H] BuTX is not exchangeable with excess unlabelled BuTX applied subsequently (Table 3). In summary, these observations show that there are components outside the synaptic receptors which also take up BuTX, but apparently much more slowly, although in practice irreversibly. This slow uptake may be due to a slower intrinsic reaction rate with the toxin, so that it represents a lower affinity than that of the true ACh receptors, although still high enough to give pseudo-irreversible behaviour. Alternatively, the various rates may merely reflect differences in accessibility, such that the first reactive sites available to the toxin protein molecules are those at synaptic membranes,

TABLE 3. *Uptake of [³H] α-bungarotoxin in diaphragm muscles, measured by extraction*

| Expt | Labelling conditions | No. of hemi-diaphragms | Mean c.p.m. per hemidiaphragm (±S.E.) Whole | EP | Non-EP | Total uptake as % theoretical |
|---|---|---|---|---|---|---|
| 1 | *In vivo*, 1·5 μg/g | 11 | 870±23 | | | 100 |
| | | | | 736± 21 | 99± 18 | 96 |
| 2 | *In vitro*, 1·0 μg/ml | 12 | | 1021± 59 | 295± 57 | 150 |
| 3 | *In vitro*, 10 μg/ml, (+ unlabelled toxin wash) | 4 | | 3621±225 | 3521±232 | 820 |
| 4 | Unlabelled toxin *in vivo*, (3·0 μg/g), then *in vitro*, [³H] toxin, 10 μg/ml | 1 | | 1735 | 2445 | 480 |
| 5 | (Rat) *In vitro*, 1·0 μg/ml | 4 | | 3326± 91 | 1445±143 | 182 |

All muscles were from mice, except in experiment 5. Labelling *in vitro* was at 24° C, 3 h, in Tyrode medium. All specimens were subsequently washed with Tyrode (10 changes, stirred) for 24 h at 4° C. Each was dissolved in 'Soluene' (Packard) and its total radioactivity was measured by liquid scintillation counting. Each diaphragm was divided into endplate-containing (EP) and apparently endplate-free (non-EP) regions, which were equalized in wet weight (to ±10%). The last column shows the relation of the total c.p.m. for the whole hemidiaphragm to the theoretical value for the uptake of the toxin at 6000 endplates per hemidiaphragm, using the autoradiographically determined (Table 2) value for the number of endplate receptor sites. In experiment 3, the labelling was at once followed with several rinses in Tyrode, and stirring for 30 min in unlabelled toxin (20 μg/ml), prior to the 24-h Tyrode washes.

including their infoldings, with much slower penetration to sites in the muscle fibres. If the latter process occurs, as with decamethonium (Creese & MacLaglan, 1970), it would become significant at concentrations above that needed for saturation of the external sites at the synaptic membrane, as is observed. In muscles thicker than the mouse diaphragm, uptake of toxin (1 μg/ml) at endplates on interior fibres can be seen, by autoradiography of [³H] BuTX, to occur slowly compared to the surface fibres (even though continual stirring is used in all cases), showing that diffusion of the toxin through the muscle is limiting. These observations lead to the conclusion that the uptake of labelled BuTX to saturation in a muscle (Miledi & Potter, 1971), followed by extraction, is not a reliable procedure for the isolation of the synaptic ACh receptor material. Due to the diffusion phenomena noted, it is difficult to ensure that the toxin, at any concentration, will react at junctional sites throughout a thick muscle without reacting at extraneous sites in the outer parts of it. The component due to the latter reaction can become, in terms of the total radioactivity present, the predominant one in the muscle. When the labelled muscle is extracted in 1% Triton X-100 solution, this extrajunctional component is solubilized as a macromolecular complex with [$^3$H] BuTX, as an experiment illustrated in Fig. 8 shows. It is seen thus that this extrajunctional radioactivity is not due to free [$^3$H] BuTX in the muscle, although the free toxin is readily soluble in 1% Triton X-100. It is of interest that the extrajunctional toxin-bound complex has a Stokes' radius corresponding to 200 000 molecular weight, compared to about 550 000 for the junctional complex (Fig. 8). It is known that the relationship of Stokes' radius to apparent molecular weight in such complexes of membrane components in 1% Triton X-100 solution is not a simple one (Meunier, Olsen, Menez, Fromageot, Boquet & Changeux, 1972), so these values are only relative. It is not clear whether the junctional and the extrajunctional binding sites involve different molecules, or the same subunits in a different state of aggregation. Care must be taken to remove this extrajunctional component, present in excess, if a whole muscle is to be used for the receptor isolation.

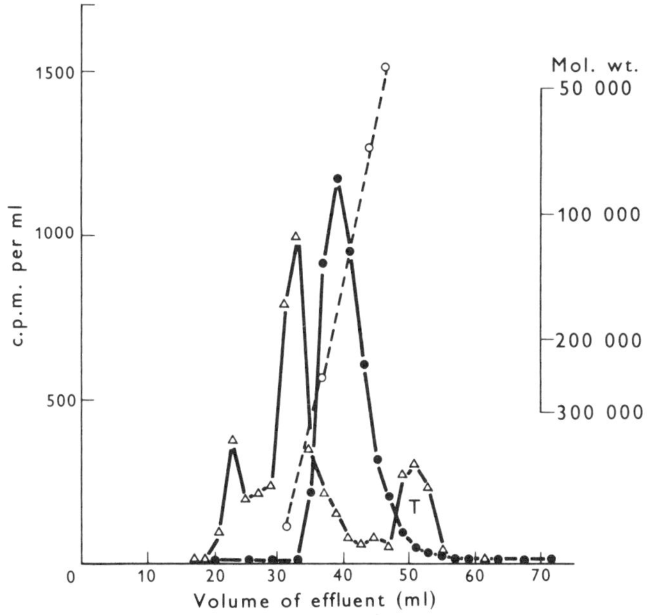


FIG. 8. Gel filtration on Sepharose 6B (68 × 1 cm column; 1 ml fractions) of the complex of [$^3$H] BuTX with extrajunctional components of mouse muscle (●——●). The endplates were first blocked *in vivo* with unlabelled toxin and then labelled *in vitro*, as in experiment 4 of Table 3. The muscle was extracted by stirring in 10 times its weight of 1·5% Triton X-100/0·05 M Tris, pH 8·0, and the soluble extract (75% of the total radioactivity in the specimen) gel-filtered in that medium. Calibration of the column with marker proteins (○-----○) is shown by the broken line. T marks the elution position for free BuTX. Void volume is 22 ml. A parallel gel-filtration (△——△) of the extract of specifically endplate-labelled diaphragm (experiment 1 of Table 3) gives a different, major peak, corresponding to apparent molecular weight 550 000, plus a heavier component.

## 6. *Conclusions*

We draw the following conclusions, with respect to the vertebrate skeletal muscle motor endplate.

(1) At each junction, there are $1–10 \times 10^7$ BuTX-binding sites (varying with the muscle type), and about the same number of active centres of ChE or closely-related molecules. The two types of sites are distinct and independent.

(2) In rodent muscles, for example, 35% of these latter sites are active AChE, the remainder being of unknown function. In the same endplates, about 50% of the BuTX-binding junctional sites have an affinity for TC, as shown by experiments such as that illustrated in Fig. 9. This indicates that these, at least, are the classical ACh receptor sites. Since TC at the concentrations used entirely blocks the indirectly-elicited endplate potential, it is not yet clear what is the identity of the remaining, TC-insensitive, toxin-binding sites. We see that there is an approximate equality of the AChE and true ACh receptor sites, but not necessarily an exact correspondence. In other species where AChE comprises a different fraction of the ChE-type sites (Barnard *et al.*, 1971a), the ratio of AChE to ACh receptors may differ.

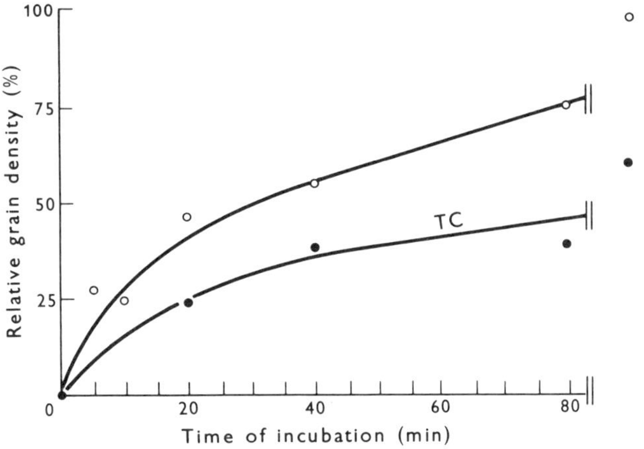


FIG. 9. Partial protection from toxin reaction by saturation with TC. Mouse hemidiaphragms were labelled with [$^3$H] BuTX, 2 $\mu$g/ml, 24° C, in Tyrode solution, alone (○). or with $1{\cdot}4 \times 10^{-4}$ M TC present (●) before (10 min) and during the reaction. Labelling was arrested by addition of unlabelled toxin (10 $\mu$g/ml) and washing, and measured by autoradiography (values expressed as % of the grain density over the endplates at saturation). The last pair of points on the right were obtained similarly, in conditions shown to label the unprotected specimen to saturation at the endplates. (From Porter *et al.*, 1973.)

(3) The *surface density* of these components on the synaptic membranes is probably constant, at about $1{\cdot}1 \times 10^4$ per $\mu m^2$. For skeletal muscle fibres that are larger, the area of contact surface with the nerve ending increases, so that, at a constant surface density, the total number of molecules of ChE, and of ACh receptor, at the synapse increases.

(4) The location of the BuTX-binding sites is, from all available evidence, the postsynaptic membrane (although a minor fraction on the presynaptic side is not excluded). The observed density there corresponds to a mean separation of the centres of about 10 nm. If the subunit binding one BuTX molecule has a minimum diameter of 4 nm (there is no direct evidence yet on its size, but for the electroplax ACh receptor, Miledi & Potter (1971) deduced a monovalent subunit of molecular weight 80 000), this means that at least 14% of the postsynaptic membrane is occupied by ACh receptors, a rather high density. Since it seems implausible that in some areas all or most of the membrane would constitute this one component, this suggests that a lattice of ACh receptors (each oligomeric in structure) at this density stretches across the entire postsynaptic membrane. The problem of also accommodating in this membrane the ChE sites is perhaps relieved by the recent finding (Hall & Kelly, 1971; Betz & Sakmann, 1971) that AChE can be removed from muscle endplates by proteolytic digestion, without impairing the receptor properties. This digestion was observed to remove the ectolemma, the mucopolysaccharide-containing layer in the cleft, suggesting that this holds the AChE. We can, in that case, suggest a mosaic as shown in Fig. 10. In this, the lattice of AChE is in a plane above the receptor lattice. (The 'silent' subunits—35% for ChE and 50% for BuTX-binding sites—are assumed arbitrarily to be other subunits, of as yet unestablished function, in the same structures.)

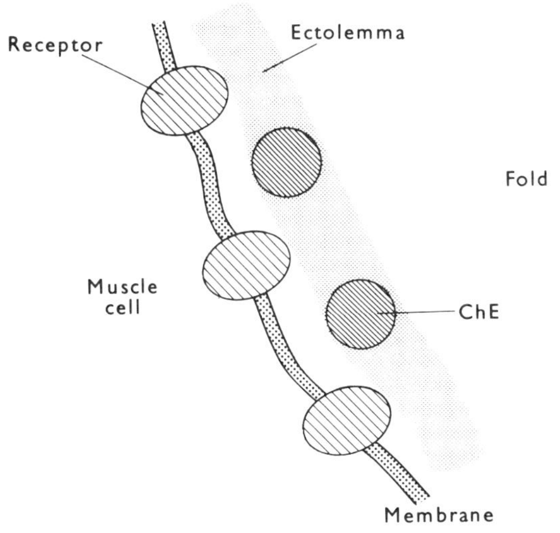


FIG. 10. A model for the possible arrangement of the ACh-receptor complex (which includes the ionophoric component) in the postsynaptic membrane (Membrane). The ChE sites (both active AChE and the inactive subunits of unknown significance) are bound in the surface coat, giving a mosaic arrangement. ACh molecules, after interaction at the receptor sites, are either lost by diffusion from the folds, or are hydrolysed by the adjacent enzyme, which prevents any concentration of ACh accumulating in the vicinity of the receptors.

(5) The receptors blocked by BuTX are required for the impulse transmission to the muscle (Fig. 4), and there is little margin for 'spare receptors' in this system (Barnard *et al.*, 1971b). The margin of safety at the neuromuscular junction is largely that due to the threshold potential for firing, without an additional large reserve of excess receptors. AChE is required, however, only for the passage of rapid volleys (Barnard & Wieckowski, 1970). The relations between ACh output, AChE active centres (number and turnover) and receptor numbers can be approached from the data now available, as discussed by Barnard (1973).

The work discussed herein was supported by Grant GM-11754 from the National Institutes of Health, and by the Muscular Dystrophy Associations of America. C.W.P. is an N.I.H. predoctoral trainee in Experimental Pathology, and J. J. held a Henry and Bertha Buswell Research Fellowship.

## REFERENCES

BARNARD, E. A. (1970). *Int. Rev. Cytol.*, **29**, 213.
BARNARD, E. A. (1973). In: *The Peripheral Nervous System*, ed. Hubbard, J. I. In press. New York: Plenum Press.
BARNARD, E. A. & WIECKOWSKI, J. (1970). In: *Fundamental Concepts in Drug Receptor Interactions*, ed. Danielli, J. F. & Triggle, D. J., p. 229. New York: Academic Press.
BARNARD, E. A., RYMASZEWSKA, T. & WIECKOWSKI, J. (1971a). In: *Cholinergic Ligand Interactions*, ed. Triggle, D. J., Moran, J. F. & Barnard, E. A., p. 175. New York: Academic Press.
BARNARD, E. A., WIECKOWSKI, J. & CHIU, T. H. (1971b). *Nature, Lond.*, **234**, 207.
BETZ, W. & SAKMANN, B. (1971). *Nature, New Biol., Lond.*, **232**, 94.
BUDD, C. G. (1970). *Int. Rev. Cytol.*, **29**, 244.
CHANG, C. C. & LEE, C. Y. (1963). *Arch. Int. Pharmacodyn.*, **144**, 241.
CHANGEUX, J.-P., KASAI, M. & LEE, C. H. (1970). *Proc. natn. Acad. Sci., U.S.A.*, **67**, 1241.
CREESE, K. & MACLAGAN, J. (1970). *J. Physiol., Lond.*, **210**, 363.
ELDEFRAWI, M. E., ELDEFRAWI, A. T., GILMOUR, C. P. & O'BRIEN, R. D. (1971). *Mol. Pharmac.*, **7**, 420.
FELTZ, A. & MALLART, A. (1971). *J. Physiol., Lond.*, **218**, 85.
HALL, S. W. & KELLY, R. B. (1971). *Nature, Lond.*, **232**, 62.
KATZ, B. & MILEDI, R. (1964). *J. Physiol., Lond.*, **170**, 379.
KRUCKENBURG, P. & BAUER, H. (1971). *Pflügers Arch.*, **326**, 184.
LEE, C. Y. & CHANG, C. C. (1966). *Mem. Inst. Butantan, Simp. Internac.*, **33**, 555.
MEUNIER, J.-C., OLSEN, R. W., MENEZ, A., FROMAGEOT, P., BOQUET, P. & CHANGEUX, J.-P. (1972). *Biochemistry*, **11**, 1200.
MILEDI, R. & POTTER, L. T. (1971). *Nature, Lond.*, **233**, 599.
MILEDI, R., MOLINOFF, P. & POTTER, L. T. (1971). *Nature, Lond.*, **229**, 544.
OSTROWSKI, K., BARNARD, E. A., STOCKA, Z. & DARZYNKIEWICZ, Z. (1963). *Exp. Cell Res.*, **31**, 89.
OSTROWSKI, K., BARNARD, E. A., SAWICKI, W., CHORZELSKI, T., LANGNER, A. & MIKULSKI, A. (1970). *J. Histochem. Cytochem.*, **18**, 490.
PADYKULA, H. A. & GAUTHIER, G. F. (1970). *J. cell Biol.*, **46**, 27.
PORTER, C. W., CHIU, T. H., WIECKOWSKI, J. & BARNARD, E. A. (1973). *Nature, New Biol.*, **241**, 3.
ROGERS, A. W., DARZYNKIEWICZ, Z., SALPETER, M. M., OSTROWSKI, K. & BARNARD, E. A. (1969). *J. cell Biol.*, **41**, 605.
SALPETER, M. M. (1969). *J. cell Biol.*, **42**, 122.
WASER, P. (1967). *Ann. N.Y. Acad. Sci.*, **144**, 737.
WASER, P. (1970). In: *Molecular Properties of Drug Receptors*, ed. Porter, R. & O'Connor, M., p. 59. London: Churchill.
WERKHEISER, W. C. (1961). *J. Biol. Chem.*, **236**, 888.
WILSON, I. B., GINSBURG, S. & QUAN, C. (1958). *Archs Biochem. Biophys.*, **77**, 286.

# THE ISOLATION OF FUNCTIONAL ACETYLCHOLINE RECEPTOR

R. D. O'BRIEN, M. E. ELDEFRAWI AND A. T. ELDEFRAWI

*Section of Neurobiology and Behavior, Cornell University, Ithaca, N.Y. 14850, USA*

## *Introduction: the reversible ligand technique*

In current studies on the purification of acetylcholine receptor, efforts have been directed towards purification of that component of the receptor which bears the recognition site or sites. Consequently, we do not use the term 'functional' in the sense that we propose to describe purification of receptor macromolecules which contain the whole apparatus of recognition and (after insertion into an appropriate membrane) transduction. Instead we mean 'functional' to imply only that the purified macromolecule can recognize and bind its own transmitter. In particular, we are concerned to contrast the use of the technique which we shall call the reversible ligand technique, and which generally employs acetylcholine as the ligand, with techniques in which 'irreversibly' bound α-bungarotoxin (BuTX) is used as a label.

The fundamental problem in using irreversibly bound label in purification attempts, is that the purification procedure might well have the effect of profoundly denaturing the receptor, and perhaps even of separating lipid and protein components (should they be present), without the experimenter even being aware of it. To make a comparison with another field, if acetylcholinesterase were labelled with [$^{32}$P] diisopropyl phosphorofluoridate ([$^{32}$P] DFP), and purification then attempted, it would be quite possible to finish up with a polypeptide to which the $^{32}$P was firmly attached, but which would provide only limited information about the neighbouring amino-acid groups in the primary structure of the enzyme. Even the ability of the fragment, after removal of $^{32}$P, to recombine with more DFP might quite well be lost.

Similarly, the use of labelled BuTX can lead to the purification of material which we would call functionally inactive. For instance, holding preparations under conditions typical of electrofocusing (that is, pH 4·5 in the cold) can reduce the acetylcholine binding by 95% in 24 h, though previously attached

BuTX is not affected. Similarly, the BuTX-labelled receptor can be very conveniently solubilized with sodium dodecyl sulphate (SDS) but we have found that SDS virtually eliminates the ability of the soluble material to bind acetylcholine.

It was in anticipation of this kind of problem that we developed assay techniques based upon the ability of fractions to bind with appropriate reversible ligands. We have used, in particular, muscarone, nicotine, dimethyl-(+)-tubocurarine, atropine, decamethonium and in all our recent work, acetylcholine.

### *Studies on the* Torpedo *electric organ*

Most of the work that we shall describe was done with lyophilized fractions from the electric organ of *Torpedo*, and we have normally used an equilibrium dialysis technique. In this technique, the tissue or fraction is enclosed in a cellophane dialysis bag which is immersed in a bath containing the radioactive ligand, and allowed to come to equilibrium. Donnan effects are minimized because the salt concentration is very much higher than the ligand concentration. Also, the bath volume is large in relation to the dialysis bag so that the ligand concentration in the bath is not sensibly depleted. The system is allowed to come to equilibrium in the cold, and then the radioactivity within the bag and in the bath is determined, the difference giving the amount of radioactivity that is bound to the sample.

The early work showed that muscarone, a very close structural analogue of acetylcholine, was bound by electroplax fractions in the manner predicted for binding to the acetylcholine receptor, in that the amount bound was small and the binding was blocked by drugs that act on cholinergic receptors, but not by other drugs. We were then able to show that concentrations of organophosphates, which were high enough to block the acetylcholinesterase completely, did not interfere with muscarone binding, and this finding enabled us to study the binding of acetylcholine by the same technique, without interference from cholinesterase. Fig. 1 shows results obtained with the organophosphate Tetram on a particulate electroplax preparation. The top part shows that the acetylcholinesterase is fully inhibited by 0·1 mM Tetram, and the bottom part shows that acetylcholine binding is blocked by Tetram only at concentrations much above 0·1 mM, while binding is not seen at low concentrations of Tetram, because of the activity of acetylcholinesterase. But there is a range of concentrations of Tetram which allows the acetylcholine binding to be measured. Working with preparations from housefly head, *Electrophorus*, and *Torpedo*, we were able to show that the particular organophosphate and concentration range which is suitable for this purpose differs for each tissue. The blocking effect of high concentrations of organophosphate is reversible, as was shown by Bartels & Nachmansohn (1969) for physiological preparations of eel electroplax.

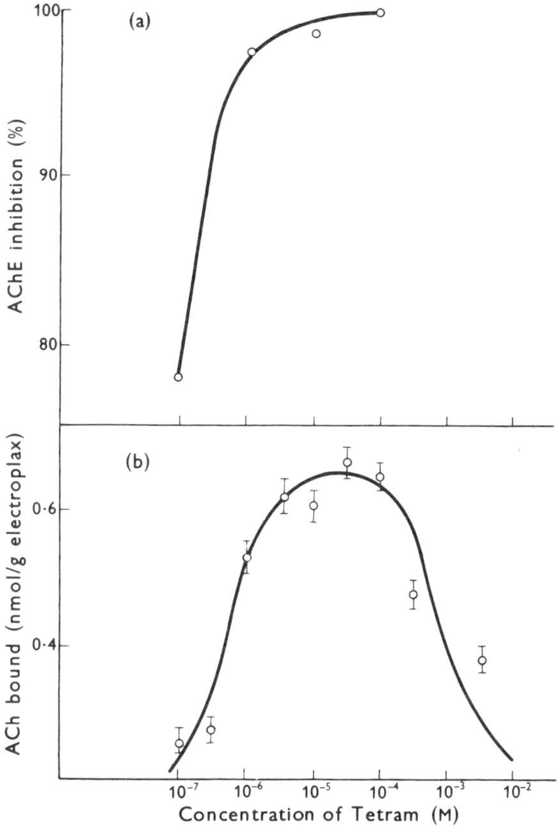


FIG. 1. Effect of increasing Tetram concentration on (a), the inhibition of acetylcholinesterase (AChE) in *Torpedo* electroplax, and (b), the binding of acetylcholine (ACh) (at 0·25 $\mu$M) to *Torpedo* electroplax. The circles and vertical bars represent the mean and standard deviation for three experiments, five samples each. (From Eldefrawi, Britten & O'Brien, 1971.)

We were therefore able to study acetylcholine binding as an index of acetylcholine receptor activity. Some of the properties of acetylcholine binding macromolecules from electroplax are as follows.

With the *Torpedo* membrane fraction, there is more than one kind of acetylcholine binding, as Fig. 2 shows by the nonlinearity of the Scatchard plot. For all the ligands studied in *Torpedo*, it was found that there are multiple binding sites, which for any one ligand differ greatly in affinity and amount (Table 1). For acetylcholine, there are two sites which differ 8-fold in their amount, as indicated by the values of *B* (expressed in nmol bound per g of original tissue). The sites differ about 10-fold in affinity, as measured by *K*, the dissociation constant. Muscarone and nicotine also have dual binding sites, and in each case the low affinity site is relatively large in amount,

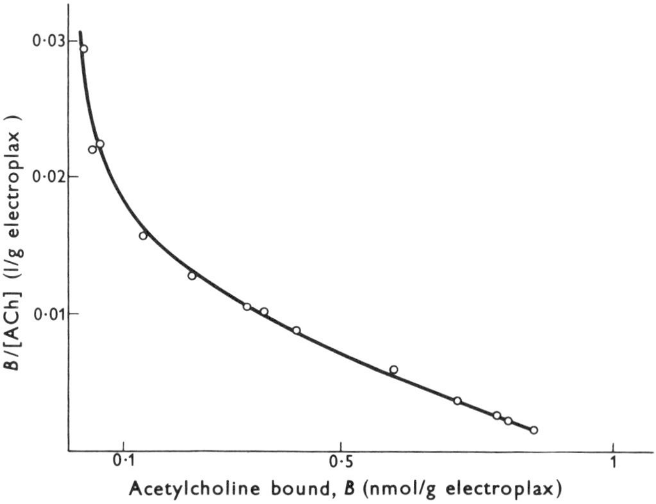


FIG. 2. Scatchard plot of binding of acetylcholine to a particulate preparation of *Torpedo* electroplax; [ACh], acetylcholine concentration in nM; *B*, amount of acetylcholine bound in nmol/g electroplax. Each point represents the average of two experiments, three samples each. (From Eldefrawi, Britten & Eldefrawi, 1971.)

TABLE 1. *Dissociation constants (K) and concentrations of binding sites (B) in a particulate preparation of* Torpedo *electroplax for five cholinergic ligands (from Eldefrawi, Britten & Eldefrawi, 1971 and Eldefrawi, Eldefrawi, Gilmour & O'Brien, 1971)*

| Ligand | *K* μM | *B* (nmol/g electroplax) | % error* |
|---|---|---|---|
| Acetylcholine | $K_1=0{\cdot}008$ | $B_1=0{\cdot}1$ | |
| | $K_2=0{\cdot}068$ | $B_2=0{\cdot}83$ | 7 |
| Muscarone | $K_1=0{\cdot}065$ | $B_1=0{\cdot}08$ | |
| | $K_2=0{\cdot}55$ | $B_2=0{\cdot}38$ | 21 |
| Nicotine | $K_1=0{\cdot}2$ | $B_1=0{\cdot}06$ | |
| | $K_2=2{\cdot}5$ | $B_2=0{\cdot}75$ | 9 |
| Dimethyl-(+)-tubocurarine | $K_1=0{\cdot}037$ | $B_1=0{\cdot}18$ | |
| | $K_2=1{\cdot}0$ | $B_2=3{\cdot}6$ | 17 |
| Decamethonium | $K_1=0{\cdot}3$ | $B_1=0{\cdot}6$ | |
| | $K_2=0{\cdot}59$ | $B_2=1{\cdot}4$ | |
| | $K_3=8{\cdot}0$ | $B_3=3{\cdot}2$ | 14 |

Data were derived from iterative treatment of Scatchard plots. * Root-mean-square percentage error.

about 1 nmol/g, the high affinity sites being less abundant, about 0·1 nmol/g. Decamethonium has three binding sites, the lowest affinity site being more abundant than any of the other binding sites shown in Table 1. Table 2 shows comparable data (but lacking values for acetylcholine, which are not

TABLE 2. *Dissociation constants (K) and concentration of binding sites (B) in a particulate preparation of* Electrophorus *electroplax for four cholinergic ligands (from Eldefrawi, Eldefrawi & O'Brien, 1971)*

| Ligand | K μM | B (nmol/g electroplax) | % error* |
|---|---|---|---|
| Muscarone | 0·055 | 0·021 | 11·8 |
| Nicotine | 0·063 | 0·033 | 7·1 |
| Decamethonium | $K_1$= 0·0025 | $B_1$= 0·03 | |
| | $K_2$= 0·055 | $B_2$= 0·02 | |
| | $K_3$= 2·5 | $B_3$= 0·25 | |
| | $K_4$=100 | $B_4$= 4·0 | 17·0 |
| Dimethyl-(+)-tubocurarine | $K_1$= 0·08 | $B_2$= 0·05 | |
| | $K_2$= 40 | $B_3$=14·0 | 6·5 |

Data derived from iterative treatment of Scatchard plot. * Root-mean-square percentage error.

yet available) for eel electroplax. In this case only one binding site for muscarone or nicotine was observed, but four decamethonium binding sites were found. Thus it appears that decamethonium behaves in an anomalous way and that the binding which occurs at high concentrations does not appear to correspond to the binding of any other ligand. Comparison of Table 1 and 2 also shows that the number of binding sites for muscarone and nicotine, which are thought, from other evidence, to be acetylcholine receptors, is about twenty-five times as great in *Torpedo* as in *Electrophorus*, and therefore *Torpedo* is a better source of receptor material.

Fig. 3 shows the effects of various sulphydryl and disulphide agents upon acetylcholine binding in particulate fractions from *Torpedo* tissue. In general, the effects observed are comparable to the results obtained by Karlin, Prives, Deal & Winnik (1971) on physiological preparations of eel electroplax. The binding of acetylcholine was substantially inhibited by *p*-chloromercuribenzoate (PCMB), by dithiothreitol (DTT) and *p*-(trimethylammonium) benzenediazonium fluoroborate (TDF). The effect of DTT was reversed by the Ellman reagent (DTNB) or potassium ferricyanide. It appears that acetylcholine binding requires SH groups (as seen by the blocking by PCMB) and also intact S–S groups as seen by the inhibitory effect of the reducing agent, DTT.

### *Solubilization and characterization of binding material*

Acetylcholine binding material was readily solubilized by cholates, by Lubrol WX and by Triton X-100; but SDS destroyed activity. The Lubrol-solubilized material could be fractionated chromatographically, and Fig. 4 shows that the peak of acetylcholinesterase activity was readily separated

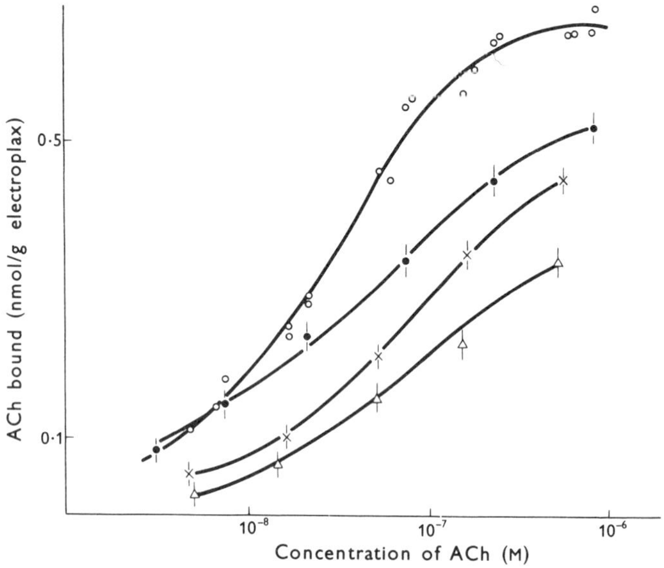


FIG. 3. Binding of acetylcholine (ACh) to a particulate preparation of *Torpedo* electroplax and reduction of this binding by pretreatment of the preparation with different reagents. (○——○), Control; (●——●), PCMB; (×——×), DTT; (△——△), TDF. The vertical lines at each point represent the standard deviation of nine test points. (From Eldefrawi & Eldefrawi, 1972.)

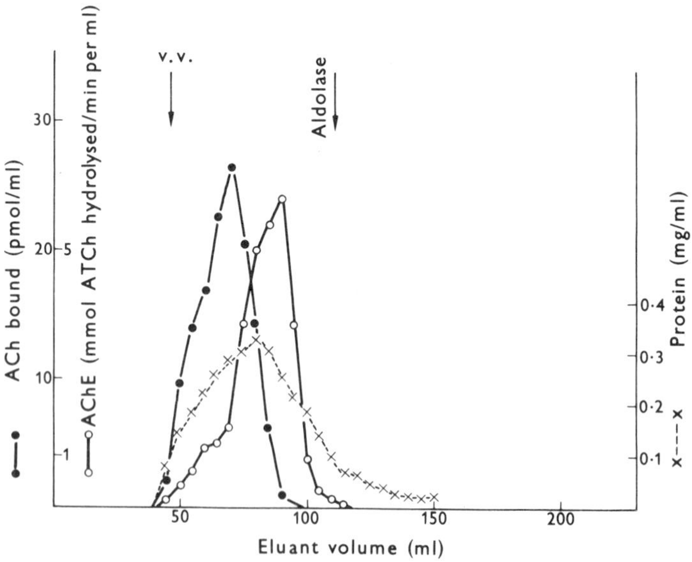


FIG. 4. Gel chromatography on Sepharose 6B of Lubrol-solubilized preparation of *Torpedo* electroplax (v.v. is void volume; aldolase mol. wt. 158 000; ATCh, acetylthiocholine). (From Eldefrawi *et al.*, 1971.)

from the peak of acetylcholine binding activity, providing additional evidence that the enzyme and the receptor are quite different macromolecules.

One of the most important questions which can be answered by use of the reversible ligand technique is, whether or not the properties of the receptor changed in the course of purification. It has been suggested by others that purification can lead to 'a loss of stereospecificity', but our results show that no major change in binding properties occurs when the material is solubilized with Lubrol. Table 3 shows that the binding of acetylcholine is still inhibited in the presence of nicotinic cholinergic agents, and only slightly affected by muscarinic drugs; and it is still insensitive to drugs that do not act on cholinergic receptors. However, solubilization does modify the affinity of the *Torpedo*

TABLE 3. *Inhibition of binding of ACh (at 0·1 μM) to the Lubrol-solubilized receptor, from* Torpedo *electroplax by different drugs (from Eldefrawi, Eldefrawi, Seifert & O'Brien, 1971)*

| Drug (10 μM) | % block of ACh binding ± % error | Significance ($P$) |
|---|---|---|
| Butyrylcholine | 91 ± 37 | 0·01 |
| Carbachol | 74 ± 16 | 0·01 |
| Benzoylcholine | 12 ± 3 | <0·05 |
| Choline | 6 ± 1 | N.S. |
| Succinylcholine | 75 ± 19 | <0·01 |
| Decamethonium | 54 ± 8 | 0·01 |
| Hexamethonium | 12 ± 1 | 0·01 |
| (+)-Tubocurarine | 60 ± 6 | 0·01 |
| Gallamine | 32 ± 5 | 0·01 |
| Nicotine | 41 ± 7 | 0·01 |
| Anabasine | 19 ± 3 | 0·01 |
| Hemicholinium-3 | 19 ± 2 | 0·01 |
| Physostigmine* | 30 ± 6 | 0·01 |
| Neostigmine* | 82 ± 20 | 0·01 |
| Pyridostigmine* | 20 ± 2 | 0·01 |
| Edrophonium* | 100 ± 25 | 0·01 |
| Paraoxon* | 15 ± 2 | 0·01 |
| α-Bungarotoxin† | 99 ± 12 | 0·01 |
| Cobra toxin‡ | 98 ± 10 | 0·01 |
| L(+)-Muscarine | 4 ± 2 | N.S. |
| Arecoline | 3 ± 1 | N.S. |
| Pilocarpine | 12 ± 1 | 0·05 |
| Atropine | 10 ± 1 | 0·05 |
| Hyoscine | 1 ± 0·2 | N.S. |
| Acetyl-β-methylcholine | 9 ± 12 | 0·05 |

Amongst the stimulants, strychnine blocked 25 ± 3% of ACh binding but amphetamine, methylamphetamine, caffeine and picrotoxin had no effect. Dibenamine was the only adrenergic drug which blocked ACh binding significantly (14 ± 2%). Ineffective adrenergic ligands were adrenaline, noradrenaline, dopamine, L-dopa and ergotamine. No blocking was observed by local anaesthetics (procaine, piperocaine, amethocaine, cocaine), hypnotics (barbitone sodium) or hallucinogens (LSD 25, mescaline). Other ineffective compounds were 5-hydroxytryptamine, histamine, glutamate, glutamine, and γ-aminobutyrate. N.S. signifies that $P > 0·05$. * Drug used at 1 mM. † Toxin used at 0·1 μM. ‡ Toxin used at 1 μM.

electroplax receptor for acetylcholine. There are still two binding sites apparent, but the affinity of the high affinity site is increased 5-fold (to 1·4 nM) while that of the low affinity site is decreased 3-fold (to 0·22 μM). Furthermore, a Hill plot of the binding data (Fig. 5) shows that whereas the receptor in particulate preparations (P) shows no cooperativity (that is, the Hill coefficient is 1·0) the solubilized material (S) shows evidence of a negative cooperativity (Hill coefficient 0·66).

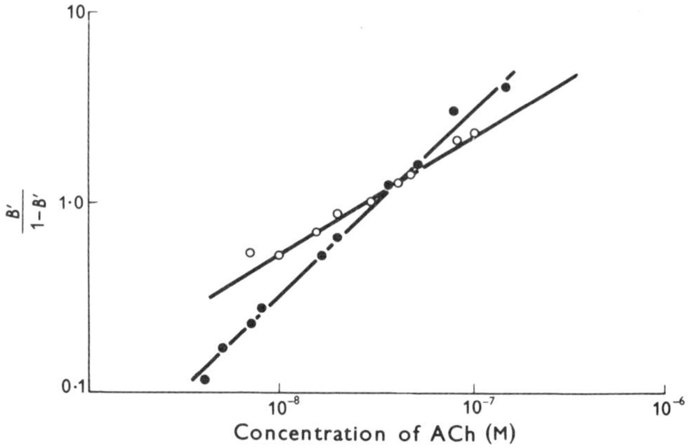


FIG. 5. Hill plot of binding of acetylcholine (ACh) to acetylcholine receptor from *Torpedo* electroplax (*B′*, ACh bound as fraction of maximal binding; (●), particulate; (○), Lubrol-solubilized). (From Eldefrawi *et al.*, 1972.)

TABLE 4. *Effect of enzyme treatment on binding of cholinergic ligands to* Torpedo *electroplax (from Eldefrawi, Eldefrawi, Gilmour & O'Brien, 1971)*

| Ligand | Concentration μM | % reduction of binding* | | |
|---|---|---|---|---|
| | | Trypsin | Chymotrypsin | Phospholipase C |
| Muscarone | 0·01 | 64 | 72 | 64 |
| | 0·1 | 78 | 65 | 42 |
| | 1·0 | 67 | 80 | 48 |
| Nicotine | 0·01 | 74 | 71 | 41 |
| | 0·1 | 87 | 78 | 54 |
| | 1·0 | 49 | 58 | 16 |
| Dimethyl-(+)-tubocurarine | 0·01 | 50 | 47 | 22 |
| | 0·1 | 44 | 47 | 21 |
| | 1·0 | (7)† | 12 | (5)† |
| Decamethonium | 0·001 | 71 | 69 | 27 |
| | 0·01 | 76 | 71 | 21 |
| | 0·1 | 81 | 75 | 24 |
| | 1·0 | 80 | 80 | 25 |

* Controls showed significant binding of decamethonium to the three enzymes, and of dimethyl-(+)-tubocurarine to trypsin and phospholipase C. Values in the table were corrected accordingly. † Values in parentheses are not significantly different from controls as judged by the Student's *t* test.

Another property which is retained after solubilization and subsequent fractionation is sensitivity to phospholipase C and proteolytic enzymes. Table 4 shows some data upon the loss of binding activity of *Torpedo* particulate preparations for a number of ligands, following treatment with trypsin, chymotrypsin, and phospholipase C. Similar results were obtained with tissue from *Electrophorus*. Our tentative conclusion is that functional receptor activity involves either a phospholipoprotein or a complex of protein and phospholipid.

Purification of *Torpedo* electroplax material by electrofocusing indicates that the acetylcholine binding activity is associated with an acid fraction of pI about 4·5. Fig. 6 shows the narrow precipitation bands which occur in this region, and the high resolution of columns of this type Fig. 7 shows the distribution of acetylcholinesterase, acetylcholine binding material and protein in such an experiment. Although acetylcholine binding activity is retained with this technique, the recoveries from such columns are generally very low. As mentioned above, acetylcholine binding activity is sensitive

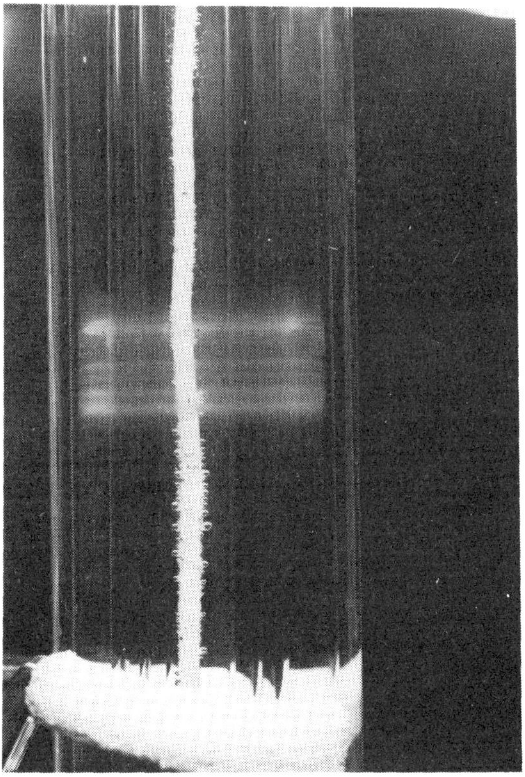

FIG. 6. Part of an electrofocusing column (using ampholytes (3–10)) showing several precipitated bands at pH range 4–5·2 at the end of a run of a 1 % Triton extract of *Torpedo* electroplax. (From Eldefrawi and Eldefrawi, 1972.)

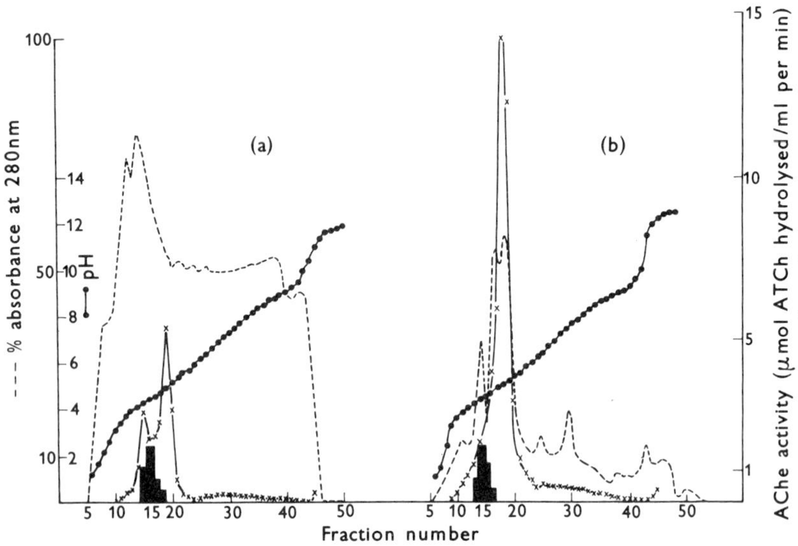


FIG. 7. Isoelectric focusing of (a), 1% Triton extract and (b), 1% Lubrol extract of *Torpedo* electroplax, showing the distribution of protein, AChE and acetylcholine binding activity (solid histograms). The absorption at 280 nm is due mostly to the Triton in (a), but to the protein in (b). (From Eldefrawi & Eldefrawi, 1972.)

to low pH, and consequently electrofocusing which is effective in fractionating material labelled with BuTX, is of limited usefulness in the purification of functional acetylcholine receptors. Affinity chromatography columns offer more promise, because they are quick, and do not involve extremes of pH, and we have achieved a 10-fold purification by means of an agarose column with a phenyltrimethylammonium side-chain.

An important consideration is whether the macromolecules that bind reversible ligands are the same as those that bind irreversible ligands. The only evidence available relates to the amount of 'receptor' which the different techniques indicate. For electric eel electroplax, excellent agreement has been found: Karlin *et al.* (1971) studied the irreversible binding of tritiated 4-(*N*-maleimido)-α-benzyltrimethylammonium to reduced receptor, and found* between 7 and 21 pmol/g wet weight. Raftery, Schmidt, Clark & Wolcott (1971) examined the irreversible binding of $^{125}$I-labelled BuTX and found 35 pmol/g. We found (Table 2) a value of 21 pmol/g with muscarone and 33 with nicotine.

For *Torpedo* electroplax, we have reported (Table 1), for combined high- and low-affinity bindings, 930 pmol/g electroplax for acetylcholine, 460 for muscarone and 810 for nicotine. These measures of the amount of receptor agree well with the value† of 1100 pmol/g based on binding of BuTX (Miledi,

* Specifically, 'A 35 mg electroplax contains $1 \cdot 6 \times 10^{11}$ to $3 \cdot 0 \times 10^{11}$ binding sites per cell.'

† Specifically, 'there seems to be $6 \cdot 6 \times 10^{14}$ binding sites per gram of tissue.'

Molinoff & Potter, 1971). But La Torre, Lunt & De Robertis (1970) observed a completely different value* of 8400 pmol/g, based on the ability of a proteolipid to carry [$^{14}$C] methylhexamethonium through a Sephadex LH20 column being eluted with chloroform–methanol.

This discrepancy could have been due to the fact that La Torre *et al.* (1970) measured binding in an organic phase. We therefore extracted the proteolipid fraction from *Torpedo* electroplax with chloroform–methanol, and examined the possibility that acetylcholine bound to it in an organic phase. We performed equilibrium dialysis experiments in chloroform–methanol, and explored acetylcholine binding and the effects upon it of several drugs. Dialysis tubing was washed thoroughly in water and then with chloroform–methanol (2 : 1) before use according to the method employed by Tenenbaum & Folch-Pi (1966). We readily saw such binding, but the binding showed no saturation and there was a linear relationship between ligand concentration and amount bound. The amount bound at 1 $\mu$M showed no block by 0·1 mM concentrations of drugs such as (+)-tubocurarine, decamethonium, succinylcholine and gallamine. On the basis of the nonsaturation and the insensitivity to competing drugs, we conclude that binding in an organic phase represents a nonspecific partitioning of polar ligands out of the organic phase and into the polar components of the macromolecules. This appears to be a nonspecific reflection of the polar character of the macromolecules relative to chloroform–methanol, and not to be an index of receptor activity.

### *Receptor-like activity in axonal membranes*

We have recently been studying receptor-like activity in a membrane preparation derived entirely from axons, obtained from the walking leg nerves of lobsters. We had expected that acetylcholine receptors would be absent from this tissue, and indeed we could not detect the binding of radioactive acetylcholine. However, we were able to measure quite easily the binding of radioactive nicotine, and then by studying the inhibitory effect of acetylcholine, we were able to detect an acetylcholine binding site with a sufficiently low affinity that it had escaped detection by the radioactive acetylcholine technique. The nicotine binding site displayed a drug specificity that was surprisingly similar to the nicotinic cholinergic receptor from synapses (Table 5). BuTX was an effective inhibitor. The material behaved like a phospholipoprotein or a protein phospholipid complex, as judged by enzyme studies (Table 6). The amount of material was about 0·8 nmol/g of original tissue, which is fairly close to the figure found for the low-affinity site of acetylcholine or nicotine binding to *Torpedo* electroplax. However, it

* Specifically, '. . . from about 2 g of fresh tissue . . . we could separate some 130 $\mu$g of proteolipid, having high affinity for [$^{14}$C] MHM' and 'the amount of [$^{14}$C] MHM bound to the proteolipid was $1 \cdot 3 \times 10^{-10}$ moles per microgram protein.'

TABLE 5. *Inhibition of binding of nicotine* (0·1 μM) *to axon membranes by drugs (from Denburg, Eldefrawi & O'Brien, 1972)*

| Drug (10 μM) | % inhibition |
|---|---|
| (+)-Tubocurarine | 94 |
| Atropine | 67 |
| Decamethonium | 58 |
| Physostigmine | 78 |
| Procaine | 61 |
| Benzoylcholine | 11 |
| Tetram | 60 |
| Tetraethylammonium | 11 |
| 5-Hydroxytryptamine | (5) |
| Noradrenaline | (3) |
| γ-Aminobutyrate | (0) |
| α-Bungarotoxin (3 μM) | 60 |

Numbers in parentheses represent nonsignificant inhibition.

TABLE 6. *Effects of enzyme treatment of axon membranes on nicotine binding* (0·1 μM) (from Denburg *et al.*, 1972)

| Enzyme | % reduction in binding |
|---|---|
| Pronase | 77 |
| Trypsin | 53 |
| Chymotrypsin | 50 |
| Papain | 0 |
| Collagenase | 0 |
| Ribonuclease | 0 |
| Deoxyribonuclease | 0 |
| Lipase | 19 |
| Phospholipase A | 90 |
| Phospholipase C | 12 |
| Phospholipase D | 47 |

differed from the receptor activity of electroplax in its lower affinity for acetylcholine ($K_i = 43$ μM) and its sensitivity to procaine, which inhibited binding competitively with a $K_i$ of 3 μM. Radioactive procaine binds to the preparation with an affinity virtually identical to that with which it inhibits nicotine binding, but the binding capacity for procaine is 3 times as great as for nicotine. Procaine is entirely inactive against electroplax receptor. The nicotine binding component of lobster nerve was insensitive to tetrodotoxin and DTT. We conclude that there is in axons a macromolecule whose pharmacological properties resemble the synaptic acetylcholine receptor. Its functional significance is not yet clear, but it appears to be a possible candidate for the site of action of local anaesthetics in peripheral nerve.

The presence of this material raises once again the question of whether acetylcholine may have a role in axonal transmission as postulated by Nachmansohn (1970).

### *The physiological significance of acetylcholine binding activity*

The binding affinities measured for acetylcholine tend to be higher than those estimated by physiological methods. For example, one can calculate acetylcholine concentrations required for half-maximal response as follows: for blocking of action potential in eel electroplax, 3 μM (Rosenberg, Higman & Nachmansohn, 1960); for depolarization of eel electroplax, 9 μM (Bartels & Nachmansohn, 1965). These values are about 10 times higher than the low-affinity dissociation constant (0·22 μM) for acetylcholine binding to solubilized *Torpedo* receptor. However, such dissociation constants in soluble preparations are often lower than those measured in the whole cell; for example, Webb & Johnson (1969) found that the dissociation constants of five anticholinesterases were, on average, 300 times lower for solubilized acetylcholinesterase, than for the enzyme *in situ* in the eel electroplax.

If we suppose that the low-affinity binding (which in the soluble form comprises 69 % of the total binding) accounts for the normal response of receptor to acetylcholine, what is the role of the high-affinity site? One intriguing possibility is that miniature potentials are produced by binding to the high-affinity site. One can compute that in muscle preparations the miniature potentials occur with acetylcholine concentrations in the range 2–200 nM. These values are roughly comparable with the high affinity dissociation constants obtained for acetylcholine (1·4 nM for the soluble material and 8 nM for the particulate fraction of *Torpedo* electroplax).

Alternatively, the two acetylcholine sites we find might represent two interchangeable forms of receptor, so that higher acetylcholine concentrations, in the μM range, might induce a change in the form of the receptor, much as Koshland (1970) has proposed for enzymes. In this connection, it is notable that the high- and low-affinity sites both show the typical nicotinic drug sensitivity as shown by the fact that (a) the drug sensitivity is measured with acetylcholine concentrations which result in binding to both low- and high-affinity binding; and (b) studies with muscarone and nicotine at low and at high concentrations show similar drug sensitivities (Eldefrawi, Eldefrawi, Gilmour & O'Brien, 1971), which would not be the case if the two sites were affected differently by the various inhibitors tested.

By contrast, the low-affinity binding of (+)-tubocurarine and decamethonium differs from the high-affinity binding in both susceptibility to inhibitors and sensitivity to hydrolytic enzymes. We conclude that whereas nicotine, muscarone, and (especially) acetylcholine binding provide faithful indicators of receptor activity, the binding of decamethonium or (+)-tubocurarine at concentrations in the μM range is due largely to nonreceptor sites.

In conclusion, we have provided evidence that the optimal index of nicotinic receptor activity for use in receptor purification is binding of acetylcholine or perhaps muscarone or nicotine. Unfortunately, this measure of what we call 'functional receptor' activity leads us to recognize that loss of activity during purification is just as common in this sensitive phospholipoprotein as it is in the most delicate enzymes, and progress towards full purification has been correspondingly slow.

Financial support for the work reported herein is gratefully acknowledged from U.S. Public Health Service grants NS 09144 and GM 07804.

## REFERENCES

BARTELS, E. & NACHMANSOHN, D. (1969). *Archs Biochem. Biophys.*, **133**, 1.
BARTELS, E. & NACHMANSOHN, D. (1965). *Biochem. Z.*, **342**, 359.
DENBURG, J. L., ELDEFRAWI, M. E. & O'BRIEN, R. D. (1972). *Proc. natn. Acad. Sci., U.S.A.*, **69**, 177.
ELDEFRAWI, M. E., BRITTEN, A. G. & ELDEFRAWI, A. T. (1971). *Science, N.Y.*, **173**, 338.
ELDEFRAWI, M. E., BRITTEN, A. G. & O'BRIEN, R. D. (1971). *Pesticide Biochem. Physiol.*, **1**, 101.
ELDEFRAWI, M. E. & ELDEFRAWI, A. T. (1972). *Proc. natn. Acad. Sci., U.S.A.*, **69**, 1776.
ELDEFRAWI, M. E., ELDEFRAWI, A. T., GILMOUR, L. P. & O'BRIEN, R. D. (1971). *Mol. Pharmac.*, **7**, 420.
ELDEFRAWI, M. E., ELDEFRAWI, A. T. & O'BRIEN, R. D. (1971). *Proc. natn. Acad. Sci., U.S.A.*, **68**, 1047.
ELDEFRAWI, M. E., ELDEFRAWI, A. T., SEIFERT, S. & O'BRIEN, R. D. (1972). *Archs Biochem. Biophys.*, **150**, 210.
KARLIN, A., PRIVES, J., DEAL, W. & WINNIK, M. (1971). *J. Mol. Biol.*, **61**, 175.
KOSHLAND, D. E., JR. (1970). In: *The Enzymes. Structure and Control*, ed. Boyer, P. D. **1**, 3rd ed., p. 341. New York: Academic Press.
LA TORRE, J. L., LUNT, G. S. & DE ROBERTIS, E. (1970). *Proc. natn. Acad. Sci., U.S.A.*, **65**, 716.
MILEDI, R., MOLINOFF, P. & POTTER, L. T. (1971). *Nature, Lond.*, **229**, 554.
NACHMANSOHN, D. (1970). *Science, N.Y.*, **168**, 1059.
RAFTERY, M. A., SCHMIDT, J., CLARK, D. G. & WOLCOTT, R. G. (1971). *Biochem. biophys, Res. Comm.*, **45**, 1622.
ROSENBERG, P., HIGMAN, H. & NACHMANSOHN, D. (1960). *Biochim. biophys. Acta*, **44**, 151.
TENENBAUM, D. & FOLCH-PI, J. (1966). *Biochim. biophys. Acta*, **115**, 141.
WEBB, G. D. & JOHNSON, R. L. (1969). *Biochem. Pharmac.*, **18**, 2153.

## DISCUSSION

*Olsen* (*Paris*)

What preparation of phospholipase C was used to inhibit ligand binding? Can you comment on the phospholipid content of receptor macromolecules?

*O'Brien* (*Ithaca*)

For particulate preparations from *Torpedo* and eel, we used Worthington enzyme from *Cl. perfringens* (see O'Brien *et al.*, 1970, *Proc. natn. Acad. Sci., U.S.A.*, **65**, 438 for details); later, with soluble preparations from *Torpedo*, we used Sigma enzyme from *Cl. Welchii* under more appropriate conditions (see Eldefrawi *et al.* (1972) for details). Since commercial enzymes were used, we must confirm these findings with purified enzymes. The phospholipid content of the receptor will not be known until better purification of functional receptor is achieved. It is possible that the highly purified α-bungarotoxin-binding proteins which others study may lack phospholipid and may recognize α-bungarotoxin but not acetylcholine.

# THE ISOLATION AND MOLECULAR PROPERTIES OF RECEPTOR PROTEOLIPIDS*

E. DE ROBERTIS

*Instituto de Anatomía General y Embriología, Facultad de Medicina, Universidad de Buenos Aires, Buenos Aires, Argentina*

The existence of specific receptor macromolecules incorporated within the structural framework of the cell membrane is implicit in any theory dealing with the action of drugs. Until recently our knowledge of receptors has been mainly indirect, resulting from the study of the responses observed at the cellular or organ level, namely metabolic changes, contraction of muscle, secretion of glands, and so forth. The primary interaction, which is at the initiation of a chain of events leading to the physiological response, can only be sought at a macromolecular level and true progress can only be achieved after isolation of the chemical entity involved in the interaction with the drug.

Our approach to the investigation of this problem has been based in the following premises. (1) Receptors should be macromolecules present at the chemosensitive sites of the cell membrane; in the case of nervous tissue, this means that they should be present at the postsynaptic membrane. (2) They should be intrinsic proteins of the membrane, intimately bound or embedded within the lipoprotein framework of the cell membrane. (3) They should show high affinity and specific binding for neurotransmitters and other active drugs. (4) By interacting with the drug these macromolecules should be able to undergo conformational changes, capable of inducing the translocation of ions and producing a corresponding bioelectric change.

In the course of this short exposition I will mainly refer to studies from our laboratory leading to the isolation of a family of hydrophobic proteins having high affinity for cholinergic or adrenergic ligands and to the demonstration that, once incorporated into artificial membranes, such proteins are able to initiate a bioelectrical response.

* The original work has been supported by Grants of Instituto de Farmacología, Leg. 4699/70 (Consejo Nacional de Investigaciones Científicas y Técnicas, Argentina and National Institutes of Health (5 RO1 NS 06953-05 NEUA), U.S.A.

## *I. Studies on the isolation of receptor proteolipids*

Interest in receptors arose very early in our laboratory when we found that during the process of cell fractionation of the brain the postsynaptic membrane remained attached to the nerve ending (De Robertis, Pellegrino de Iraldi, Rodríguez de Lores Arnaiz & Salganicoff, 1962). Later on, by osmotically disrupting the isolated nerve ending, we could separate the synaptic vesicles and the nerve-ending membranes (De Robertis, Rodríguez de Lores Arnaiz & Pellegrino de Iraldi, 1962) and by gradient centrifugation it was possible to isolate and purify several populations of nerve-ending membranes (De Robertis, Alberici, Rodríguez de Lores Arnaiz & Azcurra, 1966). We studied the binding *in vitro* of cholinergic agents such as dimethyl-[$^{14}$C] (+)-tubocurarine (DMTC), methyl-[$^{14}$C] hexamethonium (MHM) and [$^{3}$H] alloferine, at low concentrations (that is, $10^{-7}$–$10^{-6}$ M), and found that these drugs were preferentially bound to the nerve-ending membranes that were rich in acetylcholinesterase (AChE) (Azcurra & De Robertis, 1967). These cholinergic agents could be displaced from the binding sites by acetylcholine (ACh) and atropine. [$^{14}$C] 5-hydroxytryptamine (5-HT) was also found to bind to the nerve-ending membranes, a binding that could be inhibited by desmethylmipramine, reserpine and butanolamine of lysergic acid (Fiszer & De Robertis, 1969). Also some adrenergic blocking agents such as [$^{14}$C] SY28 (Fiszer & De Robertis, 1968), [$^{14}$C] dibenamine and [$^{14}$C] propranolol (De Robertis & Fiszer, 1969) showed high affinity binding to nerve-ending membranes from the hypothalamus and basal ganglia (for a review on the binding of these and other drugs see De Robertis, 1971). Using Triton X-100 at low concentrations, we could proceed further in the dissection of the synaptic membranes by dissolving most of the limiting membrane of the nerve ending and leaving intact the subsynaptic membrane. In these membranes we found that the binding of [$^{14}$C] DMTC and [$^{14}$C] MHM remained intact indicating that the receptor properties were localized in the subsynaptic membrane (De Robertis, Azcurra & Fiszer, 1967).

### *1. Isolation of brain receptor proteolipids*

In 1967 we tried to find out which of the molecular components of the membrane were responsible for the binding of the ligands. We used the rather unorthodox procedure of extracting with organic solvents nerve-ending membranes previously incubated with [$^{14}$C] DMTC (De Robertis, Fiszer & Soto, 1967), [$^{14}$C] 5-HT (Fiszer & De Robertis, 1969) or with [$^{14}$C] dibenamine (De Robertis & Fiszer, 1969) and we found that the label was present in the organic phase (Table 1.) Further investigations using thin layer chromatography and column chromatography with Sephadex LH20 led to the demonstration that these drugs were bound to the small amount of hydrophobic protein—the so called proteolipid—present in the organic extract.

TABLE 1. *Binding of drugs to nerve-ending membranes of rat brain. Effect of extraction in organic solvents and partition with water*

| Sample | Content | d.p.m./g tissue | % of total |
|---|---|---|---|
| dimethyl-[14C] (+)-tubocurarine $1 \cdot 5 \times 10^{-6}$ M* | | | |
| Nerve-ending membranes | | 17632 | 100 |
| Residual pellet | proteins | 897 | 5 |
| Water phase | gangliosides | 891 | 5 |
| Chloroform–methanol phase | lipids and proteolipids | 15424 | 87 |
| [14C] 5-hydroxytryptamine $3 \cdot 3 \times 10^{-6}$ M† | | | |
| Nerve-ending membranes | | 73020 | 100 |
| Residual pellet | proteins | 9770 | 13·4 |
| Water phase | gangliosides | 9555 | 13·1 |
| Butanol phase | lipids and proteolipids | 53700 | 73·5 |
| [14C] dibenamine $1 \times 10^{-6}$ M‡ | | | |
| Nerve-ending membranes | | 45972 | 100 |
| Residual pellet | proteins | 2972 | 6·5 |
| Water phase | gangliosides | 575 | 1·5 |
| Chloroform–methanol phase | lipids and proteolipids | 43000 | 93·5 |

* Data from De Robertis, Fiszer & Soto (1967).
† Data from Fiszer & De Robertis (1969).
‡ Data from De Robertis & Fiszer (1969).

Proteolipids constitute a special group of lipoproteins present in biological membranes that are characterized by their hydrophobic nature. First isolated from white matter (Folch-Pi & Lees, 1957) they have since been found in mitochondria, chloroplasts, microsomes and in different subcellular membranes of the cerebral cortex (Lapetina, Soto & De Robertis, 1967). In the nerve-ending membranes proteolipids represent only 6–7% of the total protein content. These special proteolipids from the nerve-ending membrane were found to bind with high affinity [14C] DMTC, and also [3H] atropine (De Robertis, González Rodríguez & Teller, 1969) as well as 5-hydroxytryptamine (Fiszer & De Robertis, 1969) and some adrenergic blocking agents (Fiszer & De Robertis, 1968; De Robertis & Fiszer, 1969).

The early studies on brain receptor proteolipids were done by first allowing the drug to bind to the membrane and then extracting with organic solvents, but the high affinity binding could also be demonstrated directly on the organic extract or on the isolated receptor proteolipid and this procedure was then more generally adopted.

## 2. *Isolation of cholinergic receptor proteolipids from the electroplax*

A tissue having a rich cholinergic innervation is provided by the electric organs of fishes such as *Torpedo* and *Electrophorus*. The so-called *electroplax* is a large sheet-like modified muscle cell physiologically adapted to the generation of transcellular current. A single electroplax of *Electrophorus* weighing 30–50 mg has some 30–50 000 cholinergic nerve endings impinging only on one side. In 1970, we described the isolation of the proteolipid cholinergic receptor from the electroplax (De Robertis, Fiszer, La Torre & Lunt, 1970; La Torre, Lunt & De Robertis, 1970). We extracted lyophilized electric tissue from *Torpedo* and *Electrophorus* with chloroform–methanol (2 : 1) and treated the organic extract with low concentrations of [$^{14}$C] ACh, [$^{14}$C] MHM or [$^{3}$H] *p*-(trimethylammonium)-benzene diazonium fluoroborate ([$^{3}$H] TDF). After column chromatography on Sephadex LH20 and elution in organic solvents of increasing polarity several protein peaks were isolated only one of which was labelled (Fig. 1). The three cholinergic ligands used gave similar patterns of elution.

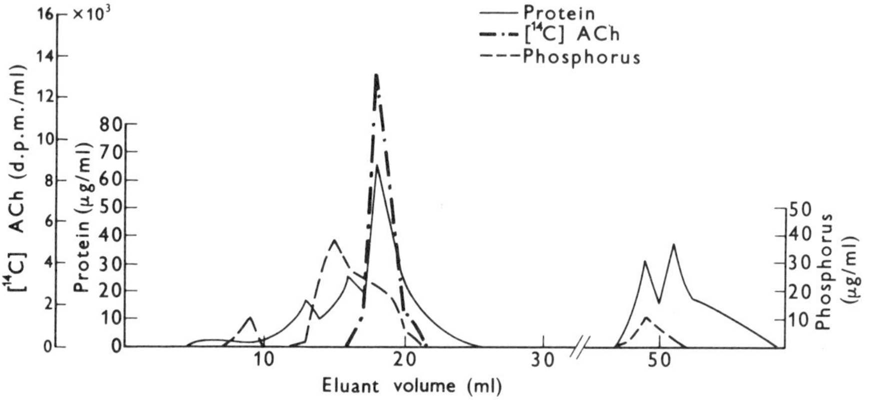


FIG. 1. Chromatographic pattern of the proteolipids from electroplax of *Electrophorus*. The chloroform–methanol extract (2 : 1 by volume) was treated with $5 \times 10^{-7}$ M [$^{14}$C-methyl]-acetylcholine ([$^{14}$C] ACh) and passed through a column of Sephadex LH-20 (2·1 × 18 cm). The bound radioactivity appeared together with peak 3 of proteolipid protein. The elution of lipid phosphorus is also shown. (From De Robertis, Lunt & La Torre, 1971.)

A study of the saturation curve for acetylcholine suggested that this proteolipid had multiple sites of binding with one site of high affinity (apparent dissociation constant $K_1 = 10^{-7}$ M) and some 9 sites of low affinity ($K_2 = 10^{-5}$ M) per molecule of protein of molecular weight 40 000 (De Robertis, Lunt & La Torre, 1971). The quantitative findings were of great interest in view of recent studies on the binding of α-bungarotoxin (α-BuTX) to the electric tissue. Changeux, Kasai & Lee (1970) found some $2{\cdot}4 \times 10^{14}$ binding sites per g in *Electrophorus* and Miledi & Potter (1971) some $6{\cdot}6 \times 10^{14}$ α-BuTX sites per g of *Torpedo* electroplax. From our studies we calculated that some $6{\cdot}8 \times 10^{14}$ cholinergic proteolipid molecules may be extracted from 1 g of electroplax in *Torpedo* and $2{\cdot}7 \times 10^{14}$ from *Electrophorus*. La Torre, Lunt & De Robertis (1970) suggested that the higher content of receptor proteolipid in *Torpedo* could be due to the richer innervation and related to the fact that bioelectrogenesis originates only from postsynaptic potentials (Bennett, Wierzel & Grundfest, 1961).

In other experiments we isolated the membranes of the electroplax and studied the binding of several cholinergic drugs as well as the effect of S–S and SH reagents on the binding (De Robertis & Fiszer, 1970). Considerable inhibition of binding was found when the membranes were treated with dithiothreitol (DTT) followed by N-ethylmaleimide, a treatment that first reduces the S–S-groups and then permanently blocks the resulting SH. Such treatment has been shown to block the response of the electroplax to depolarizing drugs (Karlin & Bartels, 1966). It was interesting to find that DTT alone did not interfere with the binding and that the SH reagents only produced a small reduction (Table 2). Treating the electroplax membrane

TABLE 2. *Action of drugs on the binding of* [$^{14}$C] *acetylcholine to electroplax membranes from* Electrophorus

| Drug | Drug. conc. (mM) | d.p.m./mg protein Control | Treated | Inhibition % |
|---|---|---|---|---|
| *p*-Hydroxymercuribenzoate | 50 | 6071 | 5000 | 18 |
| *p*-Chloromercuribenzoate | 50 | 6539 | 4714 | 28 |
| Dithiothreitol } N-Ethylmaleimide } | 10<br>10 | 2500 | 816 | 67 |

Membrane fractions were incubated with *p*-hydroxymercuribenzoate and *p*-chloromercuribenzoate in a 0·1 M glycylglycine buffer (pH 8). After 20 min they were sedimented and submitted to binding with $1 \times 10^{-6}$ M [$^{14}$C] acetylcholine in distilled water with Tris buffer (pH 7) containing $2 \times 10^{-5}$ M physostigmine to inhibit acetylcholinesterase. Other membranes were successively treated with dithiothreitol and N-ethylmaleimide and then with acetylcholine. Data from De Robertis and Fiszer (1970).

with 1 M NaCl, we were able to confirm the finding of Silman & Karlin (1967) that most of the acetylcholinesterase became solubilized. These AChE-deprived membranes showed the same binding capacity for the cholinergic ligands (Fig. 2) and from them the same amount of cholinergic receptor proteolipid could be extracted. These results provide definite evidence that the cholinergic receptor proteolipid and acetylcholinesterase are two different macromolecules present in the electroplax membrane (De Robertis & Fiszer, 1970).

### *3. Isolation of a cholinergic receptor proteolipid from skeletal muscle. Effect of denervation*

A cholinergic proteolipid has recently been isolated from rat diaphragm (Lunt, De Robertis & Stefani, 1970; Lunt, Stefani & De Robertis, 1971; De Robertis, Mosquera & Fiszer, 1972). As shown in Fig. 3 only peak 2-R

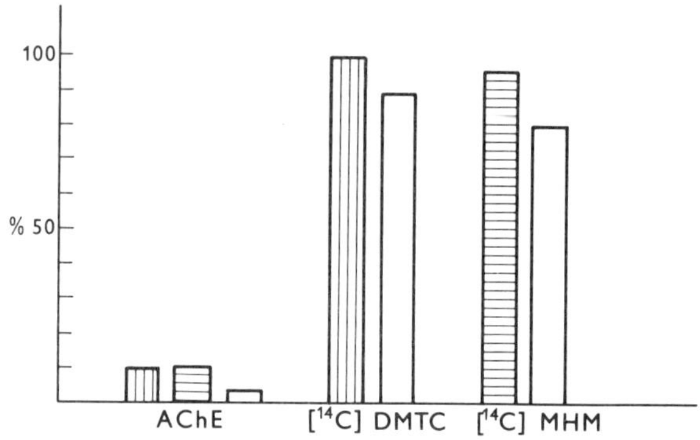


FIG. 2. Acetylcholinesterase and binding of dimethyl-[$^{14}$C] (+)-tubocurarine and methyl-[$^{14}$C] hexamethonium in electroplax membranes after treatment with 1 M NaCl. The results are expressed as % of the corresponding control in three different experiments. AChE, acetylcholinesterase; [$^{14}$C] DMTC, dimethyl-[$^{14}$C] (+)-tubocurarine; [$^{14}$C] MHM, methyl-[$^{14}$C] hexamethonium. The column shadings denote different experiments. (From De Robertis & Fiszer, 1970.)

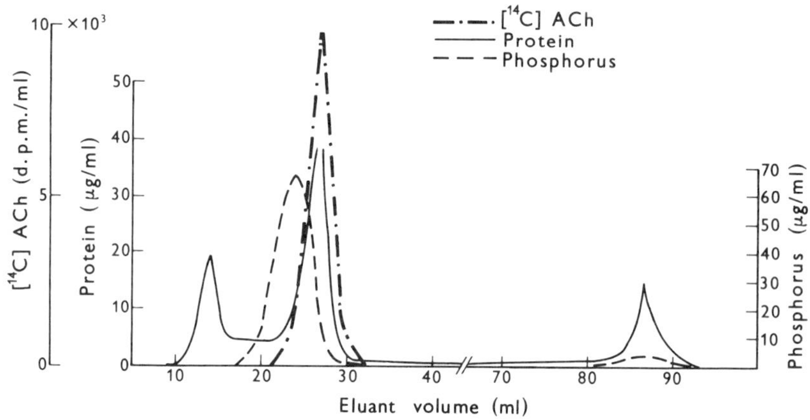


FIG. 3. Chromatographic pattern in Sephadex LH20 of a lipid extract from rat diaphragm treated with $7 \cdot 8 \times 10^{-7}$ M [$^{14}$C] acetylcholine. The elution patterns of protein, lipid phosphorus and radioactivity are indicated. Observe that all [$^{14}$C] acetylcholine appears in relation to a single peak (2-R) of protein. (From De Robertis, Mosquera & Fiszer, 1972.)

of proteolipid was found to bind with high affinity [$^{14}$C] ACh, [$^{14}$C] MHM, [$^{14}$C] (+)-tubocurarine and [$^{14}$C] decamethonium. This peak appears in the chromatogram in the same region as the receptor proteolipid isolated from the electroplax.

It is well known that while normally the ACh-receptors of skeletal muscle are confined to the myoneural junction, after denervation the chemosensitivity spreads to cover the entire muscle fibre (Ginetzinsky & Shamarina, 1942; Axelsson & Thesleff, 1959; Miledi, 1960). One mechanism of the ACh hypersensitivity could be the activation of normally latent receptors. Another possible explanation is that receptors are not permanent entities but that they are continuously being produced and degraded.

Our work favours the existence of the two mechanisms. We found that 20 days after denervation there is an increase in the amount of the proteolipid of peak 2-R and that this increment is slightly higher in the non-innervated portion of the muscle fibre. Furthermore with denervation there is an increase in the binding of [$^{14}$C] ACh to the receptor proteolipid which in the nonplate region is of the order of 3 times with respect to the control. Lunt, Stefani & De Robertis (1971) found that the incorporation of [$^{3}$H] leucine into the proteolipid of peak 2-R increased after denervation reaching a ratio of about ten with respect to the normal control in the non-innervated region. These results support the hypothesis that hypersensitivity was produced by an increase in turnover of the receptor macromolecules. However, a quantitative consideration of the results indicates that the mechanism of unmasking latent receptors may also play a role. In the normal non-innervated region there is also a proteolipid peak in 2-R, which has the same binding for ACh as that of the plate region. Furthermore, by assuming a molecular weight of 40 000 for this cholinergic receptor, we found that the number of molecules of proteolipid per muscle fibre far exceeds the values obtained by the binding of α-bungarotoxin applied *in vivo* or *in vitro* to the whole diaphragm. In fact while Barnard, Wieckowski & Chiu (1971), calculated $3{\cdot}0 \times 10^{7}$ molecules per endplate and Miledi & Potter (1971) found $4{\cdot}7 \times 10^{7}$ per single muscle fibre we obtain figures of $1{\cdot}5 \times 10^{10}$ proteolipid molecules by the content of protein of peak 2-R and $8{\cdot}4 \times 10^{9}$ by the binding of acetylcholine under normal conditions. After denervation the number of binding sites for ACh in peak 2-R increased only to $1{\cdot}7 \times 10^{10}$ per fibre. We have attempted to explain these contradictory results by suggesting that in the normal fibre most of the proteolipid receptor macromolecules are held in a latent unreactive form and that these receptors may be activated either by denervation or by their extraction from the cell membrane (De Robertis, Mosquera & Fiszer, 1972).

### *4. The binding of α-bungarotoxin to the cholinergic receptor proteolipid*

Lee and co-workers have found that α-BuTX, a basic polypeptide of molecular weight 8000 extracted from the venom of the elapid snake *Bungarus multicinctus*, produces a permanent block of the neuromuscular junction (Lee & Chang, 1966) and of the electroplax (Changeux, Kasai & Lee, 1970). The binding of α-BuTX has recently been used to isolate a protein–toxin complex from *Electrophorus* (Changeux, Kasai, Huchet & Meunier, 1970) and *Torpedo* (Miledi, Molinoff & Potter, 1971). The extraction procedures used by both groups of investigators, which involve strong detergents, suggest that they are concerned with a rather hydrophobic protein (or lipoprotein).

We used several methods to study the binding of [$^{131}$I] α-BuTX or [$^{3}$H] α-BuTX to the receptor proteolipid of *Electrophorus*. By means of a partition method based on the technique developed by Weber, Borris, De Robertis, Barrantes, La Torre & Llorente de Carlin (1971) for a fluorescent ligand, it was found that the binding curve was hyperbolic and that saturation was reached with 215 ng of α-BuTX per μg of proteolipid. From this result it was calculated that one molecule of α-BuTX binds to one molecule of proteolipid protein of molecular weight of approximately 37 000. This finding suggests that, unlike ACh which shows multiple sites of binding (De Robertis, Lunt & La Torre, 1971), α-BuTX binds only to one site per molecule of proteolipid. These and other results that are published elsewhere (Fiszer & De Robertis, 1972b) suggest that the special proteolipid extracted by us with organic solvents and the α-BuTX–protein–detergent complexes isolated by the other groups of investigators are probably the same receptor macromolecule. Furthermore we have preliminary evidence that after isolation the cholinergic proteolipid can be dissolved in a water solution in the presence of a detergent.

## 5. *Isolation of adrenoreceptor proteolipids*

Recently Fiszer & De Robertis (1972a) have reported on the isolation of a proteolipid from the spleen capsule having adrenergic properties. By the use of methods similar to those employed for the cholinergic proteolipid several peaks of protein were eluted in the chloroform and one in chloroform–methanol (4 : 1) at the end of the chromatogram (Fig. 4). Addition of (±)-[$^{3}$H] noradrenaline in concentrations varying between $1{\cdot}6\times10^{-8}$ M and $5\times10^{-5}$ M resulted in the elution of the label together with the first peak of protein while the free [$^{3}$H] noradrenaline was retained by the column. As in the case of the cholinergic proteolipid, the binding curve suggested the presence of multiple sites with different affinities (namely, $K_1=3{\cdot}3\times10^{-7}$ M and $K_2=1{\cdot}8\times10^{-5}$ M). The binding curve for [$^{3}$H] noradrenaline was displaced by various adrenergic blocking agents which inhibited the high affinity binding to the proteolipid.

The amount of adrenoreceptor proteolipid that may be extracted from 2 g of lyophilized tissue is of the order of 80–100 μg. From this value and assuming a molecular weight of 200 000 for this proteolipid we calculated a content of $1{\cdot}5\times10^{11}$ receptor molecules per mg dry tissue. Such a figure is not far from the estimates done for the binding sites of [$^{3}$H] phenoxybenzamine in the rat seminal vesicle (that is, $2\times10^{11}$ sites per mg dry tissue, Lewis & Miller, 1966) and of [$^{3}$H] SY28 bound to aortic strips ($1{\cdot}5\times10^{12}$ sites per mg dry tissue, Moran & Triggle, 1970).

A study of the β-adrenergic receptor of bovine ventricle was carried out using (±)-[$^{3}$H] noradrenaline and (±)-[$^{3}$H] isoprenaline (Ochoa, Llorente de Carlin & De Robertis, 1972).

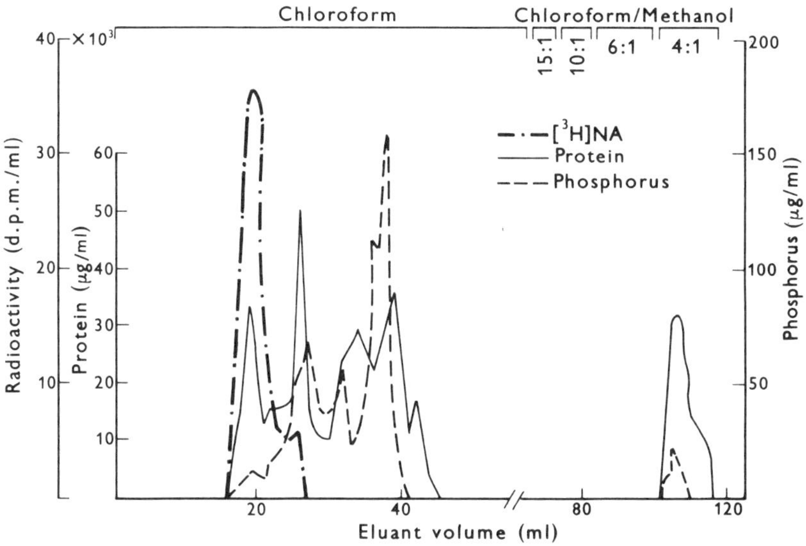


FIG. 4. Chromatographic pattern in Sephadex LH20 of a lipid extract from spleen capsule. The extract was submitted to binding with $1 \cdot 6 \times 10^{-8}$ (±)-[$^3$H] noradrenaline. The radioactivity appears together with a single peak of proteolipid protein. (From Fiszer & De Robertis, 1972a.)

After column chromatography of the extract two peaks of protein were eluted with chloroform and three peaks in more polar solvents. Both the [$^3$H] isoprenaline and the [$^3$H] noradrenaline appeared in a single peak coinciding with the first peak of proteolipid, which was eluted in the same volume as the adrenoreceptor of the spleen capsule (Fig. 4). In this work an attempt was made to establish the subcellular localization of this adrenergic proteolipid. It was found that the binding of catecholamines was mainly associated with a microsomal fraction which contains the membranes of the muscle cells. This binding was inhibited by propranolol but not by phentolamine. The proteolipids extracted from such a fraction had a simpler pattern in which peak 1, binding the [$^3$H] isoprenaline, was the most conspicuous. This finding suggests that the adrenergic receptor proteolipid of the heart ventricle is localized in the membrane of the muscle cells. In this case the number of proteolipid receptor molecules per mg dry tissue was calculated to be $0 \cdot 4 \times 10^{11}$ (Ochoa, Llorente de Carlin & De Robertis, 1972).

## *II. Studies on proteolipid receptor responses*

All the above mentioned studies refer to the separation of the different proteolipid receptors, the demonstration of the high affinity and specificity of the binding and the localization of the receptor proteolipids in the corresponding cell membranes. The second step in the drug–receptor interaction, that of eliciting a response was approached in our laboratory with the use of ultrathin (that is, black) artificial lipid membranes. Since receptor proteolipids are hydrophobic proteins they can easily be incorporated into the membrane-forming solution which contains cholesterol and different phospholipids. These membranes are essentially similar to those first described by Mueller, Rudin, Ti Tien & Westcott (1963) and are made across a 1-mm hole in a Teflon septum separating two chambers containing solutions of ions. With the apparatus shown in Fig. 5 current voltage curves were determined and the conductance was measured under control conditions and after application of the drug with a fine capillary tube (Parisi, Rivas & De Robertis, 1971). Furthermore a technique was developed which permits the fixation of the membrane and its study under the electron microscope (Vásquez, Parisi & De Robertis, 1972) (Fig. 5).

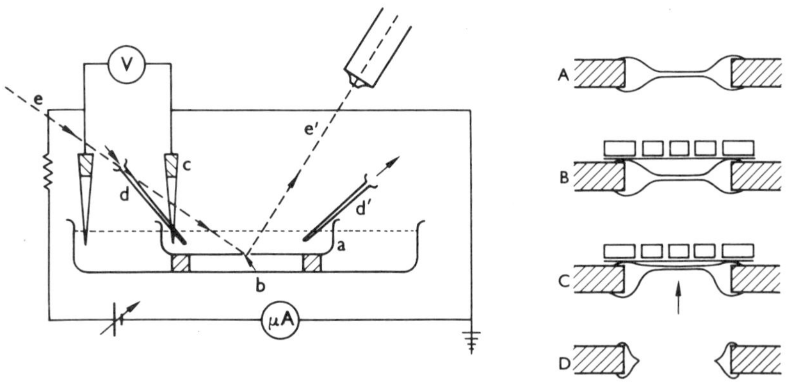


FIG. 5. Left: diagram of the apparatus used to study the electrical properties of artificial membranes. A Teflon cup (a) is immersed in a Petri dish. The membrane is formed in a 1-mm hole at the bottom (b). The electrical measurements are made via calomel electrodes (c). For fixation with glutaraldehyde the solution of the upper chamber is changed with the aid of two syringes (d, d′). A light beam (e, e′) reflects on the membrane which is observed with a stereomicroscope. Right: the hole in the Teflon septum is represented at a larger scale and the different steps to remove the membrane for the electron microscope are shown. A, artificial membrane; B, grid placed on the hole; C, a hydrostatic pressure sticks the membrane to the grid; D, after removal of the grid some material from the 'torus' remains at the edge. (From Vásquez, Parisi & De Robertis, 1971.)

## *1. Cholinergic proteolipid and acetylcholine*

The introduction of 5–80 μg/ml of cholinergic proteolipid from *Electrophorus* into the membrane-forming solution which contains 10 mg/ml of cholesterol and 10 mg/ml of phospholipids, produces a reduction in resistance (that is, from $1{\cdot}25 \times 10^6$ ohm cm$^2$ in the control to $2{\cdot}3 \times 10^5$ ohm cm$^2$ with 16 μg/ml of proteolipid). This change is accompanied by a decrease in electron density of the membrane and a smoother texture, suggesting that the hydrophobic protein has produced a molecular reorganization of the membrane. In the case of the cholinergic proteolipid from *Electrophorus* this effect was accompanied by the appearance of a cationic selectivity favourable to potassium and sodium and the development of bi-stable conductance changes. These findings are reminiscent of those previously observed with a proteinaceous material released by *Aerobacter clocae* called the Excitability Inducing Material (EIM) (Mueller & Rudin, 1967), or with various polypeptide macrocyclic antibiotics particularly alamethicin (Mueller & Rudin, 1968), which are also rather hydrophobic. These substances induce an increase in conductance with ionic selectivity and discrete current jumps, which have been interpreted as due to the opening and closing of conducting channels (Ehrenstein, Locar & Nossal, 1970). Another interesting finding is that the increase in conductance is proportional to the fourth power of the proteolipid concentration in the membrane-forming solution (Parisi, Reader & De Robertis, 1972). This finding supports the tetrameric model proposed by us for the organization of cholinergic receptor within the postsynaptic membrane (see De Robertis, 1971, Fig. 6).

The most important finding in these investigations was that the injection of acetylcholine produced a considerable and transient increase in conductance (Parisi, Rivas & De Robertis, 1971). In Fig. 6 it may be observed that the injection of choline has no effect and the previous injection of (+)-tubocurarine produces blocking of the reaction to acetylcholine. Further investigations have shown that gallamine and hexamethonium modify the reaction produced by acetylcholine and that α-bungarotoxin interacts with the cholinergic proteolipid and can change the type of reaction given by acetylcholine (Parisi, Reader & De Robertis, 1972). The electron microscope study of the membranes fixed at the height of the conductance showed a striking change in fine structure. These 'activated' membranes showed a more uneven or 'corrugated' appearance with the presence of dense spots having a maximal diameter of 2 nm, into which the osmium tetroxide, used in vapours as fixative, was deposited (Fig. 7). These changes, which are transient and disappear when the membrane regains the normal conductance, suggest that the translocation of ions may be accompanied by the incorporation of osmium at certain points of the membrane. It may be concluded that the presence of minute amounts of cholinergic proteolipid from the electroplax in artificial lipid membranes results in a decrease in resistance, cationic selectivity and sometimes in a bistable state. Furthermore the presence of the receptor confers to the membrane a special 'chemical excitability' which is specific for acetylcholine.

### 2. *Adrenergic proteolipid and (−)-noradrenaline*

Similar studies have been carried out by incorporating into the artificial membrane the adrenergic proteolipid of the spleen capsule isolated by Fiszer

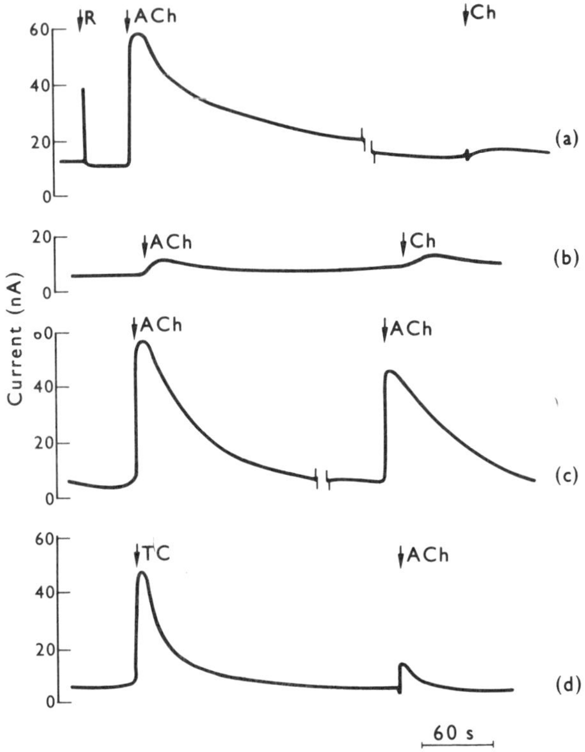


FIG. 6. Records of current across artificial lipid membranes containing proteolipids from *Electrophorus*. (a), (c), and (d) correspond to peak 3, and (b) to peak 1 (see Fig. 1). ACh, acetylcholine; Ch, choline; TC, (+)-tubocurarine; R, control; the artifact is due to the injection of the bath solution. (From Parisi, Rivas & De Robertis, 1971.)

& De Robertis (1972a). It was found that the addition of (−)-noradrenaline produced a transient conductance change whose amplitude was related to the dose. (−)-Isoprenaline gave a smaller response and (+)-noradrenaline had no effect. Furthermore the response toward (−)-noradrenaline could be blocked with phentolamine (Fig. 8). Evidence was obtained that the conductance responses are due to the protein moiety and not to the lipids attached to the proteolipid (Ochoa, Fiszer & De Robertis, 1972).

### *III. Possible integration of receptor proteolipids within the cell membrane*

The hydrophobic nature of the proteolipids poses very interesting problems regarding the possible integration of the receptor within the lipoprotein framework of the membrane. In recent years the importance of hydrophobic proteins and hydrophobic interactions in biological membranes has been

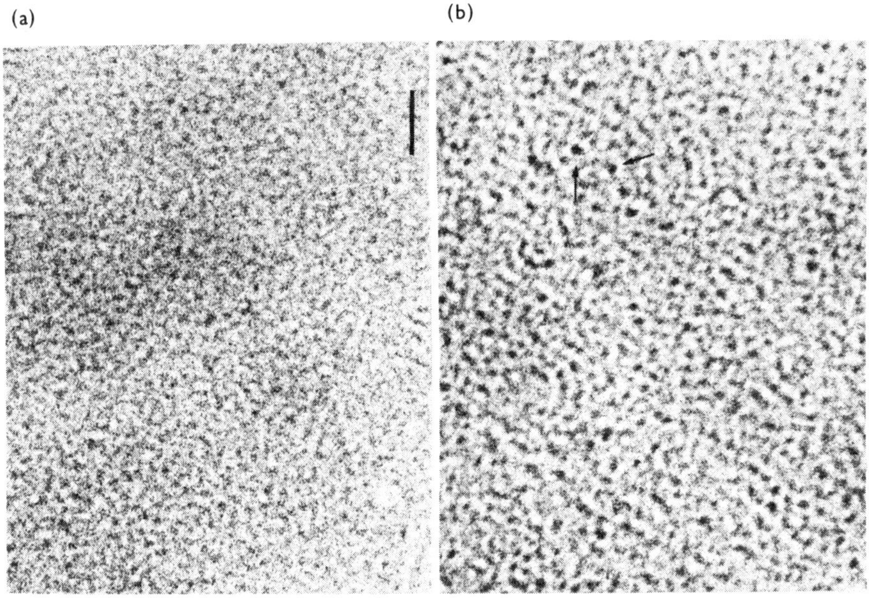


FIG. 7. Electron micrographs of lipid–proteolipid (peak 3 of *Electrophorus*, see Fig. 1) membranes after fixation in 2% glutaraldehyde and exposure to osmium vapours. The bar indicates 20 nm. (a), Control membrane, observe that the surface structure is rather smooth and uniform. (b), Membrane 'activated' with acetylcholine. The surface structure is rougher and shows the presence of dense spots of 2 nm with a darker centre. Arrows point to some of these spots. (From Vásquez, Parisi & De Robertis, 1971.)

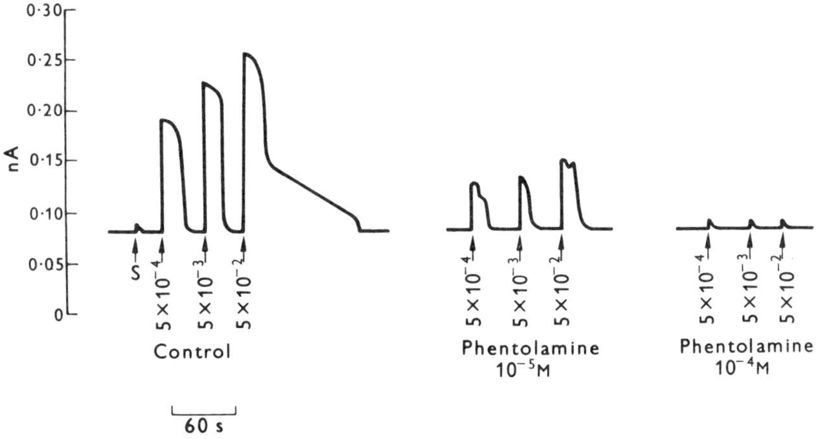


FIG. 8. Records of current across artificial membranes containing the adrenergic proteolipid from spleen capsule (see Fig. 4) produced by (−)-noradrenaline in the concentrations shown and inhibition of the response by phentolamine. The arrows indicate the time of injection. S, injection of the bath solution. (From Ochoa, Fiszer & De Robertis, 1972.)

increasingly stressed and models having protein segments penetrating across the membrane have been produced (Wallach & Zahler, 1966; Lenard & Singer, 1966). The unique properties of some structural membrane proteins were found in the hydrophobic character of the monomer units (Hatch & Bruce, 1968) and their ability to exist in a variety of conformational states (Green, Haard, Lenaz & Silman, 1968; see Triggle, 1971). Proteolipids from myelin contain a high content of alpha helix (Sherman & Folch-Pi, 1970). Electron microscope observations have shown that the brain receptor proteolipid is made of rod shaped macromolecules (1·5 nm × 15 nm), which, with addition of small amounts of atropine sulphate ($10^{-8}$ M), aggregate into paracrystalline ordered arrays (Vásquez, Barrantes, La Torre & De Robertis, 1970). Similar arrays of macromolecules were observed with the cholinergic proteolipid from *Electrophorus* interacting with acetylcholine and with that of skeletal muscle interacting with hexamethonium (see De Robertis, 1971, Fig. 5. These findings, as well as the electron microscope observations of the artificial membranes activated with acetylcholine (Vásquez, Parisi & De Robertis, 1972), may throw light on the possible organization and function of the receptor proteolipid within the membrane. We think that the hydrophobic surface of the proteolipid protein, with the associated lipids, could serve to anchor the macromolecules to the lipid layer of the membrane. Penetration of these layers would be facilitated by the elongated shape of these macromolecules. In the model of the cholinergic receptor postulated by us the proteolipid molecules are thought to adopt an oligomeric arrangement, probably tetrameric (see De Robertis, 1971, Fig. 6). We mentioned before that support for this model has been recently obtained in our laboratory from biophysical measurements in artificial membranes. Furthermore a tetrameric organization of the receptor has been postulated in the past from pharmacological results (see Khromov-Borisov & Michelson, 1966). In our model each proteolipid molecule has a binding site of high affinity for ACh. Four molecules in parallel constitute the ionophoric portion of the receptor used for the translocation of ions across the membrane. The increased conductance may result from a change in the degree of interaction between the monomeric units resulting from the binding of the transmitter to the receptor site. Such a reversible effect would be facilitated by the fact that the proteolipid molecules are held in place by hydrophobic interactions within the framework of the membrane.

## REFERENCES

AXELSSON, J. & THESLEFF, S. (1959). *J. Physiol., Lond.*, **149**, 178.

AZCURRA, J. M. & DE ROBERTIS, E. (1967). *Int. J. Neuropharmac.*, **6**, 15.

BARNARD, J. A., WIECKOWSKI, J. & CHIU, T. H. (1971). *Nature, Lond.*, **234**, 207.

BENNETT, M. V. L., WIERZEL, M. & GRUNDFEST, H. (1961). *J. gen. Physiol.*, **44**, 757.

CHANGEUX, J.-P., KASAI, M., HUCHET, M. & MEUNIER, J.-C. (1970). *C. R. Acad. Sci., Paris*, **270**, 2864.

CHANGEUX, J.-P., KASAI, M. & LEE, C. Y. (1970). *Proc. natn. Acad. Sci., U.S.A.*, **67**, 1241.

De Robertis, E. (1971). *Science, N.Y.*, **171**, 963.
De Robertis, E., Alberici, M., Rodríguez de Lores Arnaiz, G. & Azcurra, J. M. (1966). *Life Sci.*, **5**, 577.
De Robertis, E., Azcurra, J. M. & Fiszer, S. (1967). *Brain Res.*, **5**, 45.
De Robertis, E. & Fiszer, S. (1969). *Life Sci.*, **8**, 1247.
De Robertis, E. & Fiszer, S. (1970). *Biochem. biophys. Acta*, **219**, 388.
De Robertis, E., Fiszer, S. & Soto, E. F. (1967). *Science, N.Y.*, **158**, 928.
De Robertis, E., González-Rodríguez, J. & Teller, D. (1969). *F.E.B.S. Letters*, **4**, 4.
De Robertis, E., Fiszer, S., La Torre, J. L. & Lunt, G. S. (1970). In: *Drugs and Cholinergic Mechanisms in the CNS*, ed. Heilbronn, E. & Winter, A., p. 505. Res. Inst. National Defense, Stockholm.
De Robertis, E., Lunt, G. S. & La Torre, J. L. (1971). *Mol. Pharmac.*, **7**, 97.
De Robertis, E., Mosquera, M. T. & Fiszer, S. (1972). *Life Sci.*, **11**, 1155.
De Robertis, E., Pellegrino de Iraldi, A., Rodríguez de Lores Arnaiz, G. & Salganicoff, L. (1962). *J. Neurochem.*, **9**, 23.
De Robertis, E., Rodríguez de Lores Arnaiz, G. & Pellegrino de Iraldi, A. (1962). *Nature, Lond.*, **194**, 794.
Ehrenstein, G., Lecar, H. & Nossal, R. (1970). *J. gen. Physiol.*, **55**, 119.
Fiszer, S. & De Robertis, E. (1968). *Life Sci.*, **7**, 1093.
Fiszer, S. & De Robertis, E. (1969). *J. Neurochem.*, **16**, 1201.
Fiszer, S. & De Robertis, E. (1972a). *Biochim. biophys. Acta*, **266**, 246.
Fiszer, S. & De Robertis, E. (1972b). *Biochim. biophys. Acta*, **274**, 258.
Folch-Pi, J. & Lees, M. (1957). *J. Biol. Chem.*, **191**, 807.
Ginetzinsky, A. G. & Sharmarina, N. M. (1942). *Adv. Mod. Biol.* (*USSR*) *Usp. Sovrem. Biol.*, **15**, 283.
Green, D. E., Haard, N. F., Lenaz, G. & Silman, H. I. (1968). *Proc. natn. Acad. Sci., U.S.A.*, **60**, 277.
Hatch, F. T. & Bruce, A. L. (1968). *Nature, Lond.*, **218**, 1166.
Karlin, A. & Bartels, E. (1966). *Biochim. biophys. Acta*, **126**, 525.
Khromov-Borisov, N. V. & Michelson, M. J. (1966). *Pharmac. Rev.*, **18**, 1051.
Lapetina, E. G., Soto, E. F. & De Robertis, E. (1967). *Biochim. biophys. Acta*, **135**, 33.
La Torre, J. L., Lunt, G. S. & De Robertis, E. (1970). *Proc. natn. Acad. Sci., U.S.A.*, **65**, 716.
Lee, C. Y. & Chang, C. C. (1966). *Mem. Inst. Butuntan*, **33**, 555.
Lenard, J. & Singer, S. J. (1966). *Proc. natn. Acad. Sci., U.S.A.*, **56**, 1828.
Lewis, J. E. & Miller, J. W. (1966). *J. Pharmac. exp. Ther.*, **154**, 46.
Lunt, G. S., De Robertis, E. & Stefani, E. (1970). *Biochem. J.*, **121**, 23.
Lunt, G. S., Stefani, E. & De Robertis, E. (1971). *J. Neurochem.*, **18**, 1545.
Miledi, R. (1960). *J. Physiol., Lond.*, **151**, 1 and 24.
Miledi, R., Molinoff, P. & Potter, L. T. (1971). *Nature, Lond.*, **229**, 554.
Miledi, R. & Potter, L. T. (1971). *Nature, Lond.*, **233**, 599.
Moran, J. F. & Triggle, D. J. (1970). In: *Drug Receptor Interactions*, ed. Danielli, J., Morán, J. F. & Triggle, D. J., p. 133. New York: Academic Press.
Mueller, P. & Rudin, D. O. (1967). *Nature, Lond.*, **213**, 603.
Mueller, P. & Rudin, D. O. (1968). *Nature, Lond.*, **217**, 713.
Mueller, P., Rudin, D. O., Tien, T. H. & Wescott, W. C. (1963). *J. phys. Chem.*, **67**, 534.
Ochoa, E., Fiszer, S. & De Robertis, E. (1972). *Mol. Pharmac.*, **8**, 215.
Ochoa, E., Llorente de Carlin, M. C. & De Robertis, E. (1972). *Eur. J. Pharmac.*, **18**, 367.
Parisi, M., Reader, T. & De Robertis, E. (1972). *J. gen. Physiol.*, **60**, 454.
Parisi, M., Rivas, E. & De Robertis, E. (1971). *Science, N.Y.*, **172**, 56.
Sherman, G. & Folch-Pi, J. (1970). *J. Neurochem.*, **17**, 597.
Silman, H. I. & Karlin, A. (1967). *Proc. natn. Acad. Sci., U.S.A.*, **58**, 1664.
Triggle, D. J. (1971). *Neurotransmitter Receptor Interactions.* New York: Academic Press.
Vásquez, C., Barrantes, J. F., La Torre, J. L. & De Robertis, E. (1970). *J. Mol. Biol.*, **52**, 221.
Vásquez, C., Parisi M. & De Robertis, E. (1971). *J. Memb. Biol.*, **6**, 353.

WALLACH, D. F. H. & ZAHLER, P. H. (1966). *Proc. natn. Acad. Sci., U.S.A.*, **56**, 1552.
WEBER, G., BORRIS, D. P., DE ROBERTIS, E., BARRANTES, F. J., LA TORRE, J. L. & LLORENTE DE CARLIN, M. C. (1971). *Mol. Pharmac.*, **7**, 530.

# STUDIES ON THE MODE OF ACTION OF CHOLINERGIC AGONISTS AT THE MOLECULAR LEVEL

J.-P. CHANGEUX, J.-C. MEUNIER, R. W. OLSEN, M. WEBER, J.-P. BOURGEOIS, J.-L. POPOT, J. B. COHEN, G. L. HAZELBAUER AND H. A. LESTER

*Unité de Neurobiologie Moléculaire, Département de Biologie Moléculaire, Institut Pasteur, Paris 15e, France*

Electrophysiological methods have provided a phenomenological description of the ionic permeability changes underlying cholinergic excitation. In order to decipher the sequence of molecular events involved, it appears necessary to combine the more traditional electrophysiological and pharmacological techniques with new approaches and perhaps new concepts.

This work has been guided by the idea that the regulation of the permeability of an excitable membrane by acetylcholine presents analogies with the control of a regulatory enzyme by its specific metabolic signal (Changeux, 1966; Changeux, Thiéry, Tung & Kittel, 1967; Changeux & Thiéry, 1968). Indeed, it is well established that the increase of permeability caused by acetylcholine arises neither from the transport of acetylcholine as a permeant ion (Fatt & Katz, 1951) nor from its chemical transformation. In addition data from various preparations have uncovered no structural analogy between the ion transported and acetylcholine. Acetylcholine thus acts in an 'indirect' manner. It triggers the change of membrane property by its reversible binding to a receptor site, the cholinergic receptor site, where it acts as a *regulatory ligand.*

It was therefore postulated that the most elementary membrane unit under the control of acetylcholine comprises two, at least partially distinct, elements of structure: the *receptor protein*, which carries the receptor site, and an *ionophore* involved in the selective translocation of ions through the membrane (Changeux, Podleski & Meunier, 1969). Coupling between acetylcholine and the permeant ion, that is, between receptor protein and ionophore, was viewed as an indirect, and thus allosteric, interaction mediated by a structural transition (Monod, Wyman & Changeux, 1965). In other words, receptor and ionophore would play a role similar to that of the regulatory and catalytic subunit in a regulatory enzyme like aspartate transcarbamylase (Gerhart & Schachman, 1965).

In the simplest formulation of the theory the ionophore–receptor complex was assumed to exist in at least two conformational states in reversible equilibrium ($T \rightleftharpoons S$). In the resting state, T, the receptor would present a high affinity for antagonists but little affinity for agonists. In the active state, S, the receptor would bind agonists preferentially and thus be stabilized by them, and, in addition, the ionophore would selectively transport cations. The excitation process would then consist of the displacement of the $T \rightleftharpoons S$ equilibrium in favour of the active state by acetylcholine or the cholinergic agonists. The antagonists would shift the equilibrium in the opposite direction. A plausible but not unique explanation for the different maximal responses caused by partial agonists would be an incomplete shift of the conformational equilibrium caused by the non-exclusive binding of the agonist to *both* T and S states (Rubin & Changeux, 1966).

These ideas have been extended to a variety of cases and systems (Karlin, 1967; Colquhoun, this symposium). A crucial finding, in favour of the theory is that the permeability of purified membrane fragments is affected by cholinergic agonists in the absence of any source of energy or electrochemical gradient across the membrane (del Castillo & Katz, 1955; Kasai & Changeux, 1970, 1971). The capacity for control is thus built into the membrane structure just as the capacity for control of a regulatory protein by its specific allosteric effector is built into its three-dimensional organization. However, the direct demonstration of a conformational transition associated with acetylcholine binding is still lacking.[1]

These ideas have been pursued experimentally by using a biological material rich in homogeneous synaptic elements: the electric organs of *Electrophorus electricus* and *Torpedo marmorata* (Nachmansohn, 1959, 1971). An *Electrophorus* electric organ weighing several hundred grams might contain $10^9$–$10^{10}$ identical synapses. Single cells or electroplax can be isolated and dissected from the same electric organ, and electrophysiological measurements can be performed under controlled conditions (Schoffeniels & Nachmansohn, 1957; Higman, Podleski & Bartels, 1964a). Thus the comparison between *in vivo* and *in vitro* data required for the 'reduction' of a physiological mechanism to the molecular level became feasible. Experiments were carried out with systems corresponding to three levels of organization (Fig. 1). (a), The isolated electroplax: measurements of steady state membrane potentials in the presence of given concentrations of agonists and antagonists have been used to establish concentration–effect curves. Measurements of conductance and ionic fluxes can also be made (Higman, Podleski & Bartels, 1964b; Podleski & Changeux, 1969). (b), The excitable microsacs (Kasai & Changeux, 1970, 1971): ion fluxes from membrane fragments from the innervated caudal face of the electroplax have been estimated by a simple

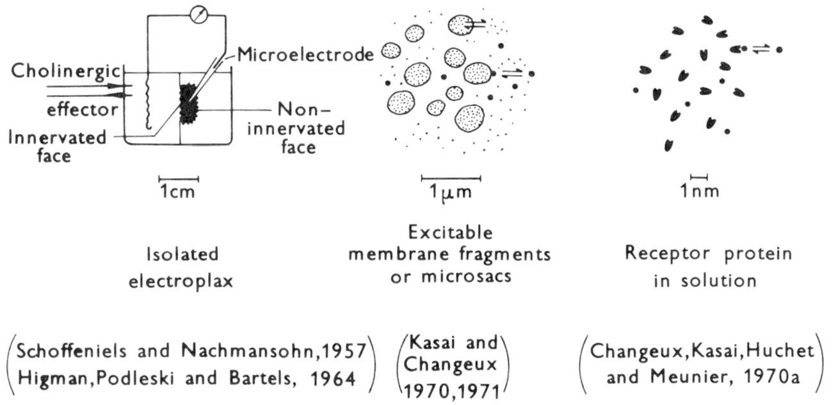


FIG. 1. Diagrammatic representation of the three preparations from *Electrophorus electricus* electric tissue used in the study of the response of an excitable membrane to cholinergic agents.

filtration assay in a controlled environment. Binding of radioactive cholinergic ligands and other pharmacological agents can be measured with the same preparation. (c), The receptor protein: direct binding curves at equilibrium for a variety of agonists and antagonists have been made with a protein solubilized from excitable microsacs by Na-cholate or deoxycholate (Changeux, Kasai, Huchet & Meunier, 1970a; Changeux, Meunier & Huchet, 1971; Olsen, Meunier & Changeux, 1972).

### *A. The characterization of the physiological receptor site for acetylcholine by cholinergic ligands and α-toxins from snake venoms*

Characterization of the membrane site to which acetylcholine binds as the first step in its electrogenic action required a specific assay for that site. Binding of cholinergic agonists and antagonists was not sufficient since several of these compounds have a high affinity for the catalytic and allosteric sites of acetylcholinesterase, for presynaptic transport sites for acetylcholine, and perhaps for several other sites in addition to the cholinergic receptor. A complementary and totally independent test of specificity was therefore needed.

If our experimental material had been the bacterial cell, the use of genetics would have provided such a test. Obviously, it cannot be used with *Electrophorus*. An alternative solution was provided by the small toxic proteins from snake venoms which appear to react in a highly specific way with the cholinergic receptor protein, although they do not show any structural analogy with cholinergic effectors. The best known substances are the α-toxins from *Bungarus multicinctus* (Lee & Chang, 1966; Lee, 1970; Changeux, Kasai & Lee, 1970b), *Naja n. siamensis* (Karlsson, Arnberg & Eaker, 1971;

Lester, 1970, 1971), *Naja n. naja* (Karlsson, Eaker & Ponterius, 1972), *Naja nigricollis* (Boquet, Izard, Jouannet & Meaume, 1966, 1967; Boquet, Izard & Ronsseray, 1970; Karlsson, Eaker & Porath, 1966), *Laticauda semifasciata* (Arai, Tamiya, Toshioka, Shinonaga & Kano, 1964; Sato & Tamiya, 1971). All act as blocking agents at the vertebrate neuromuscular junction with different degrees of irreversibility, and (+)-tubocurarine gives good protection against the effect of several of them.

Both α-bungarotoxin and *N. nigricollis* α-toxin block, almost irreversibly under our experimental conditions, the electrical response of the electroplax to carbachol or decamethonium (Changeux, Kasai & Lee, 1970b; Changeux *et al.*, 1971). They also block *in vitro* the permeability response of excitable microsacs to cholinergic agonists (Changeux *et al.*, 1970b; Kasai & Changeux, 1971). Moreover, (+)-tubocurarine efficiently protects against their effect. One of the most striking features of the *in vitro* effect of these toxins is that they displace a large amount of [$^{14}$C] decamethonium, a potent cholinergic agonist reversibly bound to excitable membrane fragments or to a deoxycholate extract of these fragments (Changeux *et al.*, 1970b). The maximum amount of bound decamethonium displaced by α-toxin is the same as that displaced by low concentrations of (+)-tubocurarine or gallamine. The residual binding, which is resistant to α-toxin as well as to those antagonists, is displaced by carbachol and other cholinergic ligands which are known to be inhibitors of acetylcholinesterase (Changeux *et al.*, 1971). This latter class of site is eliminated by heat treatment under conditions which inactivate acetylcholinesterase and thus probably corresponds to the catalytic site of acetylcholinesterase (Meunier, Huchet, Boquet & Changeux, 1971a). The similarity of the effects of the snake venom toxins and of typical cholinergic agonists suggested to us that the fraction of decamethonium displaced by the toxins was indeed bound to the cholinergic receptor site. The general agreement observed (Fig. 2) between the 'intrinsic' binding constants, measured using the binding assay, and the 'apparent' binding constants, estimated from measurements on intact cells estimated *in vivo* and *in vitro* (Changeux & Podleski, 1968) and on microsac preparations, (Kasai & Changeux, 1971) gave strong support to this conclusion.

The use of α-toxins thus reveals various classes of [$^{14}$C] decamethonium sites present in the excitable membrane but, then, the same question was raised for the toxin. Did several classes of α-toxin binding sites exist in our membrane fragments? In order to test this, tritiated *Naja nigricollis* α-toxin was prepared. This was achieved by a two-step procedure consisting of the iodination of a readily accessible histidine of the pure toxin followed by a catalytic dehalogenation in the presence of tritium gas (Menez, Morgat, Fromageot, Ronsseray, Boquet & Changeux, 1971). The recovered tritiated toxin possessed all the pharmacological properties on mice or electroplax of the native toxin and had a specific radioactivity of 10–15 Ci/mmol. Almost 90% of the freshly labelled material was active toxin and approximately

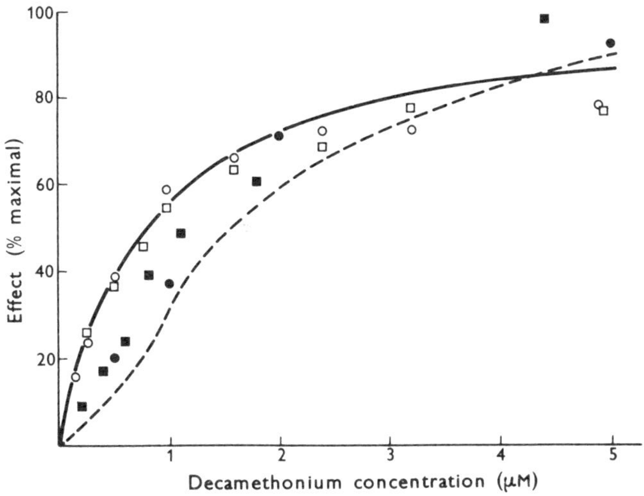


FIG. 2. Comparison of the concentration–effect curves and of the binding curves obtained with decamethonium *in vivo* and *in vitro*. (-----), Steady state depolarization of the isolated electroplax (from Changeux & Podleski, 1968). (■), Increase of permeability to $^{22}Na^+$ of excitable microsacs (from Kasai and Changeux, 1971). (●), Binding of [$^{14}$C] decamethonium to the same microsacs (from Kasai and Changeux, 1971). (○), (□), Decrease of rate of binding of *N. nigricollis* [$^{3}$H] α-toxin to membrane fragments (Weber *et al.*, 1972).

40% of the toxin molecules were labelled. By means of a simple filtration technique the rate of binding of toxin to excitable membrane fragments can be measured easily (Weber, Menez, Fromageot, Boquet & Changeux, 1972): all the kinetic data are consistent with the hypothesis of a bimolecular mechanism of toxin binding to a homogeneous class of binding sites. At room temperature and in the presence of 0·13 M sucrose in physiological salt solution, the 'association' rate constant $k$ is $(1{\cdot}7 \pm 0{\cdot}5) \times 10^7$ $M^{-1}$ $min^{-1}$. Interestingly, in the presence of physiological concentrations of cholinergic agonists or antagonists the initial rate of toxin binding decreases markedly and becomes negligible at saturating levels of effector. A simple formal treatment of the protection by cholinergic agents shows that the decrease in the initial rate of binding in the presence of an effector is simply proportional to the fractional occupancy of the receptor site by the effector. The curve of protection against effector concentration can thus be taken as a binding curve for the cholinergic agent. Superimposition of the curve of protection by decamethonium with the actual binding curve of the same compound to excitable microsacs and with the concentration–effect curves measured on whole cells and on microsacs (Fig. 2) strongly supports this conclusion. The same conclusion was reached with a variety of cholinergic agonists and antagonists. In contrast with the findings of Miledi, Molinoff & Potter (1971) on *Torpedo* electroplax, and of Lester (1971) on the motor endplate, agonists and antagonists do not appear to differ in the manner in which they protect. The measured dissociation constants always fall close to the apparent dissociation constants (Fig. 3). These observations, along with the result that complete protection occurs at saturating levels of effector, clearly show that, under the present experimental conditions (ionic strength = 0·18 and purified membrane fragments) the tritiated toxin binds *exclusively* to the cholinergic receptor site.

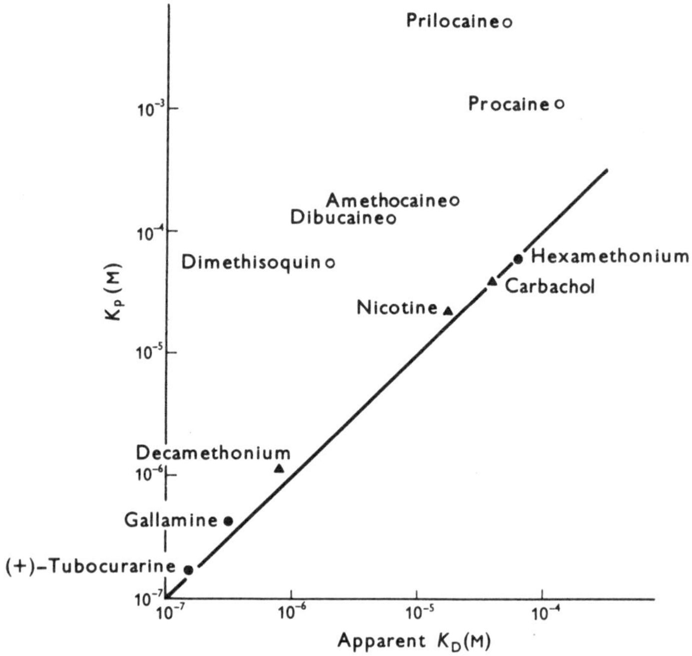


FIG. 3. Comparison of the dissociation constants ($K_P$) measured *in vitro* by inhibition of [$^3$H] α-toxin binding and of the apparent dissociation constants ($K_D$) measured with the isolated electroplax for a variety of cholinergic agonists, antagonists and local anaesthetics (from Weber *et al.*, 1972).

Local anaesthetics such as amethocaine or procaine block the electrical response of the electroplax to cholinergic agonists in a *noncompetitive* manner, in contrast to the typical *competitive* antagonists like (+)-tubocurarine or gallamine. Interestingly, with the local anaesthetics, the curves of protection against toxin binding do not coincide with their concentration–effect curves. They act as anaesthetics at concentrations much lower (often one order of magnitude or more) than those at which they protect. The local anaesthetics presumably bind as anaesthetics on the receptor protein to sites that are different from the site to which agonists and antagonists bind and also, with a much lower affinity, to the cholinergic receptor (Weber *et al.*, 1972).

Studies on the reversibility of the binding of toxin to membrane fragments gave additional support to the specificity of its association with the cholinergic receptor site. In the absence of effector the dissociation of *Naja nigricollis* α-toxin is slow: $\overleftarrow{k}=(2{\cdot}1 \pm 0{\cdot}2)\times 10^{-4}\ \text{min}^{-1}$. However, high concentrations of decamethonium and (+)-tubocurarine considerably enhance this rate. Displacement also is observed at equilibrium (Fig. 4) and becomes complete in the presence of an excess of effector. Knowing the binding constant of the effector, an estimate of the dissociation constant of the toxin bound to the receptor can be calculated from the amount of toxin displaced at a given concentration of effector. The value found is $(2\pm 1)\times 10^{-11}$ M (Weber *et al.*, unpublished results), which is compatible with the values of the association and dissociation rate constants measured directly with the toxin in the absence of effector. The mechanism by which decamethonium accelerates dissociation of the toxin is under study.

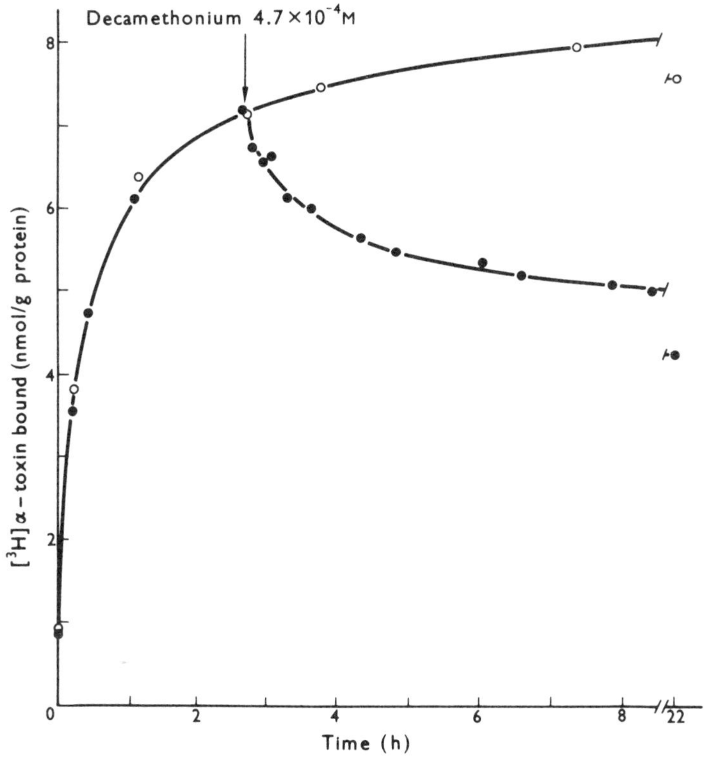


FIG. 4. Displacement by decamethonium of *N. nigricollis* [$^3$H] α-toxin bound to membrane fragments. 250 μl of membrane suspension (14·5 g protein per l, 5·5 nmol receptor per g protein) was diluted 20-fold with physiological salt solution containing 0·02% $NaN_2$, at room temperature. The reaction was started by adding 300 μl of [$^3$H] α-toxin ($8{\cdot}9\times 10^{-8}$ M). 200 μl aliquots were withdrawn at intervals and rapidly filtered on Millipore filters, which were then washed with physiological salt solution and counted. At the time indicated by the arrow, the decamethonium was added to give a concentration of $4{\cdot}7\times 10^{-4}$ M (●——●). (○——○), Results obtained when no decamethonium was added.

All the currently available data support our earlier conclusion that the α-toxin bound to the membrane is indeed exclusively bound to the cholinergic receptor site. The [$^3$H] α-toxin thus constitutes a reliable and versatile probe of the cholinergic receptor site and of the macromolecule which carries this site.

### *B. The localization of the cholinergic receptor sites in* Electrophorus *electroplax*

Since the snake α-toxins constitute highly specific and slowly reversible markers of the receptor site, they can be used to localize the receptor at the cellular and subcellular level (Lee & Tseng, 1966; Sato, Abe & Tamiya, 1970). In a first series of experiments we used the $\alpha_1$-isotoxin from *Naja nigricollis*. The bound toxin was revealed by a combination of rabbit antiserum directed against the toxin and fluorescent γ-globulins directed against the rabbit antibodies. Only the innervated membrane became fluorescent, suggesting an exclusive localization of the receptor protein on this face of the cell (Bourgeois, Tsuji, Boquet, Pillot, Ryter & Changeux, 1971) (Plate 1a).

This finding was confirmed by autoradiography with the tritiated α-toxin. After exposure of a slice of electroplax to the [$^3$H] α-toxin, more than 99% of the grains were present on the innervated face. In addition, as expected for a specific binding to the receptor site, no radioactivity was bound after exposure to an irreversible antagonist or after contact with an excess of unlabelled toxin (Bourgeois, Ryter, Menez, Fromageot, Boquet & Changeux, 1972) (Plate 1b).

In order to obtain fine localization which would distinguish labelling on membrane areas underlying the nerve terminals (subsynaptic areas) from labelling on extrasynaptic areas, we used high resolution autoradiography with the electron microscope. After exposure of the whole electroplax to the tritiated toxin, grains appeared both between and under the synapses but were much more numerous under than between. We calculated the absolute density of receptor sites per unit of surface area on the basis of assumptions as to the actual area of the surface of the cytoplasmic membrane, the yield of grains in relation to radioactive disintegrations, and the thickness of the sections (Table 1). The most critical aspect was the estimate of the real surface of the cytoplasmic membrane. Under the nerve terminals the subsynaptic membrane is rather smooth and closely follows the presynaptic membrane. On the other hand, between the nerve terminals the surface is highly convoluted and has two kinds of villosities: large villosities, irregular in shape, which give an approximately 3-fold apparent surface increase, and micro-villosities (average diameter 0·18 μm, depth 1·7 μm) which give an approximately 10-fold surface increase. Because of these factors, the subsynaptic membrane constitutes between 1 and 2% of the total surface of the cell. There are approximately 33 000 ± 10 000 toxin binding sites per $\mu m^2$ in the

TABLE 1. *Number of cholinergic receptor sites in* Electrophorus *electroplax*

| | | Grains per $\mu$m of cell section* | [$^3$H] $\alpha$-toxin molecules bound per $\mu m^2$ of membrane surface† |
|---|---|---|---|
| Innervated face | Subsynaptic | $3 \cdot 10 \pm 0 \cdot 9$ | $33\,000 \pm 10\,000$ |
| | Extrasynaptic | $0 \cdot 34 \pm 0 \cdot 3$ | $400 \pm 300$ |
| Non-innervated face | | $0 \cdot 09 \pm 0 \cdot 08$ | $39 \pm 20$ |

* Uncorrected for microvillosities. † Taking into account an increase of cell surface by the microvillosities of 10-fold on the innervated face and of 30-fold on the non-innervated one. From Bourgeois *et al.* (1972).

synaptic regions; between the synapses the density is approximately 100 times lower and the density on the noninnervated surface is a further 10 times smaller. According to these values, about 60% of the total number of toxin molecules would be bound to the subsynaptic areas and 40% to the extra-synaptic ones. The total number of toxin molecules bound per cell would be $(3 \pm 2) \times 10^{11}$, a number which falls within the range found by direct counting of the [$^3$H] $\alpha$-toxin or an affinity labelling reagent (Karlin, this symposium) (see Table 2).

A striking difference in receptor density between subsynaptic and extra-synaptic areas has also been reported with muscle (Barnard, Wieckowski & Chiu, 1971; Miledi & Potter, 1971; Berg, Kelly, Sargent, Williamson & Hall, 1972; Fambrough & Hartzell, 1972; Barnard, this symposium). Interestingly, the densities of $\alpha$-toxin binding sites in subsynaptic areas fall close to ours. Assuming that the smallest unit of the receptor protein to which the $\alpha$-toxin binds has a molecular weight of 50 000 (Meunier, Olsen, Menez, Morgat, Fromageot, Ronsseray, Boquet & Changeux, 1971b) and a density of 1·37, then the maximum density of receptor molecules in a single layer is approximately 40 000 per $\mu m^2$. If all our assumptions are correct, then the subsynaptic membrane surface is occupied almost exclusively by the receptor protein. There is little room left for acetylcholinesterase unless the enzyme is not integrated in the membrane framework in the same manner as the cholinergic receptor (Barnard, 1973). An alternative, at least in the case of the electroplax, would be that the acetylcholinesterase does not show the same distribution between subsynaptic and extrasynaptic areas of membrane as the receptors. Evidence of this latter interpretation is offered by the centri-fugation experiment shown on Fig. 5. Membrane fragments which prefer-entially bind the $\alpha$-toxin appear to have, under the present experimental con-ditions, a density higher than those which contain the highest amounts of acetylcholinesterase activity (Bourgeois *et al.*, 1972; Cohen *et al.*, 1972).

In any case, all the currently available data indicate that the density of receptor is much higher under than between the synapses. The factors

TABLE 2. *Comparison of the densities of cholinergic receptor sites reported in the literature*

| | *Electrophorus* electroplax | *Electrophorus* microsacs | *Torpedo* electroplax | Rat motor endplate | Mouse motor endplate | Frog motor endplate |
|---|---|---|---|---|---|---|
| Number of receptors per synapse | — | — | — | $1–4 \times 10^7$ (5) | $1–4 \times 10^7$ (5, 6) | $10^9$ (5)<br>$10^7$ (7) |
| Number of receptors per $\mu m^2$ of cytoplasmic membrane | 3400 (1)<br>sub-synaptic: 33 000 (2)<br>extra-synaptic: 400 (2) | 30–450 (3) | 10 000 (4) | — | 12 000 (6)<br>10 000 (7) | 100 000 (5) |
| Number of receptors per cell | $1·6–3 \times 10^{11}$ (1)<br>$1–4 \times 10^{11}$ (2) | — | $5 \times 10^{10}$ (4) | — | — | — |

(1) Karlin, Prives, Deal & Winnick (1971): affinity labelling reagent after treatment of the cell by a disulphide bonds reducing agent.
(2) Bourgeois *et al.* (1972): tritiated α-toxin from *Naja nigricollis* irreversible binding.
(3) Kasai & Changeux (1971): [$^{14}$C] decamethonium reversible binding.
(4) Miledi *et al.* (1971): iodinated α-bungarotoxin.
(5) Miledi & Potter (1971): iodinated α-bungarotoxin.
(6) Barnard *et al.* (1971): tritiated α-bungarotoxin.
(7) Barnard (1972): tritiated α-bungarotoxin.

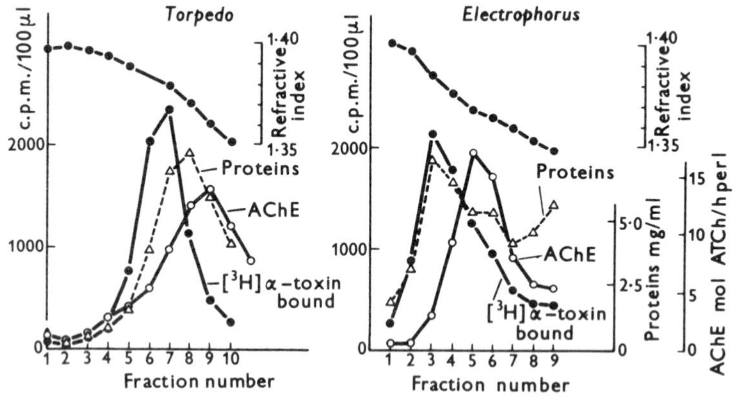


FIG. 5. Distribution of total protein, bound [$^3$H] α-toxin and acetylcholinesterase (AChE) in sucrose density gradients after ultracentrifugation of homogenates of *E. electricus* and *T. marmorata* electric organ (from Bourgeois *et al.*, 1972; Cohen *et al.*, 1972). The specific activity of cholinergic receptor sites in the peak fraction of the *Torpedo* gradient was 2000 nmol/g protein (approximately 10% of the proteins consisted of receptor material). AChE activity is expressed as the rate of hydrolysis of acetylthiocholine (ATCh). By permission of North-Holland Publishing Company, Amsterdam.

involved in this regulation are unknown, but several hypotheses can be proposed for the local enrichment in receptor protein under the nerve terminals. For instance: (1) the synthesis and liberation by nerve terminals of additional receptor molecules which become integrated in the subsynaptic membrane; (2) a differential turnover of receptor proteins in subsynaptic and extrasynaptic proteins; the ionic fluxes in spike propagation might, for instance, increase the susceptibility to degradation of the receptor protein in extrasynaptic areas; (3) the presence in the synaptic cleft or in the presynaptic membrane of molecules which show a high affinity for the receptor protein, and which might act as cross-linking agents (Allison, 1972). Denervation experiments with *Electrophorus* electric organ are in progress to test these possibilities.

### *C. Physical properties of the receptor protein in detergent solution*

Early experiments mentioned above showed that the molecule which carries the cholinergic receptor site can be extracted in a soluble form by anionic detergents like Na-deoxycholate or cholate or non-ionic detergents like Triton X-100. The solubilized receptor molecule still binds the cholinergic agonists and antagonists and the snake α-toxins. This molecule does not pass through Diaflo membranes which retain spherical proteins with a molecular weight greater than 50 000, and it is digested by pronase. It is thus a protein or, at least, it contains a protein moiety. Moreover, the receptor protein readily separates from acetylcholinesterase on a column made of Sepharose beads to which *Naja nigricollis* α-toxin was covalently coupled (Meunier *et al.*, 1971a).

The tritiated α-toxin from *Naja nigricollis* was used to follow the hydrodynamic behaviour of the receptor protein. The receptor was either labelled before solubilization or the free receptor sites of the solubilized protein were assayed with the [$^3$H] α-toxin by taking advantage of the fact that the receptor–toxin complex precipitates with ammonium sulphate while the unbound toxin remains in solution. Extraction of labelled membrane fragments by 1% Na-deoxycholate, Na-cholate or Triton X-100 preserves the association of the toxin to a macromolecule which precipitates in the absence of detergent but migrates as a single band, in the presence of 1% Na-deoxycholate, on gel electrophoresis. The toxin–receptor complex as well as the free receptor protein sediments as a single peak in sucrose gradients containing one of the above mentioned detergents. It is eluted again as a single peak from a Sepharose 6B column. Under the present experimental conditions and according to the criteria used, the protein species to which the toxin binds appears to be homogeneous (Meunier *et al.*, 1971b; Meunier, Olsen, Menez, Fromageot, Boquet & Changeux, 1972a).

An interesting paradox arises when one compares sedimentation and gel filtration data. In the presence of 1% Triton X-100 the receptor complex sediments slightly more slowly than beef liver catalase (7·4*s*, mol. wt. = 240 000) but is eluted from a Sepharose 6B column slightly ahead of *E. coli* β-galactosidase (16*s*, mol. wt. 540 000). In other words the receptor–toxin complex, and this is also true for the free receptor protein, sediments more slowly than expected from its Stokes' radius (*a*) assuming the receptor protein to be a sphere with a density close to that of regular proteins. Two properties might account for the observed unusual behaviour, a nonglobular shape and/or a density different from that of the soluble proteins used as standards.

Ultracentrifugation of the receptor–toxin complex in media where the density was varied by replacing $H_2O$ by $D_2O$ shows that the receptor complex has an unusual density (Meunier, Olsen & Changeux, 1972b) (Fig. 6). Increasing the density by adding $D_2O$ in the centrifugation medium is accompanied by a greater decrease of sedimentation velocity of the receptor–toxin complex than of the globular proteins used as standards. In the presence of 1% Triton X-100 the apparent density of the receptor protein is smaller, or the apparent partial specific volume ($\bar{v}$) larger, than that of a regular globular protein: $\bar{v}=0{\cdot}78$ instead of 0·73. In Table 3 are collected the data obtained

TABLE 3. *Hydrodynamic parameters of the cholinergic receptor protein in the presence of Triton X-100*

| $\bar{v}$ (ml × g$^{-1}$) | $s_{20,\,w}$ | *a* (nm) | Apparent molecular weight (g) | Apparent frictional ratio ($f/f_0$) |
|---|---|---|---|---|
| 0·78 ± 0·01 | 12·5 ± 0·01 | 7·3 ± 0·3 | 470 000 ± 30 000 | 1·39 ± 0·02 |

From Meunier *et al.* (1972b).

with Triton X-100 and the *apparent* molecular weight and frictional ratio ($f/f_0$) calculated from these values.

It appears that the anomalous behaviour observed in the presence of Triton X-100 can be accounted for by the binding of up to 21% of the total mass of the receptor–toxin complex by Triton X-100 (160–170 molecules of detergent of density close to 1·0). Under these conditions the apparent molecular weight of the protein moiety without Triton X-100 would then be 360 000.

In conclusion, there is strong evidence for considerable binding of Triton X-100 to the receptor protein, and such a conclusion might possibly extend to other membrane proteins solubilized by the same detergent with similar physical properties. It is tempting to relate this property to the fact that all these proteins are normally integrated in a biological membrane and thus may have on their surface hydrophobic loci that establish nonpolar interactions with the fatty acid hydrocarbon chains of membrane lipids. These loci would be responsible for the insolubility of the protein in aqueous solvents

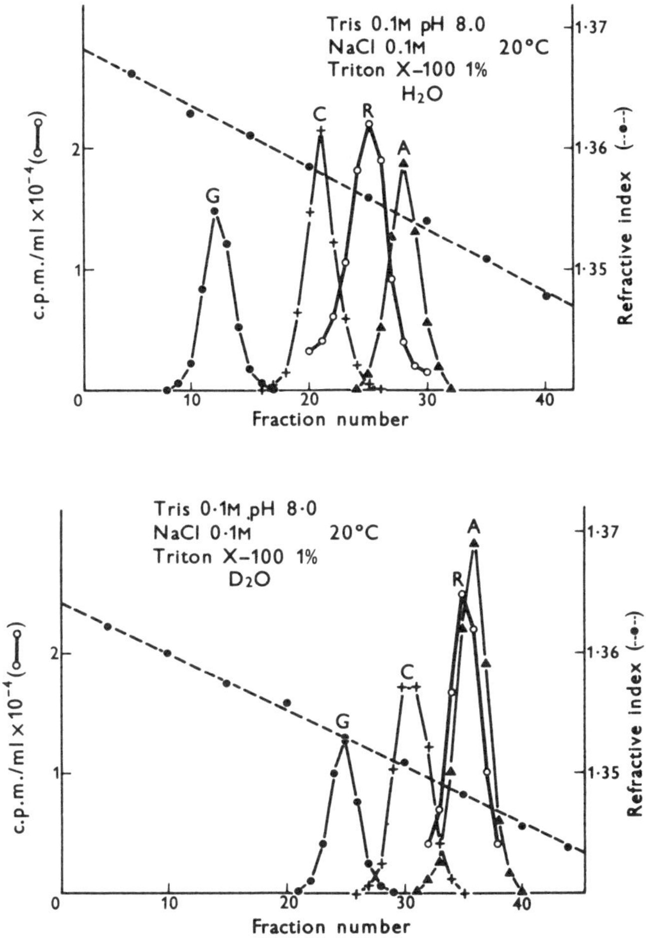


FIG. 6. Sedimentation profile of the complex receptor–α-toxin in $H_2O$ and $D_2O$ in the presence of Triton X-100. A: Alcohol dehydrogenase; C: catalase; G: β-galactosidase; R: receptor–α-toxin. (From Meunier, Olsen & Changeux, 1972b.) By permission of North-Holland Publishing Company, Amsterdam.

and would be occupied by detergent molecules during the solubilization process. The solubilized receptor protein in aqueous detergent solutions would no longer be a proteolipid but a 'proteo-detergent'.

Treatment of a deoxycholate extract of labelled membranes gives a radioactive unit of apparent molecular weight close to 50 000 by polyacrylamide gel electrophoresis in the presence of sodium dodecylsulphate. This unit is the smallest one seen before dissociation of the receptor–toxin complex. Interestingly, similar values have been found independently by Karlin and co-workers (this symposium) for the receptor protein labelled with a cholinergic affinity reagent and by Raftery (1972) and ourselves (see later section) with a purified preparation of *Torpedo* receptor protein. It thus appears plausible that the form which is solubilized by deoxycholate or Triton X-100 is a well-defined polymer made up of a finite number of smaller subunits, an oligomer of possibly 6–8 subunits. It is not possible at present to ascertain whether this polymer is made exclusively of such units and corresponds to the 'native state' of the receptor protein integrated in the membrane framework. It can only be said that, in this state, the protein is able to bind cholinergic ligands and snake venom toxins.

### *D. The purification of the receptor protein*

Since some detergents extract the receptor protein without loss of binding capacity, and since the protein is stable for days in the presence of these detergents, the receptor should be easy to purify. Indeed, it was shown that conventional purification procedures like ammonium sulphate precipitation, chromatography on DEAE cellulose columns, or filtration on gels give significant purification of the free receptor protein or of its toxin complex. However, the low specific activity of the extracts obtained from *Electrophorus* electric organs presented a serious difficulty. Usually the crude extracts contained 10–20 nmol of receptor sites per g of protein. Assuming a molecular weight per receptor site of 50 000, then the specific activity of the pure receptor protein should be close to 20 000 nmol/g protein. The purification factor required was 1000 or 2000. This is why we turned to more efficient purification procedures. Affinity chromatography was selected as giving both high purification factors and high yields.

The first columns we used consisted of *N. nigricollis* α-toxin coupled covalently to activated Sepharose beads (Meunier *et al.*, 1971a). A highly selective adsorption occurred but quantitative release of the receptor protein in its free form appeared to be difficult. In the second class of columns, cholinergic side-chains with either triethylammonium or phenyltrimethylammonium residues were coupled to Sepharose beads (Olsen, Meunier & Changeux, 1972). As shown in Fig. 7, in one step a 30-fold enrichment was obtained. The fraction with the highest purity of free receptor protein from *Electrophorus* contained 4 500 ± 500 nmol/g protein.[2]

With *Torpedo marmorata* the purification was considerably facilitated by the fact that membrane fragments with a particularly high specific activity can be used as starting material (Cohen *et al.*, 1972). Starting from a pool of membrane fragments of a specific activity of 200 nmol/g protein, 100 μg of protein was obtained with an average specific activity of 2000 nmol/g protein (peak tube 6000 nmol/g) by means of the above mentioned affinity column with a cholinergic side-chain. This last preparation gave a single band on gel electrophoresis in the presence of sodium dodecyl sulphate

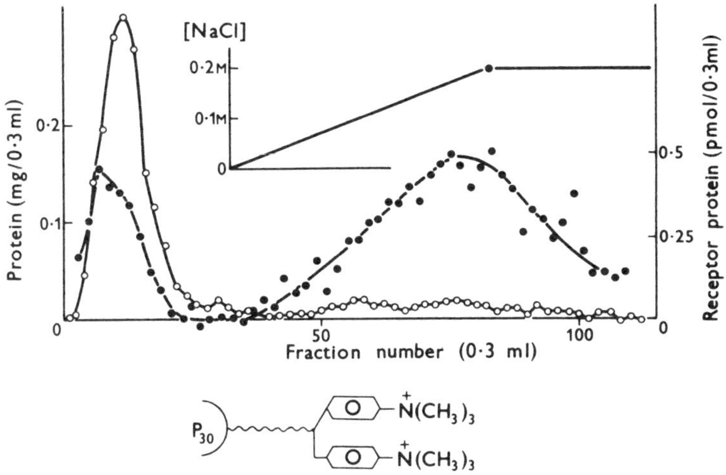


FIG. 7. Purification of receptor protein from *E. electricus* by affinity chromatography on a column of polyacrylamide beads with side-chains of the structure indicated. The column (10 ml) was equilibrated and developed in 0·01 M Tris (pH 8·0) and 2% sodium cholate The sample contained 5 mg protein, and 25 pmol of receptor sites, and was obtained from cholate-solubilized electric organ (Meunier *et al.*, 1972a). (○), Total protein; (●), receptor.

(Fig. 8). The apparent molecular weight measured was 41 500 (Olsen, Meunier & Changeux, 1972).

### *E. The cholinergic ionophore and the reconstitution of an excitable membrane after solubilization*

It is not yet known whether the cholinergic ionophore belongs to the same polypeptide chain as the receptor protein or whether it is a separate entity. However, several of its properties can be inferred from permeability studies developed with excitable microsacs and an experimental method which should lead to its identification can now be envisaged.

Microsacs at rest are permeable to $^{45}Ca^{2+}$, $^{42}K^{+}$, $^{22}Na^{+}$ and to $^{36}Cl^{-}$, but slightly or not at all to [$^{32}$S] $SO_4^{2-}$. The permeability to neutral compounds is in general very low. In agreement with conventional electrophysiological data, in the presence of carbachol the permeability to $Na^{+}$, $K^{+}$ and $Ca^{2+}$ increases, whereas the permeability to [$^{14}$C] tetraethylammonium and [$^{14}$C] choline does not change. Carbachol had no effect on the permeability to negatively charged or uncharged permeants. The ionophore in its active or open state thus appears selective for small cations (Kasai & Changeux, 1971).

By relating the increase in $^{22}$Na efflux with the binding of decamethonium in the microsac preparation it is possible to characterize the transport properties of the ionophore that is activated by a single molecule of decamethonium

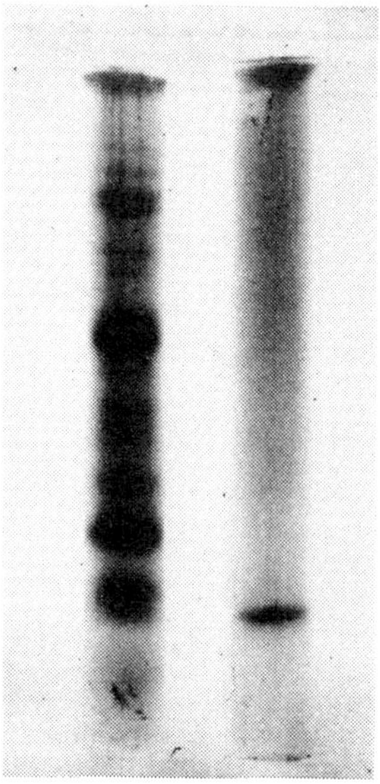

FIG. 8. Gel electrophoresis in sodium dodecyl sulphate, as described by Weber & Osborn (1969), of the purest fraction of receptor protein (specific activity > 6000 nmol/g protein) from *T. marmorata* electric organ, obtained by affinity chromatography as in Fig. 7. Left-hand gel: crude membrane fraction, prepared as in Fig. 5. Right-hand gel: receptor material obtained after passage through affinity column, with elution by salt. 400 μg protein was applied to each gel.

(Kasai & Changeux, 1971). The density of receptor sites varied among different microsac preparations between 30 and 450 per $\mu m^2$, and the increase in permeability (for both $Na^+$ and $K^+$) was about $5 \times 10^{-9}$ cm/s. With 0·17 M $Na^+$ inside the sacs, the efflux rate per molecule of decamethonium bound was found to be about 5000 ions/min. It is interesting that similar flux rates have been calculated for single transport sites in various other systems, for example, Na-pumping sites in cell membranes, the permease involved in β-galactoside transport in *E. coli*, and the increase in potassium permeability of liposomes treated with cyclic polypeptide antibiotics such as valinomycin. Microsacs treated with gramicidin also show an increased potassium permeability, and calculations show that the increase in permeability attributable to a single gramicidin molecule is within an order of magnitude the same as that associated with a single molecule of decamethonium bound to the receptor.

The calculation of the conductance of a single ionophore involves various untested assumptions. Kasai & Changeux (1971) arrived at a figure between $5 \times 10^{-17}$ and $5 \times 10^{-15}$ mho per channel.[3] This is very much lower than the value ($10^{-10}$ mho) calculated by Katz & Miledi (1971) for the magnitude of the transient conductance change required to account for the random fluctuations in membrane potential seen when cholinergic agonists were applied

TABLE 4. *Conductance change per cholinergic receptor site*

| | Conductance or flux data | Number of receptor sites | $\Delta g_{Na}$/site | Reference |
|---|---|---|---|---|
| Electroplax | $g_{Na}=0\cdot15$ mho/cm$^2$ (window area) | 900/$\mu$m$^2$ (cytoplasmic membrane) (*average*) | $5\cdot5\times10^{-14}$ mho | Ruiz-Manresa & Grundfest (1971) Bourgeois *et al.* (1972) |
| Microsacs | $10^{-6}$–$10^{-5}$ mho/cm$^2$ (for $V=0$) | 10 nmol $\alpha$-toxin per g protein | $5\times10^{-17}$–$5\times10^{-15}$ mho | Kasai & Changeux (1971) Weber *et al.* (1972) |
| Noise | | | | |
| Frog endplate | $10^{-10}$ mho/fluctuation | ? | ? | Katz & Miledi (1971) |
| Gramicidin lipid bilayer | $2\times10^{-11}$ mho/fluctuation | ? | ? | Hladky & Haydon (1970) |

to the frog motor endplate (Table 4). The large discrepancy between these estimates might be accounted for by postulating that the ionophore associated with a receptor site occupied by a decamethonium molecule is active in a discontinuous manner so that the average conductance of the channel could be very much less than the transient conductance occurring for brief periods. Experiments are in progress to test this possibility.

Objective information on the nature and properties of the ionophore will only be gained by its characterization and isolation *in vitro*. If microsacs of excitable membrane could be dissociated into their elementary components and subsequently reconstituted in a form which exhibits both the characteristic of a selective permeability to cations and the sensitivity to acetylcholine of native microsacs, it is possible that fractionation before reconstitution could lead to the identification of the components responsible for the selective permeability change caused by the cholinergic agents. Experiments carried out so far have shown that solubilization of excitable microsacs by Na-cholate or deoxycholate in adequate conditions occurs without loss of the specific binding capacity of the cholinergic receptor and of the catalytic activity of acetylcholinesterase. After extensive dialysis to remove detergents and the introduction of divalent cations, membrane fragments re-form. These reconstituted fragments bind [$^3$H] $\alpha$-toxin with a high specific activity and contain large amounts of acetylcholinesterase (Changeux, Huchet & Cartaud, 1972). Recently it has been possible to produce reconstituted microsacs loaded with $^{22}Na^+$ that are sensitive to carbachol (Hazelbauer & Changeux, unpublished). Reconstitution of an excitable membrane can thus be achieved, and experiments are in progress to identify the ionophore in the solubilized extracts and, in particular, to determine its relation to the receptor protein.

## *F. Conclusion*

Several groups of workers have developed, in parallel, methods for studying the cholinergic receptor (see the articles of De Robertis, Karlin, O'Brien and Potter, this symposium) and some of their findings agree well with ours. For instance the proteolipid of De Robertis and co-workers binds cholinergic agonists and antagonists as well as $\alpha$-bungarotoxin. However, the binding experiments are carried out in the presence of organic solvents and the dissociation constants measured can hardly be compared with the apparent dissociation constants observed *in vivo*, in the presence of physiological salt solution. Nevertheless the number of proteolipid molecules per gram of tissue and the molecular weight of the smallest proteolipid subunit are close to our values. The work of O'Brien and co-workers has been concerned almost exclusively with cholinergic ligands without the help of any additional specific reagent. As mentioned above some of these ligands, like decamethonium, bind to several classes of site in addition to the cholinergic receptor site. Moreover, some of the dissociation constants reported are several orders of magnitude different from those measured *in vivo* and *in vitro* by our methods. It is nevertheless possible that in several instances some of the binding measured occurs at the level of the cholinergic receptor site. The molecular weight reported by Karlin for the smallest subunit of the receptor protein labelled by an affinity reagent is in agreement without results on material labelled by the tritiated α-toxin from *N. nigricollis*. Thus, there seems to be a good agreement between his results and ours in this respect. Finally, Miledi, Molinoff & Potter (see Potter this symposium) have reported data from *Torpedo* electric tissue which are very similar to ours. Some difference exists, however, between their estimate of the molecular weight and ours.

In conclusion, by virtue of the exceptional properties of the electric organ of *E. electricus*, we have been able to 'reduce' an excitable system from the cellular level—the isolated electroplax—to a subcellular one—the excitable membrane fragments—and finally to reach the molecular level with the isolation of the cholinergic receptor protein. At each step of this analysis, *in vitro* data were carefully and critically compared with *in vivo* electrophysiological results. The response of an excitable membrane to a neurotransmitter can thus be studied at the molecular level. The first results obtained are in agreement with the general theory of an allosteric transition of the receptor protein. However, the essential feature of the theory, that a conformational transition is associated with the physiological mechanism, has not yet been demonstrated.

We thank Dr R. Baldwin for essential suggestions and critical comments, Drs G. Gachelin, A. Fritsch and S. Bram for helpful discussions and Drs A. Menez, P. Fromageot and P. Boquet for the gift of tritiated $\alpha_1$-isotoxin from *Naja nigricollis*. This work was supported by funds from the Centre National de la Recherche Scientifique, the Délégation Générale à la Recherche Scientifique et Technique, the Collège de France, the Commissariat à l'Energie Atomique and the National Institutes of Health.

*Notes added in proofs*

[1] Direct evidence in favour of a conformational transition has been found recently by Cohen & Changeux (1973, *Proc. natn. Acad. Sci., U.S.A.*, in press) using a fluorescent cholinergic ligand.

[2] The binding constants of the purified receptor protein for cholinergic ligands measured in the presence of 1% Triton X-100, 0·5% Na-cholate or in the absence of detergent are: $(2 \pm 1) \times 10^{-8}$ M decamethonium, $(1{\cdot}9 \pm 0{\cdot}5) \times 10^{-6}$ M carbachol, $(1{\cdot}0 \pm 0{\cdot}5) \times 10^{-6}$ M phenyltrimethylammonium; $(3{\cdot}9 \pm 1) \times 10^{-7}$ M (+)-tubocurarine, $(1{\cdot}3 \pm 0{\cdot}2) \times 10^{-7}$ M gallamine, $(6{\cdot}2 \pm 1) \times 10^{-5}$ M hexamethonium. A significant increase of the affinity for agonists occurs during purification with little change of the affinity for the antagonists. *One* interpretation of this phenomenon is that after purification the receptor protein is stabilized in its S active conformation, assuming the agonists to

be exclusive ligands and the antagonists highly non-exclusive ones. (Meunier & Changeux, in press.)

[3] A more direct method uses the maximum increase in conductance that can be produced by steady application of agonists to the innervated face of a single electroplax, causing simultaneous activation of all the receptors. This value is $5–10 \times 10^{-2}$ mho per cell (Ruiz-Manresa & Grundfest, 1971; and our own measurements); since we find $1–4 \times 10^{11}$ receptors in a single electroplax, we calculate $10^{-13}$ to $10^{-12}$ mho per receptor.

## REFERENCES


ALLISON, A. (1972). In: *Cell Interactions; Third Lepetit Symposium*, ed. Silvestri, L., p. 156. Amsterdam and London: North-Holland Co.

ARAI, H., TAMIYA, N., TOSHIOKA, S., SHINONAGA, S. & KANO, R. (1964). *J. Biochem., Tokyo*, **56**, 568.

BARNARD, E. (1973). *Neuroscience Research Program.* Work Session on Receptor Biochemistry and Biophysics, March 5–7, 1972, Boston (Mass).

BARNARD, E. A., CHIU, T. H., JEDRZEJCYZK, J., PORTER, C. & WIECKOWSKI, J. (1973). This symposium.

BARNARD, E. A., WIECKOWSKI, J. & CHIU, T. H. (1971). *Nature, Lond.*, **234**, 207.

BERG, D., KELLY, R. B., SARGENT, P. B., WILLIAMSON, P. & HALL, Z. (1972). *Proc. natn. Acad. Sci., U.S.A.*, **69**, 147.

BOQUET, P., IZARD, Y., JOUANNET, M. & MEAUME, J. (1966). *C. R. Acad. Sci., Paris*, **262** D, 1134.

BOQUET, P., IZARD, Y., JOUANNET, M. & MEAUME, J. (1967). In: *Animal toxins*, p. 293. Oxford and New York: Pergamon Press.

BOQUET, P., IZARD, Y. & RONSSERAY, A. M. (1970). *C. R. Acad. Sci., Paris*, **271** D, 1456.

BOURGEOIS, J.-P., RYTER, A., MENEZ, A., FROMAGEOT, P., BOQUET, P. & CHANGEUX, J.-P. (1972). *F.E.B.S. Letters*, **25**, 127.

BOURGEOIS, J.-P., TSUJI, S., BOQUET, P., PILLOT, J., RYTER, A. & CHANGEUX, J.-P. (1971). *F.E.B.S. Letters*, **16**, 92.

CHANGEUX, J.-P. (1966). *Mol. Pharmac.*, **2**, 369.

CHANGEUX, J.-P., HUCHET, M. & CARTAUD, J. (1972). *C. R. Acad. Sci., Paris*, **274** D, 122.

CHANGEUX, J.-P., KASAI, M., HUCHET, M. & MEUNIER, J.-C. (1970a). *C. R. Acad. Sci., Paris*, **270** D, 2864.

CHANGEUX, J.-P., KASAI, M. & LEE, C. Y. (1970b). *Proc. natn. Acad. Sci., U.S.A.*, **67**, 1241.

CHANGEUX, J.-P., MEUNIER, J.-C. & HUCHET, M. (1971). *Mol. Pharmac.*, **7**, 538.

CHANGEUX, J.-P. & PODLESKI, T. (1968). *Proc. natn. Acad. Sci., U.S.A.*, **59**, 944.

CHANGEUX, J.-P., PODLESKI, T. & MEUNIER, J.-C. (1969). *J. gen. Physiol.*, **54**, 225S.

CHANGEUX, J.-P. & THIERY, J. (1968). In: *Regulatory Function of Biological Membranes*, ed. Järnefelt, J., p. 116. Amsterdam, London and New York: Elsevier.

CHANGEUX, J.-P., THIÉRY, J., TUNG, Y. & KITTEL, C. (1967). *Proc. natn. Acad. Sci., U.S.A.*, **57**, 335.

COHEN, J. B., WEBER, M., HUCHET, M. & CHANGEUX, J.-P. (1972). *F.E.B.S. Letters*, **26**, 43.

COLQUHOUN, D. (1973). This symposium.

DE ROBERTIS, E. (1973). This symposium.

DEL CASTILLO, J. & KATZ, B. (1955). *J. Physiol., Lond.*, **128**, 396.

FAMBROUGH, D. M. & HARTZELL, H. C. (1972). *Science, N.Y.*, **176**, 189.

FATT, P. & KATZ, B. (1951). *J. Physiol., Lond.*, **115**, 320.

GERHART, J. C. & SCHACHMAN, H. K. (1965). *Biochemistry*, **4**, 1054.

HIGMAN, H., PODLESKI, T. R. & BARTELS, E. (1964a). *Biochim. biophys. Acta*, **75**, 187.

HIGMAN, H., PODLESKI, T. R. & BARTELS, E. (1964b). *Biochim. biophys. Acta*, **79**, 138.

HLADKY, S. B. & HAYDON, D. A. (1970). *Nature*, **225**, 451.

KARLIN, A. (1967). *J. Theor. Biol.*, **16**, 306.

KARLIN, A., COWBURN, D. A. & REITER, M. J. (1973). This symposium.

Karlin, A., Prives, J., Deal, W. & Winnik, M. (1971). *J. Mol. Biol.*, **61**, 175.
Karlsson, E., Arnberg, H. & Eaker, D. (1971). *Eur. J. Biochem.*, **21**, 1.
Karlsson, E., Eaker, D. & Porath, J. (1966). *Biochim. biophys. Acta*, **127**, 505.
Karlsson, E., Eaker, D. & Ponterius, G. (1972). *Biochim. biophys. Acta*, **257**, 235.
Kasai, M. & Changeux, J.-P. (1970). *C. R. Acad. Sci., Paris*, **270** D, 1400.
Kasai, M. & Changeux, J.-P. (1971). *J. Memb. Biol.*, **6**, 1.
Katz, B. & Miledi, R. (1971). *Nature, Lond.*, **232**, 124.
Lee, C. Y. (1970). *Clinical toxicology*, **3**, 457.
Lee, C. Y. & Chang, C. C. (1966). *Mem. Inst. Butantan Simp. Internac.*, **33**, 555.
Lee, C. Y. & Tseng, L. F. (1966). *Toxicon*, **3**, 281.
Lester, H. (1970). *Nature, Lond.*, **227**, 727.
Lester, H. (1971). Ph.D. Thesis, The Rockefeller University.
Menez, A., Morgat, J. L., Fromageot, P., Ronsseray, A. M., Boquet, P. & Changeux, J.-P. (1971). *F.E.B.S. Letters*, **17**, 333.
Meunier, J.-C. & Changeux, J.-P. *F.E.B.S. Letters*, in press.
Meunier, J.-C., Huchet, M., Boquet, P. & Changeux, J.-P. (1971a). *C. R. Acad. Sci., Paris*, **272** D, 117.
Meunier, J.-C., Olsen, R. W. & Changeux, J.-P. (1972b). *F.E.B.S. Letters*, **24**, 63.
Meunier, J.-C., Olsen, R. W., Menez, A., Fromageot, P., Boquet, P. & Changeux, J.-P. (1972a). *Biochemistry*, **11**, 1200.
Meunier, J.-C., Olsen, R., Menez, A., Morgat, J. L., Fromageot, P., Ronsseray, A. M., Boquet, P. & Changeux, J.-P. (1971b). *C. R. Acad. Sci., Paris*, **273** D, 595.
Miledi, R., Molinoff, P. & Potter, L. (1971). *Nature, Lond.*, **229**, 554.
Miledi, R., Potter, L. (1971). *Nature, Lond.*, **233**, 599.
Monod, J., Wyman, J. & Changeux, J.-P. (1965). *J. Mol. Biol.*, **12**, 88.
Nachmansohn, D. (1959). *Chemical and Molecular Basis of Nerve Activity.* New York and London: Academic Press.
Nachmansohn, D. (1971). In: *Handbook of Sensory Physiology, Vol. I, Principles of Receptor Physiology*, ed. Lowenstein, W. R., p. 18. Berlin: Springer.
O'Brien, R. D., Eldefrawi, M. E. & Eldefrawi, A. T. (1973). This symposium.
Olsen, R. W., Meunier, J.-C. & Changeux, J.-P. (1972). *F.E.B.S. Letters*, **28**, 96.
Podleski, T. R. & Changeux, J.-P. (1969). *Nature, Lond.*, **221**, 541.
Potter, L. T. (1973). This symposium.
Raftery, M. (1972). *Neuroscience Research Program.* Work Session on Receptor Biochemistry and Biophysics, March 5–7, 1972, Boston (Mass).
Rubin, M. & Changeux, J.-P. (1966). *J. Mol. Biol.*, **21**, 265.
Ruiz-Manresa, F. & Grundfest, H. (1971). *J. gen. Physiol.*, **57**, 71.
Sato, S., Abe, T. & Tamiya, N. (1970). *Toxicon*, **8**, 313.
Sato, S. & Tamiya, N. (1971). *Biochem. J.*, **122**, 453.
Schoffeniels, E. & Nachmansohn, D. (1957). *Biochim. biophys. Acta*, **26**, 1.
Weber, M., Menez, A., Fromageot, P., Boquet, P. & Changeux, J.-P. (1972). *C. R. Acad. Sci., Paris*, **274** D, 1575.
Weber, K. & Osborn, M. (1969). *J. Biol. Chem.*, **244**, 4406.

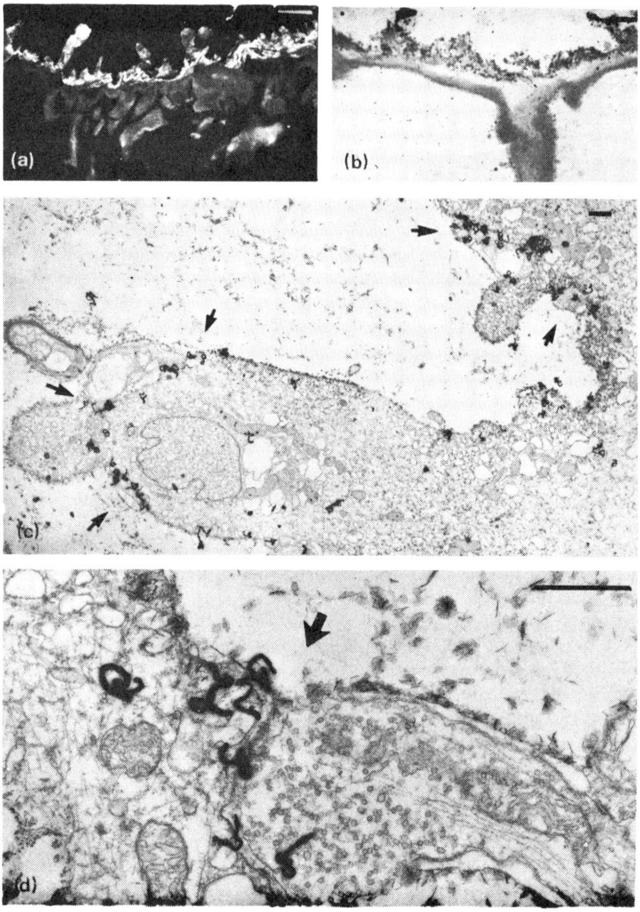


PLATE 1. Distribution of the α-toxin from *Naja nigricollis* after extensive labelling of *E. electricus* electroplax. (a), Immunofluorescence: the α-toxin is revealed by an antibody directed against the toxin (bar = 100 μm); (b), autoradiography by light microscopy (bar = 10 μm); (c) and (d), autoradiography by electron microscopy (bar = 1 μm). (From Bourgeois *et al.*, 1971 and 1972.) By permission of North-Holland Publishing Company, Amsterdam.

# ACETYLCHOLINE RECEPTORS IN VERTEBRATE SKELETAL MUSCLES AND ELECTRIC TISSUES

L. T. POTTER

*Department of Biophysics, University College London, London WC1E 6BT, England*

## *A. Introduction*

The essential features of chemical neurotransmission are as follows. (1) A nerve impulse moves along a nerve, usually of hair-thin size, as an all-or-none electrical message (action potential), being carried because of the cable properties of the axon, and because electrical depolarization of the axonal membrane permits sudden and transient increases of permeability first to sodium ions and then to potassium ions, in such a way as to make use of their electrical and concentration gradients to boost the impulse to full strength as it passes (Hodgkin, 1964). (2) Depolarization of a nerve terminal by an action potential permits calcium ions to move down an electrochemical gradient into or through the presynaptic membrane, and leads to the neuro-secretion of packages or 'quanta' of a chemical transmitter into the synaptic cleft (Katz, 1969). Circumstantial evidence indicates that release depends upon fusion of synaptic vesicles with the presynaptic membrane (Nickel & Potter, 1971; Heuser & Reese, 1973) and release of their transmitter content. Collection experiments carried out with the rat phrenic-nerve–diaphragm preparation indicate that an average of several million molecules of acetyl-choline are released for each nerve impulse and nerve terminal in this tissue (cf. Potter, 1970). (3) The transmitter diffuses to postsynaptic cells and reacts with recognition sites called 'receptors' which have high specificity for the transmitter (Paton, 1970). All known neurotransmitters are ions which do not readily diffuse through biological membranes, and since responses to them are very rapid and of short duration, it has long been assumed that receptors are membrane constituents; skeletal muscle cells respond only to the external application of acetylcholine (del Castillo & Katz, 1955), suggesting that their recognition sites are only on the outside surface of these cell membranes. (4) At most synapses the reaction between a transmitter and receptor initiates a sudden and transient increase in the permeability of the cell membrane to certain small ions, thereby producing an increase or decrease in the polarization of the membrane. At neuromuscular junctions the rate and direction of ion fluxes depend upon the electrochemical gradients present across the cell membrane (Fatt & Katz, 1951), and acetylcholine receptors appear to be coupled directly to ion channels which open for approximately 1 ms and permit the net influx of about 50 000 univalent ions per channel (Katz & Miledi, 1972). Summation of such fluxes in the electroplax of *Torpedo* electric tissue accounts for the voltage output of the electric organs of this fish (Bennett, 1971). Other receptors appear to be coupled directly to adenyl or guanyl cyclase (Sutherland, 1970; McAfee & Greengard, 1972; Lee, Kuo & Greengard, 1972), and the production of cyclic nucleotides may control subsequent ion movements. (5) In many cells synaptic potentials initiate action potentials in the remainder of the cell membrane, and these become nerve impulses or initiate muscle contraction or gland secretion. Summation of such action potentials is responsible for most of the voltage output of the electric organs of the eel, *Electrophorus electricus* (Bennett, 1971).

It is not yet known whether a single molecule or several coupled molecules are required for the conceptually distinct functions of transmitter recognition and of providing for the ion channels of synaptic potentials. There is, however, good biochemical evidence that certain receptors can be irreversibly occluded with several agents (see below), and several blocking compounds are under study which appear to independently alter synaptic potential ion channels; it should soon be possible, therefore, to determine whether blocking agents for the separate functions bind to the same or different molecules. In this regard it is pertinent to note that the ion channel of synaptic potentials in skeletal muscles differs from those which subserve action potentials, in that sodium and potassium ions move simultaneously through what behaves as a single channel, the system is chemically but not electrically excitable, responses are graded rather than all-or-none, and the channel is unaffected by toxins which block (tetrodotoxin and saxitoxin: cf. Kao, 1966) or hold open (batrachotoxin: Albuquerque, Daly & Witkop, 1971) the active sodium channel of action potentials.

Historically, research on receptors has progressed backwards in the above sequence from (5) to (3). Most of the available information about the specificity of receptors has come from pharmacological experiments in which observed cell responses (usually muscle contraction or relaxation after bath applications of drugs) were many steps removed from transmitter–receptor interactions. More direct analyses have been obtained from physiological and pharmacological studies in which synaptic potentials, or still better. current fluxes across postsynaptic membranes, have been used to monitor receptor activation. By means of intracellular recording and microionophoretic application of transmitters and similar drugs, much information has been obtained about the location and relative numbers (in terms of sensitivity) of receptive sites, their spread from the endplate region of muscles (Thesleff, 1973) after denervation (Miledi, 1962) or other interruption of nerve impulses (Lømø & Rosenthal, 1972), their desensitization during drug application (cf. Rang & Ritter, 1970), and the effects of opening a single ion channel (Katz & Miledi, 1972). It is apparent, however, that studies of coupled receptor activation and cell responses cannot give information about the actual numbers or fine-structural localization of receptors, or of the possible presence of uncoupled receptors in the membrane; in addition, no matter how plausibly 1 : 1 pharmacological competition between a transmitter and another drug suggests that both act on one molecular subunit, studies of coupled receptor–response systems cannot exclude the possibility that such agents act at different steps or sites (molecules or molecular subunits) in the course of transmitter-induced cell responses.

In order to examine transmitter recognition sites directly, particularly after solubilization of cell membranes, it is necessary to measure their presence with a binding agent. Various means for doing so have been considered, including reconstitution of receptor–ion channel systems, measurements of conformational alterations produced by agonists, and direct binding studies with more or less reversible agonists, antagonists, antibodies or even ion channel proteins (cf. Potter & Molinoff, 1972). Initially and conceptually the best approach might appear to be to measure the binding of the transmitter itself. O'Brien and his colleagues (this symposium) have been particularly successful in demonstrating that the binding of acetylcholine and similar nicotinic agents to the richly-innervated tissue of electric organs (membranes and membrane proteins) can be measured by equilibrium methods. Changeux and his co-workers (this symposium) have used another agonist, decamethonium, for the same purpose, and have demonstrated quantitatively that binding parameters correlate not only with physiological blockade in intact electroplax (eel), but with expected drug antagonisms at the level of isolated synaptic membranes and membrane proteins. Waser and others (cf. Waser, 1970) have had some success in localizing the antagonist, (+)-tubocurarine, at normal neuromuscular endplates by radioautography. And with the same intent, De Robertis and his co-workers (this symposium) have studied the irreversible binding of several transmitters and antagonists in non-ionic and nonaqueous media; so far, however, these studies have not been correlated with physiological parameters.

When it comes to the measurement of the precise localization and counting of receptors *in situ*, a specific *and* long-lasting tagging agent is required; and, excepting the use of reversible binding agents in affinity chromatography for the purification of solubilized receptors, nearly irreversible binding agents are generally more convenient than readily-reversible ligands for the handling and recognition of isolated receptors. Of the 'irreversible' agents which have been tried, the greatest success has been achieved with an alkylating derivative of benzilylcholine (for the study of muscarinic receptors: Fewtrell &

Rang, this symposium), and with several snake toxins for the study of nicotinic receptors.

Snakes of the elapid family, including cobras and kraits, and some coral and sea snakes, have developed closely related 'α-toxins' which paralyse animals by blocking nicotinic receptor-response mechanisms. Of the α-toxins which have been studied in detail, those of cobras have the advantages that they are plentiful (particularly that of the Thailand Cobra, *Naja naja siamensis*: Karlsson, Arnberg & Eaker, 1972) and slowly reversible (Lee & Chang, 1966; Lester, 1972), which makes the toxins suitable for affinity chromatography. That of the Formosan Banded Krait, *Bungarus multicinctus*, appears to be the least reversible and therefore the most suitable for studies of receptors *in situ*; it is the subject of the remainder of this summary.

The rationale for using α-bungarotoxin as a tagging agent for nicotinic receptors is based on studies by Chang & Lee (1963), Lee & Chang (1966), Lee & Tseng (1966) and Lee, Tseng & Chiu (1967). They demonstrated that the toxin rapidly and irreversibly blocked neuromuscular transmission in several vertebrate skeletal muscles, without affecting action potentials in nerves or muscles, the release of acetylcholine, or its hydrolysis by acetylcholinesterase. The irreversible effect of the toxin was reduced if (+)-tubocurarine was present during exposure of muscles to the toxin, suggesting that both act on the same molecule or macromolecular complex. By whole-mount radioautography it was shown that the toxin remained bound to blocked muscles at endplates in normal muscles, and over much of the muscle surface after denervation. It was concluded, and subsequent studies by others have confirmed (see below), that α-bungarotoxin combines specifically with nicotinic receptors.

### B. *Experiments with vertebrate skeletal muscles*

Twelve proteins were isolated from the venom of *B. multicinctus* by gel filtration on Sephadex G-50 and cation exchange chromatography on CM-Sephadex in phosphate buffer at pH 7·5. One was apparently inactive at neuromuscular junctions, one was acetylcholinesterase, six blocked acetylcholine release, and four blocked acetylcholine-induced depolarization of postsynaptic membranes (Miledi & Potter, unpublished). Although all of the latter four had the properties described by Lee and his co-workers for α-bungarotoxin, only the most prevalent, accounting for 20–25% of the protein of the venom, was used. It had no discernible effect on action potentials in nerves or muscles, on resting potentials in muscles, or on the activity of acetylcholinesterase from electric tissues. It appeared as a single component by rechromatography on Sephadex G-50 and CM-Sephadex, and by polyacrylamide gel electrophoresis with or without sodium dodecyl sulphate (SDS) and β-mercaptoethanol. By gel filtration, and by gel electrophoresis in SDS, its molecular weight was 8000. Since the toxin remained physiologically active in brown solutions of iodine, it was labelled isotopically with $^{131}I$, yielding initial specific activities of 23 Ci/mmol (Miledi, Molinoff & Potter, 1971).

When frog muscles were exposed to 1 $\mu$g/ml $\alpha$-toxin (about $10^{-7}$ M), the endplate depolarization produced in surface muscle fibres by single nerve impulses declined exponentially until it could no longer be recorded, with a half-time of 2–3 minutes (Miledi & Potter, 1971). After two hours all of the fibres in frog sartorius muscles (as in innervated and denervated rat and mouse diaphragms) were unresponsive to bath- or focally-applied acetylcholine, and remained so after repeated washing in toxin-free solutions for as long as 8 days. These studies demonstrated the extraordinary irreversibility of this toxin. Similar results have been obtained with the $\alpha$-toxin of *Naja naja siamensis* (Lester, 1972), although other evidence indicates that it is more reversible than $\alpha$-bungarotoxin.

When radioactive toxin was used, the time course of binding of the toxin in frog, rat and mouse muscles was found to correspond roughly to the time course of neuromuscular blockade; after full block, binding sites were saturated (Miledi & Potter, 1971). After section of the phrenic nerves to rat diaphragms, the number of binding sites for the toxin increased for 3 weeks up to 20-fold, with a time course roughly comparable to that for the increase in acetylcholine sensitivity. Thereafter, as muscle fibres atrophied, the total number of toxin sites decreased, although acetylcholine sensitivity is known to remain high in such muscles. A precise correlation between the number of toxin sites and sensitivity has not yet been achieved. The amount of toxin-binding material in muscles may be compared to that in electric tissues as follows (Molinoff & Potter, 1973).

TABLE 1

| Tissue | nmol $\alpha$-toxin/kg fresh tissue |
|---|---|
| *Torpedo* electric tissue | 1000 |
| *Electrophorus* electric tissue | 75 |
| Denervated rat diaphragms | 60 |
| Innervated diaphragms | 3 |
| Frog sartorius | 1 |

The location of the bound toxin in muscles was assessed quantitatively by cutting bundles of fibres transversely into short segments for assays of radioactivity (Miledi & Potter, 1971). In normal rat diaphragms 85–90% was in the endplate region; the remainder was considered to represent non-specific retention of the toxin since, after dissolution of membrane proteins in Triton X-100, this part of the total radioactivity had the sedimentation characteristics of free toxin, whereas that in the endplate region behaved as would a water-soluble protein having an $s_{20}$ value of about 9 (see below).

Similar results were obtained by Berg, Kelly, Sargent, Williamson & Hall (1972). Much finer resolution of the localization of toxin-binding sites has been achieved by Barnard and his colleagues (this symposium) and by Hartzell & Fambrough (1972) using electron microscopy and radioautography: except in frog sartorius muscles, silver grains were found almost exclusively at endplates. The numbers of toxin sites found by grain counts and by radioactivity assays were in accord for mammalian muscles (10–80 million/endplate) and as in *Torpedo* electric tissue (Miledi *et al.*, 1971) the density of sites appears roughly 10 000/$\mu m^2$ and closely matched with the number of active sites of acetylcholinesterase. In denervated rat diaphragms new toxin sites first appeared in the central third of bundles of fibres and then increased in a trimodal distribution until three equal peaks of bound toxin were found centred on the three thirds of the fibres. No obvious physiological correlate has been described to explain these peaks.

An unexpected distribution of bound toxin was found by Barnard and co-workers (this symposium) in frog sartorius muscles, in that in addition to the usual density of silver grains at endplates, grains were found throughout the muscles at a density somewhat less than a tenth that in the endplate region. This observation helps to explain why so many more toxin sites were found in such muscles by radioactivity assays (about $10^9$ for every endplate in the tissue: Miledi & Potter, 1971) than in mammalian muscles, but does not explain their distribution, which is like that expected in denervated muscles. In desensitization experiments with bath-applied carbachol or with acetylcholine and neostigmine, binding of the toxin was reduced by more than 80% during brief periods of toxin exposure. Since physiological measurements of acetylcholine sensitivity in frog muscles have not shown a distribution like that of the bound toxin, it must be concluded that the extrajunctional sites do not represent receptors coupled to ion channels in the usual way and/or that their distribution is so different from that in denervated muscles as to have a major effect on the physiological measurements. It has been claimed that an average distribution of toxin sites over denervated rat muscles at a density about one-tenth that at normal endplates is sufficient to give acetylcholine sensitivity similar to that at normal endplates (Fambrough & Hartzell, 1972). The possibility that the extrajunctional sites in frog muscles represent an entirely different kind of receptor material is not supported, either theoretically by knowledge of the specificity of protein: protein interactions having such high affinities as those between α-bungarotoxin and nicotinic receptors, or by sedimentation analyses which indicate that the dissolved toxin-binding material from different tissues, including frog muscles, is the same (Molinoff & Potter, 1973; see below). Despite these curious effects in frog muscles the general conclusion remains for mammalian muscles that receptors (toxin sites) are not present where acetylcholine sensitivity is absent.

Binding of the toxin in frog muscles was found to decrease in proportion to the development of desensitization produced by acetylcholine (Miledi &

Potter, 1971). In contrast, the binding of an alkylating derivative of decamethonium was accelerated by desensitization (Rang & Ritter, 1970). Assuming for the moment that both blocking agents affect the same molecular subunit of receptors, these observations suggest that receptors can be stabilized in two different conformations by these agents.

Chang & Lee (1963) demonstrated that (+)-tubocurarine protected muscles from the effects of the toxin, and it was to be expected that toxin-binding would be reduced in proportion to physiological blocking by (+)-tubocurarine. This was found to be the case in eel electric tissue (Weber, Menez, Fromageot, Boquet & Changeux, 1972); in addition, full block of binding was produced by (+)-tubocurarine when the toxin was mixed with soluble or membrane-bound receptors from *Torpedo* (Franklin & Potter, 1972). Surprisingly, therefore, concentrations of (+)-tubocurarine 100 times greater than those required for full physiological block of frog muscles reduced binding of the toxin by only 50%. Somewhat greater protection has been obtained with mammalian muscles (Potter, unpublished; Berg *et al.*, 1972; Barnard, this symposium), but a disproportion between block and protection persists for which no adequate explanation has been found. In experiments in which (+)-tubocurarine-protected and (+)-tubocurarine-unprotected toxin sites were separately labelled with radioactive toxin, no difference in the sedimentation velocities of the dissolved, labelled proteins was found.

### *C. Experiments with electric tissues*

#### *1.* Torpedo *Electric Tissue*

Although the electric tissue of eels has the considerable advantage of being suitable for physiological as well as biochemical experiments (cf. Changeux, this symposium), *Torpedo* electric tissue is unquestionably the most plentiful source of nicotinic receptors for biochemical experiments (Table 1). The difference lies in the fact that *Torpedo* electroplax cells are much thinner and more heavily innervated than those of the eel; in fact, as far as neurotransmission is concerned, and excepting the absence of myofibrils, *Torpedo* electric tissue appears and behaves as a concentrated mass of neuromuscular endplates.

The electric organs of *Torpedo* comprise about 25% of the body weight of the fish and can reach weights of many kilograms. Each organ is composed of about 500 columns or stacks of cells, and each column, which runs from dorsal skin to ventral skin, has several hundred to several thousand cells. These vary in thickness from 5–10 $\mu$m, and in breadth from 1–10 mm or more, depending upon the size of the fish (cf. Potter & Molinoff, 1972). The number of cells in a stack determines the voltage output of the organs which is usually only 20–60 V, but the surface area of large fish can be so great that the current output can reach 50 A. Each electroplax is innervated over approximately half of its ventral surface (Sheridan, 1965; Nickel & Potter,

1971) by cholinergic nerve terminals (Feldberg & Fessard, 1942; Israel, 1970); the total area of infolded postsynaptic membrane has been estimated as 70 $m^2$/kg of fresh tissue (Miledi *et al.*, 1971).

*2. Physiological experiments*

It is difficult to record intracellular potentials in *Torpedo* electric tissue for any length of time because the cells are so thin (Bennett, 1971); however miniature synaptic potentials due to the quantal release and reception of acetylcholine were readily recorded with extracellular micropipettes (Miledi *et al.*, 1971). While these potentials were readily blocked by the ionophoretic application of (+)-tubocurarine or α-bungarotoxin, the bath-applied drugs produced full block, even in small pieces of tissue, only after several days, presumably because access to the narrow synaptic clefts by diffusion is very slow. Because of this access limitation, biochemical studies with the toxin have generally been limited to the use of disintegrated electric tissue.

*3. Labelling of membranes*

The binding of α-bungarotoxin to homogenates of *Torpedo* and eel electric tissue, and to resuspended membranes isolated from the homogenates, was found to be dependent upon time and the concentration of the toxin, and to be slowed by carbachol and by (+)-tubocurarine (Miledi *et al.*, 1971; Franklin & Potter, 1972). The saturation levels in the two tissues differed by an average factor of 13 (Table 1). As in mammalian muscles, the calculated number of active sites of acetylcholinesterase in the *Torpedo* tissue was nearly the same as the observed number of toxin sites (Miledi *et al.*, 1971); despite early claims to the contrary, this was not the case with eel electric tissue which has the same or slightly greater esterase activity as *Torpedo* tissue, but fewer toxin sites (Molinoff & Potter, 1973).

*4. Subcellular fractionation of electric tissues*

Experiments with homogenates of both eel and *Torpedo* electric tissue showed that α-bungarotoxin did not bind to water-soluble proteins, to synaptic vesicles (peak position isodense with 13% sucrose), myelin (20% sucrose), or mitochondria (41% sucrose) (Molinoff & Potter, 1973). Subcellular fractionation of toxin-saturated membranes in sucrose density gradients showed, even after prolonged sonication of the membrane suspensions, that 70–85% of the esterase activity and bound toxin were recovered with several peaks of membrane material more dense than mitochondria. These peaks were largely composed of morphologically-identifiable dorsal electroplax membranes, which were intermixed with unidentifiable membrane fragments:

the general conclusion was that postsynaptic membranes, as shown by the presence of radioactive toxin, could not be quantitatively separated from other membranes by density differences. In the case of eel tissue, there was a peak of esterase-rich vesicles corresponding to the position (peak at 25% sucrose) of the 'microsacs' studied by Kasai & Changeux (1971), but contrary to their findings, there was a separate peak of vesicles with toxin-binding sites at 34% sucrose. With material from *Torpedo*, 15–30% of the total toxin-binding sites were found with a peak of vesicles at 38% sucrose; as a microsac preparation these had approximately 100 times the toxin capacity and one-fifth the esterase activity (per unit protein) of the microsac preparation from eel tissue. With both tissues it was clear that some toxin-binding vesicles could be isolated which had little acetylcholinesterase, and the reason for this result has not been established. One possibility is that the receptor protein and acetylcholinesterase are located, at least in part, on different pieces of membrane. Another alternative is that when postsynaptic membranes are vesiculated during sonication, acetylcholinesterase, which may be present in the basement membrane, may be pulled free and found either in solution, or as small particles.

The rate of access of the toxin to membrane fragments appeared non-uniform, in that when only 20% saturation levels of the toxin were applied to sonicated membrane suspensions, virtually all of the toxin was found in gradients associated with the vesicle peak at 38% sucrose (Potter & Molinoff, 1972). Evidence from sedimentation analyses indicated that the binding protein for the toxin in this peak of subcellular material was not different from that of the denser toxin-binding membranes (Molinoff & Potter, 1972).

### 5. *Solubilization of membrane proteins*

Prolonged sonication of toxin-labelled membranes from *Torpedo* in water, with or without EDTA, or in 2 M NaCl, did not yield any toxin which was not sedimented by centrifugation at $100\,000 \times g$ for 1 h. It was concluded that toxin-binding sites are hydrophobic membrane constituents. Several agents that are well known for their ability to dissolve membrane proteins, including 1% sodium dodecyl sulphate, 8 M urea, 2 M NaI and 2 M NaBr were found to clarify suspensions of labelled membranes from *Torpedo* and to render most of the membrane protein unsedimentable by centrifugation as above. However these agents also separated α-bungarotoxin from its binding sites: the conclusion was that the bond between the toxin and receptors is not covalent (Potter & Molinoff, 1972). Mixtures of chloroform–methanol which effectively dissolve lipoproteins were not effective in dissolving toxin–receptor complexes, and appeared to denature receptor material that had not been exposed to toxin so that subsequent binding of the toxin in aqueous media did not occur (Molinoff & Potter, 1972). However certain other mixtures of organic solvents in considerable volumes were effective dissolving agents, and cold butanol-saturated buffers had the curious property of dissolving half of the toxin-binding material of *Torpedo* electric tissue.

While anionic detergents like sodium deoxycholate and sodium dodecyl sulphate were effective in dissolving toxin–receptor complexes, the preferred method of solubilization was to use 2 mg of the non-ionic detergent, Triton X-100, per milligram of membrane protein, since the dissolved material could then be purified by separation methods depending upon molecular charge (electrophoresis, including isoelectric focusing, and ion exchange chromatography). Triton X-100 was found to dissolve most of the proteins of muscle and electric tissue membranes in 20–30 min at 4° C; however the nature of the dissolved proteins subsequently varies markedly with time and temperature after this period (see below).

### 6. *Centrifugation studies of toxin–receptor complexes*

It was first demonstrated that the sedimentation velocity of several water-soluble proteins (egg albumin, serum albumin, gamma globulin and catalase) in 1–3% Triton was directly proportional to their $s_{20,w}$ values in the absence of the detergent (Molinoff & Potter, 1973). Since hydrophobic proteins are probably coated with more detergent than these water-soluble proteins, their relative *s* values will tend to be on the high side because of increased size, and on the low side because the density of Triton (about 1·08) is less than that of pure proteins. A partial correction for these errors was obtained by determining the equilibrium buoyant density of toxin–receptor complexes from *Torpedo* (about 1·18) and other proteins in sucrose gradients containing Triton.

Freshly dissolved toxin–receptor complexes from *Torpedo* showed three prominent peaks of radioactivity after centrifugation in 5–25% sucrose gradients containing 3% Triton, with relative *s* values of 6, 9·3 and 12, and several larger and/or denser materials having *s* values of about 15 and 18. The peaks at 9·3 and 12*s* ran true after recentrifugation, while those of larger *s* generally produced considerable material of 9·3 and 12*s*. The peak at 6*s* was the least stable, often disappearing overnight after storage of extracts at 4° C and producing, again, peaks of 9·3 and 12*s*. After storage of extracts at room temperature for 24 h, approximately two-thirds of the radioactivity was found at 9·3*s* and most of the remainder at 12*s*. These studies demonstrated the polymeric or aggregated nature of toxin–receptor complexes and suggested that their relative sizes were in the ratio 1, 2, 3 etc. (Molinoff & Potter, 1973). Other workers have noted the predominant form at about 9·3*s* (Raftery, Schmidt, Clark & Wolcott, 1971; Meunier, Olsen, Menez, Fromageot, Boquet & Changeux, 1972).

Freshly-dissolved toxin–receptor material from frog sartorius muscles

(Miledi & Potter, 1971), eel electric tissue, and innervated and denervated rat diaphragm muscles showed the same multiple peaks, indicating that receptors in different tissues are very similar in composition. However the proportion of the material in the different peaks initially varied with the tissue. Those tissues with dense punctate innervation like the rat diaphragm and eel electric tissue initially showed a high proportion of 15 and 18*s* material, whereas those with more diffuse toxin-binding sites, like frog muscle and *Torpedo* electric tissue showed a predominance of 9·3 and 12*s*. With prolonged storage the smaller forms became predominant with all the tissues. That the effect was not simply due to experimental artifact was suggested by the results of comparing the endplate regions of the right and left hemidiaphragms of one rat, one week after section of the left phrenic nerve (when the hemidiaphragm weights are still equal): again the normal endplate region showed a much higher proportion of 15 and 18*s* radioactivity. These results implied that there is a different state of packing of receptor molecules in different membranes, with possibly patches of highly aggregated molecules at certain synapses (Molinoff & Potter, 1973).

Triton-dispersed membrane proteins from *Torpedo* bound as much radioactive toxin as the equivalent membrane suspension, and the sedimentation profile of receptors labelled before and after extraction from the membranes was the same, indicating that no new binding sites were disclosed by dissolving the membranes, as is the case with insulin receptors (Cuatrecasas, 1972). Receptor material not previously exposed to toxin which had been stored in Triton for several days, and which yielded mostly 9·3*s* complexes after labelling, was found to bind toxin at the rate of $2 \times 10^7$ l. mol$^{-1}$ min$^{-1}$ in 0·1 % Triton at 4° C (Franklin & Potter, 1972). After part of a Triton extract of *Torpedo* membranes was exposed to carbachol before and during exposure to radioactive toxin, sedimentation analysis showed the same profile of peaks as without carbachol, but quantitatively only 15 % as much bound toxin (Molinoff & Potter, 1973). This result showed that the protective effect of agonists persists in solution (possibly because of a conformational change in the receptors as is believed to occur in membranes), and that protection occurs with receptor molecules no larger than 150 000 daltons (see below).

### 7. *Gel filtration*

It was first shown that the retention of several water-soluble proteins (egg albumin, serum albumin, ferritin, β-galactosidase and thyroglobulin) during gel filtration on Sepharose 6B in the presence of 1–3 % Triton X-100 was directly proportional to the known effective radii (Stokes' radius = *a*) for these proteins in the absence of detergents (Molinoff & Potter, 1973). Changes in Stokes' radius due to coating by the detergent must therefore be proportional to the size of the uncoated protein. Since hydrophobic proteins are probably associated with more detergent than are these standards, the *a* values given below probably overestimate the effective radii of toxin–receptor complexes.

As with the results of sedimentation analyses, elution profiles of radioactive receptor complexes from Sepharose 6B were complex and depended upon the age of the Triton extracts. Freshly-dissolved membrane proteins from *Torpedo* showed three major peaks having relative *a* values of 4·2, 6·9 and 8·5 nm, and variable amounts of larger material of indeterminate size. The peak at 4·2 nm was the least stable, producing $a=69$ and 85 material when rerun; it probably corresponded to that having an *s* value of 6. The largest material slowly disaggregated (unless treated with 2 M NaCl or left at room temperature for a day, when the change was rapid) into $a=69$ and 85 forms. After prolonged storage approximately two-thirds of the radioactivity was associated with $a=69$ (9·3*s*) material and most of the remainder was $a=85$ (12*s*). These studies further demonstrated the aggregated or polymeric structure of toxin–receptor complexes. Again, other workers have noted the major peak, with electric tissue from *Torpedo* (Raftery *et al.*, 1971) and eels (Meunier *et al.*, 1972).

### 8. *Isoelectric focusing*

Purified radioactive toxin–receptor protein from *Torpedo* (see below) was found to have an isoelectric point of 5·1 in an Ampholyte and sucrose gradient of pH 3–6, containing 3% Triton. Similar values have been found by others with receptor material from eel and *Torpedo* electric tissue (Raftery *et al.*, 1971; O'Brien, this symposium; Changeux, this symposium). Although the ion exchange behaviour of toxin–receptor complexes (Molinoff & Potter, 1972), and their ready precipitation with ammonium sulphate near pH 5 (Franklin & Potter, 1972) are in keeping with these results, it may be noted that Triton X-100 also focuses near pH 5 and may alter the apparent pI of toxin–receptor complexes.

### 9. *Ion-exchange chromatography*

The most suitable conditions found for ion-exchange studies were the use of the anion-exchange resin, DEAE-Sephadex-A50, sodium phosphate buffer, pH 6·4, and 3% Triton (cf. Potter & Molinoff, 1972). In the course of elution with a gradient of NaCl (0–1 M), partially purified toxin–receptor material from *Torpedo* (9·3*s*) was eluted as a single symmetrical peak in 0·3–0·4 M NaCl.

### 10. *Purification and polyacrylamide gel electrophoresis*

Although the procedure of choice for the purification of nicotinic receptors is probably affinity chromatography because of the varied sizes, shapes and total charges of different receptor polymers, considerable information has been gained from small samples of toxin–receptor material purified by the techniques of protein characterization noted above. One kg of *Torpedo* electric tissue binds 1 μmol of toxin and has approximately 10 g of membrane protein, so if each molecule of toxin binds to one receptor subunit of 42 000 daltons (see below), full purification and recovery of the toxin-binding protein should yield 8 mg of toxin plus 42 mg of receptor protein, and require a 200-fold purification. Starting with an aged Triton extract of toxin-saturated membranes from 500 g of *Torpedo* electric tissue, sequential application of: (a) zonal centrifugation with recovery of the peak of the 9·3*s* material, (b) precipitation with ammonium sulphate at pH 5·1 (20–30% saturation) and redissolution in 3% Triton at pH 7·4, (c) gel filtration on Sepharose 6B with retention of the peak material of $a = 69$, (d) anion-exchange chromatography with recovery of the peak of labelled material, and (e) precipitation by ultracentrifugation, yielded a protein pellet with 48 μg of toxin (recovery = 1·2%) plus 680 μg other protein. No attempt was made to achieve higher recovery. The ratio of toxin to membrane protein suggested that the purified material was either only 44% pure, or that not all the receptor subunits bind α-toxin (for example, the purity would be 88% if half had binding sites). When this labelled protein was disaggregated with 1% SDS and 1% β-mercaptoethanol, and 200 μg were subjected to polyacrylamide gel electrophoresis, only 2 stained protein bands were found, one with the mobility of egg albumin (molecular weight = 42 000) and the other, which was radioactive, with the mobility of free α-toxin (Potter, unpublished). Other workers have used affinity ligands for sulphydryl groups on nicotinic receptors in eel electric tissue to demonstrate a receptor subunit in SDS and dithiothreitol having a molecular weight of 42 000 (Reiter, Cowburn, Prives & Karlin, 1972), and a cobra toxin-labelled subunit in SDS alone of about 50 000 daltons (Meunier *et al.*, 1972). Taken together, these results show that nicotinic receptors are composed of subunits of about 42 000 daltons, at least a third to a half of which bind acetylcholine, α-toxins and other ligands.

### *11. Molecular weight calculations*

The molecular weight ($M$), frictional ratio and axial ratio of a water-soluble protein may be determined from knowledge of $a$, $s_{20}$, the density ($p$) and viscosity ($\eta$) of the media used for centrifugation, the partial specific volume of the hydrated protein ($\bar{v}$), and the Avogadro constant ($N$). $M = 6\,N\eta as/(1-\bar{v}p)$ and appears close to 150 000, 300 000, and 450 000 for the three most prominent toxin–receptor complexes seen in Triton X-100; when taken with the measured size of the subunits, these figures obviously suggest that nicotinic receptors are aggregates of trimers, of which the most prevalent form has 6 single subunits (Molinoff & Potter, 1973). Because of the uncertainties of the measurements of *a*, *s* and $\bar{v}$ in the presence of detergents, and particularly since *a* is probably overestimated, precise calculations of frictional and axial ratios seem premature.

### *12. Reconstitution experiments*

As with 'microsacs' of membranes from eel electric tissues (Kasai & Changeux, 1971), microsacs from *Torpedo* electric tissue containing radio-sodium show an increased efflux of radioactivity in the presence of carbachol, which is blocked by α-bungarotoxin. Dissolution of microsacs with organic solvents or sodium deoxycholate, followed by dialysis of the extracts and sonication of the resulting membrane material leads to the recovery of vesicles which have slightly more than half the original toxin-binding capacity, and which, while they are leakier than before, still show some carbachol-induced and toxin-blocked increases in sodium efflux. (Potter, unpublished; similar results with toxin-binding have been reported by Changeux, Huchet & Cartaud, 1972, with eel microsacs and *Naja nigricollis* α-toxin.) With redissolution, full toxin-binding is restored, indicating that some of the receptor protein in reconstituted membranes is either buried in the membranes or faces inwards. Preliminary experiments with reconstituted toxin-saturated microsacs showed that carbachol-stimulated sodium efflux was lost, but that it could be restored to the usual degree, although not increased, by adding before dialysis a 20-fold excess of purified receptor protein that had not been blocked with toxin. These results not only demonstrate the feasibility of reconstitution experiments, but suggest that other molecule(s) than receptors, possibly ion channel protein(s), are required for the nicotinic receptor-response mechanism.

## *D. Conclusions*

The evidence that several elapid α-toxins bind to the recognition sites of nicotinic receptors is now convincing, however, there must be reservations about the specificity of the toxins for neuroreceptors in some tissues, and under certain conditions, particularly in homogenates. All of those who have worked with the toxins have noted considerable nonspecific binding to proteins, membranes and resins in media of low ionic strength (for example, less than 10 mmol/l), and some long-term retention in isotonic media (for example, in intact muscles) which may be due to low-affinity binding to nonspecific sites. The firm binding of α-bungarotoxin to nicotinic sites in frog muscles outside neuromuscular junctions appears to be to protein having similar characteristics to that at endplates, and the explanation for the presence of these sites, while now obscure, may prove interesting in terms of the cellular control of the numbers and location of receptors and ion channel proteins. Less understandable is the apparent protective effect of this α-toxin on nicotinic binding sites in lobster axonal membranes (Denburg, Eldefrawi & O'Brien, 1972). The most confusing results obtained with α-bungarotoxin concern its binding to detergent-dispersed mammalian brain tissue. Despite the almost total lack of binding of the toxin to rat brain membrane fragments, including highly purified synaptic membranes (Potter, unpublished), it has been reported that there is 38 times as much binding to detergent-dispersed proteins from guinea-pig cerebral cortex (Bosmann, 1972) as has been found with an equal weight of *Torpedo* electric tissue. Studies of the binding material show a protein which has very different characteristics in Triton X-100 (molecular weight = 94 000) from those found for nicotinic receptors in muscles and electric tissues.

To date it appears that nicotinic receptors in vertebrate skeletal muscles and electric tissues are very similar if not identical. They are membrane-bound, hydrophobic proteins composed of subunits having a molecular weight of 42 000; and the predominant one of several polymers seen in detergent-containing media has the size of a hexamer. Two or three of the subunits appear to have binding sites for acetylcholine and α-toxins. Without toxin, the molecular weight may be estimated as $6 \times 42\,000 \doteq 252\,000$.

Despite the fact that nicotinic receptors and active acetylcholinesterase can be separated by a variety of biochemical techniques, the two molecules in solution are nearly the same size, are present in nearly equal numbers (in skeletal muscles and *Torpedo*, but not in eel electric tissue), and are located for the most part on the same membranes. The separation of some vesicles which have each protein and little of the other may, as noted previously, be a partial exception to the general rule, or simply an artefact due to the production of vesicles. Three possibilities for the similarity in numbers are that there is a common operon for the two proteins, that they share a common subunit, or that they are normally part of one macromolecule in the membrane plus basement membrane. Whatever the explanation for the similarities of these proteins, it is clear that the two can be separately controlled after denervation of muscles, when receptors increase and the activity of acetylcholinesterase decreases (Guth, Brown & Watson, 1967).

## REFERENCES

ALBUQUERQUE, E. X., DALY, J. W. & WITKOP, B. (1971). *Science*, **172**, 995.
BARNARD, E. A., CHIU, T. H., JEDRZEJCYZK, J., PORTER, C. & WIECKOWSKI, J. (1973). This symposium.
BENNETT, M. V. L. (1971). *Fish Physiology*, **5**, 347.
BERG, D. K., KELLY, R. B., SARGENT, P. B., WILLIAMSON, P. & HALL, Z. W. (1972). *Proc. natn. Acad. Sci.*, **69**, 147.
BOSMANN, H. B. (1972). *J. biol. Chem.*, **247**, 130.
CHANG, C. C. & LEE, C. Y. (1963). *Arch. int. Pharmacodyn.*, **144**, 241.
CHANGEUX, J.-P., HUCHET, M. & CARTAUD, M. J. (1972). *C. R. Acad. Sci., Paris*, **274**, 122.
CHANGEUX, J.-P. (1973). This symposium.
CUATRECASAS, P. (1972). *Proc. natn. Acad. Sci.*, **69**, 318.
DE ROBERTIS, E. (1973). This symposium.

DEL CASTILLO, J. & KATZ, B. (1955). *J. Physiol.*, **128**, 157.
DENBERG, J. L., ELDEFRAWI, M. E. & O'BRIEN, R. D. (1972). *Proc. natn. Acad. Sci.*, **69**, 177.
FATT, P. & KATZ, B. (1951). *J. Physiol.*, **115**, 320.
FELDBERG, W. & FESSARD, A. (1942). *J. Physiol.*, **101**, 200.
FEWTRELL, C. M. S. & RANG, H. P. (1973). This symposium.
FRANKLIN, K. & POTTER, L. T. (1972). *F.E.B.S. Letters*, **28**, 101.
GUTH, L., BROWN, W. C. & WATSON, P. K. (1967). *Expl Neurol.*, **18**, 443.
HARTZELL, H. C. & FAMBROUGH, D. M. (1972). *J. gen. Physiol.*, **60**, 248.
HEUSER, J. & REESE, E. M. *J. cell. Biol.*, in press.
HODGKIN, A. L. (1964). *The Sherrington Lectures VII*, Liverpool University Press.
ISRAEL, M. (1970). *Arch. D'Anat. Microscop.*, **59**, 5.
KAO, C. Y. (1966). *Pharmac. Rev.*, **18**, 997.
KARLSSON, E., ARNBERG, H. & EAKER, D. (1971). *Eur. J. Biochem.*, **21**, 1.
KASAI, M. & CHANGEUX, J.-P. (1971). *J. Memb. Biol.*, **6**, 1.
KATZ, B. (1969). *The Sherrington Lectures X*, Liverpool University Press.
KATZ, B. & MILEDI, R. (1972). *J. Physiol., Lond.*, **224**, 665.
LEE, C. Y. & CHANG, C. C. (1966). *Mem. Inst. Butantan Simp. Internac.*, **33**, 555.
LEE, C. Y. & TSENG, L. F. (1966). *Toxicon*, **3**, 281.
LEE, C. Y., TSENG, L. F. & CHIU, T. H. (1967). *Nature*, **215**, 1177.
LEE, T.-P., KUO, J. F. & GREENGARD, P. (1972). *Proc. natn. Acad. Sci., U.S.A.*, **69**, 3287.
LESTER, H. A. (1972). *Mol. Pharmac.*, **8**, 623.
LØMØ, T. & ROSENTHAL, J. (1972). *J. Physiol.*, **221**, 493.
MCAFEE, D. A. & GREENGARD, P. (1972). *Science, N.Y.*, **178**, 310.
MEUNIER, J.-C., OLSEN, R. W., MENEZ, A., FROMAGEOT, P., BOQUET, P. & CHANGEUX, J.-P. (1972). *Biochemistry*, **11**, 1200.
MILEDI, R. (1962). In: Ciba Symposium on *Enzymes and Drug Action*, ed. Mongar, J. L. & de Rueck, A. V. S., p. 220. Boston: Little Brown & Co.
MILEDI, R., MOLINOFF, P. & POTTER, L. T. (1971). *Nature*, **229**, 554.
MILEDI, R. & POTTER, L. T. (1971). *Nature*, **233**, 599.
MOLINOFF, P. B. & POTTER, L. T. (1972). *Adv. Biochem. Psychopharmac.*
MOLINOFF, P. B. & POTTER, L. T. (1973). To be published.
NICKEL, E. & POTTER, L. T. (1971). *Phil. Trans. Roy. Soc. Lond.*, B, **261**, 383.
O'BRIEN, R. D., ELDEFRAWI, M. E. & ELDEFRAWI, A. T. (1973). This symposium.
PATON, W. D. M. (1970). In: Ciba Symposium on *Molecular Properties of Drug Receptors*, ed. Porter, R. & O'Connor, M., p. 3. J. & A. Churchill.
POTTER, L. T. (1970). *J. Physiol.*, **206**, 145.
POTTER, L. T. & MOLINOFF, P. B. (1972). In: *Perspectives in Neuropharmacology*, ed. Snyder, S. H., p. 9. Oxford University Press.
RAFTERY, M. A., SCHMIDT, J., CLARK, D. G. & WOLCOTT, R. G. (1971). *Biochem. Biophys. res. Commun.*, **45**, 1622.
RANG, H. P. & RITTER, J. M. (1970). *Mol. Pharmac.*, **6**, 383.
REITER, M. J., COWBURN, D. A., PRIVES, J. M. & KARLIN, A. (1972). *Proc. natn. Acad. Sci.*, **69**, 1168.
SHERIDAN, M. N. (1965). *J. cell. Biol.*, **24**, 129.
SUTHERLAND, E. W. (1970). *Science, N.Y.*, **177**, 401.
THESLEFF, S. (1973). This symposium.
WASER, P. G. (1970). In: Ciba Symposium on *Molecular Properties of Drug Receptors*, ed. Porter, R. & O'Conner, M., p. 59. Churchill.
WEBER, M., MENEZ, A., FROMAGEOT, P., BOQUET, P. & CHANGEUX, J.-P. (1972). *C. R. Acad. Sci., Paris*, **274**, 1575.

## DISCUSSION

*Barnard* (*New York*)

I would like to comment on the apparent discrepancy between your results and our own (Barnard, Wieckowski & Chiu, 1971, *Nature, Lond.*, **234**,

207) concerning the number of receptor sites at a single endplate. The explanation is probably that in the frog sartorius there are many sites (demonstrable by autoradiography) that bind toxin firmly but are not associated with the endplate membrane. These additional sites, which would have been included in your estimate of receptor numbers, should probably not be used to calculate the number of receptors per endplate, as they are distinct from the sites associated with the postsynaptic membrane.

*Potter* (*London*)

Your point about frog sartorius muscles is well taken, and raises a very interesting question. Let us first agree that for *mammalian* muscles there is excellent accord between the physiological localization of the receptor-response mechanism at neuromuscular endplates (Thesleff, this symposium) and the localization of bound α-bungarotoxin observed by radioassays and dissection techniques (Miledi & Potter, 1971; Berg, Kelly, Sargent, Williamson & Hall, 1972) and by radioautography (Lee & Tseng, 1966; Barnard, Wieckowski & Chiu, 1971; Fambrough & Hartzell, 1972). We have all estimated, therefore, the same number of sites per endplate and a similar average density of sites, of the order of $10^4/\mu m^2$, much as in *Torpedo* electric tissue (Miledi, Molinoff & Potter, 1971).

In contrast, the physiological localization of the receptor-response mechanism at endplates in frog muscles (Thesleff, this symposium) is different from your finding of the widespread distribution of bound α-bungarotoxin in these muscles. Judging from the radioautograph which you have shown, your estimate of the actual number of toxin molecules at frog endplates, and the very much larger number of toxin molecules which Miledi and I found in the whole muscles divided by the number of endplates, it would appear that 90% or more of the toxin sites in this tissue are extrajunctional.

An explanation for these extrajunctional sites is obviously needed, and it must account for the following observations. In desensitization experiments with bath-applied carbachol or with acetylcholine and neostigmine, it was found that binding of α-bungarotoxin to frog sartorius muscles was reduced by more than 80% during brief periods of toxin exposure (Miledi & Potter, 1971). Thus extrajunctional sites must either be protected by these agonists, or the extra sites are not labelled during short toxin exposures. Sedimentation analyses have shown the same toxin–receptor complexes after dissolution of toxin-saturated membranes from frog muscles, electric tissues and mammalian muscles. Thus the extrajunctional toxin sites in frog muscles appear similar to the junctional sites in other tissues, a conclusion in keeping with general knowledge of the specificity of protein: protein interactions having such high affinities as that between α-bungarotoxin and receptors. Assuming that most of the toxin is bound to the recognition subunits of receptors, it would appear that these are either not coupled to the ion channel which subserves synaptic potentials, or, if the molecular or subunits required for reception and ion fluxes are coupled, that their distribution on or in the cells is not such as to be quantitatively assessed by current physiological measurements.

# INDEX

# Date Due